T0133885

Essential Paediatrics in Primary Care

A. SAHIB EL-RADHI
MRCPCH, PhD, DCH
Honorary Consultant Paediatrician, Queen Mary's Hospital, Sidcup, Kent
Honorary Senior Lecturer, Medical Schools, London

STEVE GREGSON
MBBS, MRCGP, DCH, DRCOG
GP, Swanley, Kent
GP Trainer, London Deanery

NAVREET PAUL
MBBS, BSc (Hons), MRCGP, DRCOG, DFSRH, DPD
Sessional GP, Bexley, Kent

and

ASAD RAHMAN
MBBS, BSc (Hons), MRCPCH, MRCGP
GP, Sidcup, Kent

Foreword by
JOHN SPICER
Acting Dean, GP and Community Based Education
London School of General Practice
University of London

Radcliffe Publishing
London • New York

Radcliffe Publishing Ltd
33–41 Dallington Street
London
EC1V 0BB
United Kingdom

www.radcliffehealth.com

© 2013 A. Sahib El-Radhi

A. Sahib El-Radhi has asserted his right under the Copyright, Designs and Patents Act 1988 to be identified as the author of this work.

Every effort has been made to ensure that the information in this book is accurate. This does not diminish the requirement to exercise clinical judgement, and neither the publisher nor the authors can accept any responsibility for its use in practice.

All rights reserved. No part of this publication may be reproduced, stored in a retrieval system or transmitted, in any form or by any means, electronic, mechanical, photocopying, recording or otherwise, without the prior permission of the copyright owner.

British Library Cataloguing in Publication Data

A catalogue record for this book is available from the British Library.

ISBN-13: 978 184619 577 8

The paper used for the text pages of this book
is FSC® certified. FSC (The Forest Stewardship
Council®) is an international network to promote
responsible management of the world's forests.

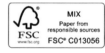

Typeset by Darkriver Design, Auckland, New Zealand
Printed and bound by TJ International Ltd, Padstow, Cornwall, UK

Contents

Foreword

The contribution of the UK general practitioner to child health is at once necessary and valued, constituting as it does such a large part of everyday primary care work. Not all healthcare systems value such a contribution, and paediatric care is often reserved in other countries for the specialist, rather than the expert generalist as in the UK.

Specialist paediatric expertise is necessary of course for the acutely ill child, the very complex child, or those children with rare pathologies, even in the UK system, and that is clearly as it should be.

So undoubtedly the expert generalist needs to acquire the skills of child health practice and arguably it should be targeted at several particular areas. We might specify the recognition of the acutely ill child, the care of long-term conditions and child developmental surveillance as core medical skills. In addition, working with his or her team, the GP will cover child safeguarding, vaccination and immunisation and health promotion, among others. This list is not meant to be comprehensive but rather illustrative of the kinds of competences a modern GP will need. Such skills and knowledge would be blended into the more generic primary care aspects including care of the family, over the long term, and in the patient's own *milieu*.

Times change, and child healthcare changes too, and it might be argued that the 'classical' view of the organisation of paediatric care as outlined above is changing too. Integrated care, where primary and secondary care practitioners work carefully together, perhaps even seamlessly, is becoming more evident on the UK scene, as well as elsewhere. There are good reasons for this: better early recognition of serious childhood disease, better care along the patient pathway and better population health outcomes, among others.

In the UK, we know there are challenges to be confronted: there is evidence that child health outcomes do not always compare well against European ones, that there is too much short-term hospital admission and that safeguarding practice is not as good as it might be. So there is work to be done.

Against this backdrop lies a clearly increasing respect among professionals for the wishes of the child in his or her care, beyond even the 'threshold' of *Gillick* competence. Much has been written of consideration of assent to treatment, rather than the formal notion of consent among children.

Into this environment, too scantily described above, comes this book, delivered by a team of expert generalists and expert specialists, all of whom are also teachers of medical practice. It uses the term 'essential' purposefully, because it is just that. Anyone practising generalist paediatrics should have the material within these chapters either hard-wired in, or at the fingertips. This book is ideal for the primary care bookshelf.

Above all, the paediatrics described in these pages comprises a manual for practising safely, a *sine qua non* of modern-day child healthcare. The words 'red flags' are often used in clinical practice as a means of identifying features that just cannot be left unconsidered, and the reader will find paediatric red flags helpfully annotated throughout the text.

Stylistically, the book is arranged in bullet points for the most part in order to maximise ease of reference rather than display elegant prose. For the latter, the reader will need to seek elsewhere, armed it is hoped with core knowledge from this book.

It has been said that the only difference between adult and child medical practice is the fact of growth: children do it, and adults don't. Reductionist as that statement may be, it has a gem of truth within it. The authors have ensured that clinicians' paediatric knowledge and skills can only grow with familiarity of their material.

John Spicer
Acting Dean, GP and Community Based Education
London School of General Practice
University of London
June 2013

Preface

In recent decades remarkable progress has been made in paediatric care, which now has a much stronger evidence base. This scientific progress on the one hand, and the lack of books specific to paediatrics in general practice on the other, gave us the impetus to write this book. There is also a huge amount of information available on the Internet which has meant that parents and carers of children we see are better informed. This information, however, is of variable quality and is difficult to keep up with. The book is written by a team comprising an experienced paediatrician together with three local GPs with regular front-line experience of the challenges and dilemmas we face in diagnosing and managing problems in children in primary care. The book is written primarily for GPs and GP trainees; however, we hope that nurse practitioners, health visitors, medical students and paediatricians considering a career in general practice will find it useful.

The book is structured in 18 clinical chapters covering the entire breadth of paediatric practice, presenting the evidence base where relevant and where this is lacking reaching a consensus view. We have also tried to give a general practice slant, concentrating on areas of relevance to a GP or other clinician working regularly with children in primary care. There is clear guidance about when children can be managed in primary care and when referral to hospital is appropriate, and how to reach a rapid diagnosis in the short time available to busy GPs. Investigations relevant to primary care have been included. We have also tried to whet your appetite for further study in areas of interest to you and have sign-posted additional resources where relevant. We are pleased to say that you can find in this book practically everything you need in general practice.

There is a chapter on neonatology, covering problems during the first few weeks of life and including the 6-week examination The current child health surveillance and immunisation programmes are included, and there is a section on child development. The book concludes with an essential chapter on safeguarding children, containing material that every GP, GP trainee or nurse practitioner should be familiar with.

The book can be read cover to cover, but is probably best used as a reference when faced with dilemmas in managing children in primary care. We hope we have produced a practical, concise and reader-friendly text suitable for use in general practice. We also hope you are inspired to study and gain further experience in this rewarding and essential part of family practice.

The authors
June 2013

About the authors

Dr A. Sahib El-Radhi, MRCPCH, PhD, DCH completed his primary medical study and PhD at the Free University of West Berlin, Germany. Currently, he is Honorary Consultant Paediatrician at Queen Mary's Hospital, Sidcup, Kent and Honorary Senior Lecturer at the Medical Schools, London. He has worked as a general paediatrician in various different countries including Germany, Finland, Iraq, Kuwait and the United Kingdom. He has served as an advisor and peer reviewer for several medical journals, including the *Archives of Disease in Childhood*.

With more than 30 papers published in indexed journals and editorials as well as several books, Dr El-Radhi has spent most of his medical career in research, performing numerous controlled and multi-centre studies.

As an undergraduate and postgraduate examiner to the Royal College of Paediatrics and Child Health, he has also had the honour of being an MRCPCH and DCH examiner for 15 years.

Dr Steve Gregson, MBBS, MRCGP, DCH, DRCOG is a GP partner in Swanley, Kent where he has practised for the last 25 years. He qualified at Guy's Hospital London and gained the Diploma in Child Health qualification while in GP training. He has worked as a Community Medical Officer in Community Paediatrics for several years alongside his GP commitments, and retains a special interest in paediatrics. He is a GP trainer in the London Deanery and remains committed to teaching and lifelong learning in general practice.

Dr Nav Paul, MBBS, BSc (Hons), MRCGP, DRCOG, DFSRH, DPD is currently a Sessional GP working in Bexley after completing her MRCGP training in Kent. She graduated from Guy's, King's and St Thomas' School of Medicine (GKT) in 2005, where she was also awarded a First Class Degree in Medical and Molecular Genetics. She then went on to train in the USA with Harvard Medical School at Boston Children's Hospital during her elective placement. She has a keen interest in advancing her own knowledge as well as developing her career in medical education.

Dr Asad Rahman, MBBS, BSc (Hons), MRCPCH, MRCGP is a GP partner in a large teaching practice in Sidcup, Kent. He qualified from Guy's, King's and St Thomas' School of Medicine where he undertook a clinical research project looking at bronchodilators in wheezy infants. He subsequently worked in a number of general and specialty paediatric posts and completed training for the MRCPCH. Having decided to pursue a career in general practice, he still maintained his interest in paediatrics and spent time working as an honorary doctor at a local hospital outpatient department. He was also appointed as Bexley's GP Children's Champion and Safeguarding lead.

Acknowledgements

The authors are grateful to their families for their encouragement and understanding while this book was being prepared. We wish to thank Sami El-Radhi (son of Sahib) and Gassan Ahmad (nephew of Sahib) for providing the excellent drawings in this book. We express appreciation and thanks to the Childhood Eye Cancer Trust (www.chect. org.uk) which very kindly supplied us with four images on eye cancer (Figures 1.3, 7.2, 13.3, 13.4). The Trust is helping to fight eye cancers, particularly retinoblastoma. We also wish to thank Meningitis UK (www.meningitisuk.org) for providing us with the images showing a meningococcal rash (Figures 4.4, 4.5). This national charity's aim is to raise awareness and fund research to eradicate all forms of meningitis and associated diseases, particularly through vaccination. We also thank the British Thoracic Society for kindly granting permission to reproduce the summaries of asthma management as shown in Figure 9.2. Finally, we acknowledge the kind permission of Richard Ashton and Barbara Leppard to reproduce the following images from *Differential Diagnosis in Dermatology*, Third Edition (Radcliffe Publishing; 2005): Figures 1.5, 4.2, 4.3, 4.7, 4.8, 6.1, 17.1–17.11, 17.13, 17.14.

CHAPTER 1

The newborn

NEONATAL HEALTH PROMOTION

(*See* Table 1.1)

TABLE 1.1 Health promotion offered to children up to 4 months of age

Age	Intervention

Soon after birth	• General examination with particular emphasis on eyes, heart, hips
	• Vitamin K administration: usually offered as a single IM dose. Some parents choose the oral preparation, in which case this is given at birth, at 7–10 days and at 28 days
	• BCG vaccination is offered to:
	  ○ All infants living in areas of the UK where the annual incidence is ≥ 40/100 000
	  ○ All infants with a parent or grandparent who was born in a country where the annual incidence is ≥ 40/100 000
	• Hepatitis B vaccine: the first dose is given to babies whose mothers or close family have been infected with hepatitis B (*see also* Chapter 8)
	• Advice regarding reducing the risk of sudden infant death

5–6 days old	• Blood spot test for hypothyroidism, phenylketonuria. Screening for sickle cell disease and cystic fibrosis
First month	• Newborn hearing screen • Hepatitis B vaccine: 2nd dose if this was given after birth
New-birth visit (around 12 days)	• Home visit by the midwife or health visitor to assess the child and family health needs, including identification of mental health needs • Distribution of 'Birth to Five' guide and the personal Child Health record
6–8 weeks	• General physical examination with particular emphasis on eyes, heart and hips • Immunisation: *see* Table 1.2 • Review of general progress and delivery of key messages about parenting and health promotion • Hepatitis B vaccine: 3rd dose
3 months	• Immunisation: *see* Table 1.2
4 months	• Immunisation: *see* Table 1.2

BCG = Bacillus Calmette-Guérin; IM = intramuscularly.

TABLE 1.2 Normal immunisation schedule for all people < 18 years in the UK

Age	Immunisation
2 months	DTaP/IPV/HiB (1st dose), *plus*
	PCV in a separate injection, *plus*
	Rotavirus (orally)
3 months	DTaP/IPV/HiB (2nd dose), *plus*
	Men C in a separate injection, *plus*
	Rotavirus (orally)
4 months	DTaP/IPV/HiB (3rd dose), *plus*
	Men C in a separate injection, *plus*
	PCV (2nd dose) in a separate injection
12–13 months	HiB/Men C (as one injection), *plus*
	MMR (as one injection), *plus*
	PCV (3rd dose) in a separate injection
3 years +	Pre-school booster of DTaP/IPV, *plus*
	MMR
12–13 years (girls)	HPV in three injections: the 2nd one is given 1–2 months after the 1st; and the 3rd is given about 6 months after the 1st
13–15 years	Td/IPV booster
	Men C booster in a separate injection

DTaP = diphtheria, tetanus and pertussis; HiB = *Haemophilus influenzae* type B; HPV = Human papillomavirus; IPV = polio; Men C = meningitis C; MMR = measles, mumps and rubella; PCV = pneumococcal conjugate vaccine; Td/IPV = Tetanus, low dose diphtheria and polio.

NEONATAL EXAMINATION (THE BABY CHECK)

GPs and midwives may be required to perform a neonatal examination soon after birth for home deliveries and where there is early discharge from obstetric units. GPs routinely perform a baby examination at 6 weeks. The examination aims to:

➤ Detect congenital abnormalities which may be present in 3–5% of infants. These should be explained to parents, recorded and referred if appropriate.
➤ Establish a baseline for subsequent examination.
➤ Ensure there are no signs of infection or metabolic disease.
➤ Perform measurements of weight and head circumference (HC) and plot them on a centile chart. A newborn's weight may decrease 10% below birthweight in the first week, but should regain or exceed birthweight by 14 days of life. Newborns should grow at approximately 25–30 g/day during the first three months.

Neonatal examination should include the following areas:

➤ Review of **family history**, including maternal diseases, sexually transmitted disease, medications (Box 1.1), and alcohol and tobacco consumption.
➤ Parental concerns should be elicited.
➤ **General examination:** Much information can be gained by simple observation without disturbing the child. Is the general appearance normal? Does the baby look well nourished? Are there any dysmorphic features?

> **BOX 1.1** Drugs which cross the placenta and may have an adverse effect, including teratogenicity on the unborn baby
>
> ● Anaesthetics and sedatives, e.g. halothane causing alteration of DNA synthesis in vitro reported to cause skeletal defects
> ● Anticoagulants (e.g. warfarin causing an embryopathy with growth retardation, skeletal and CNS abnormalities)
> ● Antibiotics (e.g. aminoglycosides causing 8th cranial nerve toxicity; tetracyclines producing dental discolouration, enamel hypoplasia)
> ● Cytotoxic drugs (e.g. methotrexate causing craniofacial anomalies)
> ● Alcohol, causing fetal alcohol syndrome
> ● Tobacco smoking, causing an increased incidence of growth retardation and developmental delay
> ● Oestrogens, causing precocious puberty and cervical/vaginal adenocarcinoma near puberty
> ● Anticonvulsants (e.g. phenytoin causing fetal hydantoin syndrome)
> ● Addicting drugs (e.g. cocaine causing eye and skeletal defects)
> ● Psychotherapeutics (e.g. lithium causing heart valve defects, Ebstein's anomaly)
> ● Analgesics (e.g. aspirin associated with skeletal and heart defects, cleft lip and palate, hypospadias)

➤ **Skin:**
  ➢ Colour is an important index of the function of the cardiorespiratory system. Normal colour in Caucasian infants is reddish pink. Infants of diabetic mothers are pinker than average.
  ➢ Evidence of jaundice, best detectable in bright natural light.
  ➢ Peripheral cyanosis, caused by peripheral circulatory instability.
  ➢ Mottling (cutis marmorata) may be due to circulatory instability.
  ➢ Capillary haemangioma (*see* 'Birthmarks' below).
➤ **Skull** (Fig 1.1):
  ➢ Palpation of the suture lines and the size and tension of the anterior fontanelle is performed. Great variation in the size of the fontanelle exists. In general, a small fontanelle enlarges during the first few months of life while a large one becomes gradually smaller. A large fontanelle should not cause any concern as long as the HC is normal and it is not tense or bulging. A persistently large fontanelle may be associated with macrocephaly, hypothyroidism or hydrocephalus. A persistently small fontanelle may suggest microcephaly, cranial synostosis or chromosomal abnormalities.
  ➢ Measure the HC around the largest occipital–frontal diameter across the forehead. If the HC measures above or below the normal for age (< 3rd or > 97th centile), the parents' HC should be measured. Macrocephaly is the most common cause of a larger than average head, usually inherited from the father.
➤ **Face:**
  ➢ Dysmorphic features are noted.
  ➢ Petechiae are common and do not blanch with pressure.
  ➢ Examine both nares to ensure their patency.

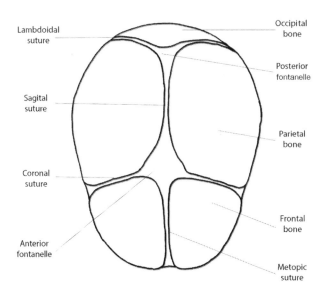

FIGURE 1.1 Skull showing the patent sutures and the two fontanelles

> Milia on the nose are a common finding.
> Snuffles, which are inspiratory noises from the upper airways. They are common and should disappear by the age of 3–6 months.
> Mouth for possible precocious dentition (incidence 1 : 2000) and for any complete or submucosal cleft palate (likely if the arch is excessively high or the uvula is bifid).
> Asymmetrical crying facies may be due to facial nerve compression (often caused by forceps use during delivery) (Fig 1.2) or to congenital hypoplastic or agenesis of the depressor anguli oris muscle which controls the downward movement of the lip. In the latter the eye and forehead muscles are unaffected. The condition may be associated with cardiac defects (Cayler's syndrome).
> **Eye:**
>> Establish that both eyes are of normal size and not microphthalmic.
>> Red reflex with ophthalmoscope. Its presence suggests the absence of cataract or of intraocular pathology. White pupillary reflex suggests cataracts, chorioretinitis, tumour, retinopathy of prematurity (Fig 1.3 – *see* Plate section).

RED FLAGS

● The presence of white pupillary reflex or a cornea > 1 cm in diameter requires prompt ophthalmological referral.
● Pre-term babies, particularly those with a birthweight of < 1500 g or < 31 weeks' gestation, should be reviewed by an ophthalmologist because of the high risk of retinopathy of prematurity, myopia, squint and cortical visual impairment.

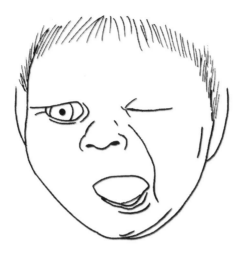

FIGURE 1.2 Right-sided facial nerve palsy. When the infant cries, there is movement only on the non-paralysed side of the face, the eye cannot be closed and the nasolabial fold is absent

➤ **Ears** are examined for:
  ➢ Structural malformation.
  ➢ Unilateral or bilateral pre-auricular skin tags or ear pits. If the tag is pedunculated, it can be ligated tightly at the base. Children are at increased risk for hearing impairment. Hearing testing is indicated.
➤ **Chest**, noting that:
  ➢ Breast hypertrophy in both sexes is common (occurs in as many as 70% of neonates) and is caused by intrauterine hormonal stimulation. Breasts should never be manipulated, as this may cause infection and abscess. Spontaneous regression is the rule within the first few weeks of life.
  ➢ Supernumerary breasts and nipples are very common, located along the 'milk line' from the axilla to the pubic symphysis, mostly just below and medial to the normal breast. They may appear as tiny pigmented macula. No treatment is required.
  ➢ Respiration in the newborn is normally irregular, with pauses that should not exceed 10 seconds. The normal respiratory rate is 30–40 breaths/min when resting.
  ➢ In heart auscultation the absence of a heart murmur does not exclude congenital heart defects. The heart rate is normally between 120 and 160 beats/min.

RED FLAGS
  ● A respiratory rate > 60 breaths/min over 1 hour of observation suggests cardiopulmonary or metabolic disease.
  ● Grunting during expiration signifies potentially serious cardiopulmonary disease.

➤ **Abdomen** is inspected for:
  ➤ Abdominal distension.
  ➤ Possible infection of the umbilical stump.
  ➤ Umbilical hernia which is common, particularly in African children.
  ➤ The abdominal muscles, which are normally weak allowing a separation between the two rectus muscles (diastasis recti).

Then palpated for:
  ➤ Any mass.
  ➤ Liver edge, which is usually palpable 1–2 cm below the right costal margin.

🏳 RED FLAG
  ● Any abdominal mass should be investigated immediately by ultrasound scan. Any inguinal hernia should be referred as soon as possible to a paediatric surgeon.

➤ **Genitalia:**
In males:
  ➤ The glans penis is normally covered completely by foreskin. Both testes should be completely descended.
  ➤ At birth, 6% of males have one or both testes undescended.
  ➤ The orifice of the urethra should be identified and any hypospadias excluded.

In females:
  ➤ Labia majora are large and cover and occlude the labia minora and vaginal introitus.
  ➤ Vaginal discharge is frequent and appears on the second or third day of life, sometimes with bleeding. It usually resolves spontaneously.

PRACTICE POINTS
  ● The foreskin is physiologically adherent to the glans and should not be retracted.
  ● Palpation of the testes with cold hands may stimulate cremasteric reflex, causing them to retract to the top of the scrotum and even into the inguinal canals. This may lead to a misdiagnosis of undescended testis.
  ● If testes are not descended at the 6–8 week examination, a review should be arranged just before 1 year of age. If still undescended, the child should be referred to a paediatric surgeon.
  ● Enlargement of the clitoris is common but has to be differentiated from congenital adrenal hyperplasia (CAH). In CAH, the enlargement is marked resembling a penis, with varying degrees of labial fusion. As the urethra opens below this clitoris, a mistaken diagnosis of hypospadias and cryptorchidism may be made.

➤ **Extremities:**
  ➤ Most newborns have mild bowing of the legs. This often becomes more pronounced during toddlerhood.

> Often there is a transient positional foot deformity caused by an intrauterine position. If the anomaly can be corrected completely by hand pressure, it is not pathological. Fixed structural deformity such as clubfoot should be referred.

> The fingers and toes should be checked for number and evidence of in-curving (clinodactyly). Palmar creases should be noted: single and unilateral palmar crease is a common finding. Clinodactyly and multiple and bilateral palmar creases may be associated with chromosomal abnormalities.

> **Back:** Many neonates (about 4%) have a simple midline sacral dimple at the lower end of the back and the top of the cleft. These dimples, also known as coccygeal dimples or pits, are the commonest cutaneous anomaly of the spine in the newborn infant. They are innocuous if they are less than 5 mm in size and localised within 25 mm of the anus.

BOX 1.2 Neonatal hip examination (Fig 1.4)

- While the baby is lying supine and relaxed, examine whether the hip is dislocated using the Barlow and Ortolani tests
- Both tests are usually useful only during the first 2–3 months of life
- Neither test detects a dislocated, irreducible hip, which is best detected by identifying limited abduction
- Clicks (resulting from soft tissues snapping over bony prominences during hip movement) and asymmetrical skin creases of the thighs are found in many normal babies and are not significant
- Babies with risk factors (breech presentation, family history of hip dislocation and foot deformity) require ultrasound examination within the first 6 weeks of life

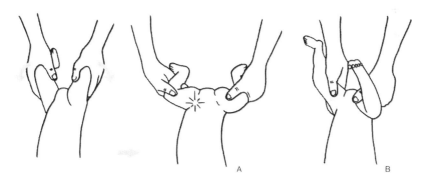

A   B

FIGURE 1.4 Hip dislocation tests

A: the Barlow test is the most important test, aimed at dislocating an unstable hip from the acetabulum. This is performed by applying the index and middle finger along the greater trochanter with the thumb on the inner thigh. Then gently adduct the hip and apply pressure posteriorly. The manoeuvre is positive if a 'clunk' or 'jerk' is felt

B: the Ortolani test aims at reducing a recently dislocated hip. With the fingers in the same position as above, gently abduct the hip while lifting the leg anteriorly

Referral is indicated if:

➣ The size is > 5 mm and situated > 25 mm from the anus.
➣ There are tufts of hair, cutaneous mass (e.g. haemangioma, lipoma), sinus tract (dermal sinuses opening into the skin surface) or skin appendage/tags over lumbosacral spine.

These cutaneous stigmata over the lower spine are associated with a higher incidence of occult spinal dysraphism (OSD) or neural tube defects. Ultrasound of the lumbosacral spine is the best screening tool for OSD.

➤ **Hip examination:** Check the hips for congenital dislocation (Box 1.2).

NEUROLOGICAL EXAMINATION

Neurological examination will focus on:

➤ The level of alertness.
➤ The quality of the baby's cry: normal, weak, high-pitched?
➤ Posture and movement of the four extremities. Do they move equally and maintain a normal posture of flexion?
➤ Muscle tone: is it normal? Assess by repeatedly flexing and extending baby's arms and legs.
➤ Head control. In ventral suspension of the infant, the head is down below the level of the body at 0–4 weeks of age and in the same plane as the body at 6 weeks.
➤ Primitive reflexes, such as:
  ➣ Rooting reflex. If the cheek is touched by a smooth object (e.g. the mother's breast), the child will turn towards that object with their mouth open to receive the nipple.
  ➣ Placing or stepping reflex. When the child is held upright, touching the dorsum of the feet to the bed or table elicits steps as if the baby is trying to walk. Parents are invariably fascinated by seeing this.
  ➣ The Moro reflex is elicited by holding the baby facing the examiner and then allowing the baby's head to gently drop back. The child symmetrically abducts and extends the arms and flexes the thumbs.
  ➣ The grasp reflex is elicited by placing a finger in the palm of each of the baby's hands.
  ➣ The asymmetric tonic neck reflex is elicited by turning the baby's head to one side and noting the arm's gradual extension on the same side of the turned head with flexion of the opposite arm.

NUTRITION

Breast-feeding

➤ Promotion of breast-feeding should be initiated pre-natally by GPs, obstetricians, midwives and obstetric nurses. Women often make decisions about breast-feeding early in pregnancy, sometimes even before they become pregnant.
➤ Healthcare providers must provide support and encouragement for breast-feeding, including provision of literature on the benefits of breast-feeding. Breast milk provides an average energy of 67 kcal/100 ml (280 kJ /100 ml). Healthy term babies grow well with intakes (breast or formula) of at least 90–100 kcal/kg/day (376–418 kJ/kg/day). This energy is provided when the intake of milk is at least 150 mL/kg/day.

Guidelines for successful breast-feeding include the following:
➤ The baby should have skin-to-skin contact with the mother and be allowed to suckle as soon as possible after birth.
➤ The baby should be initially nursed on demand or every 2–3 hours.
➤ Supplementation of breast milk with water, glucose or formula is generally not recommended.
➤ Both breasts should be used at each feeding.
➤ No artificial teats or pacifiers should be offered.
➤ Manual expression of breast milk is sometimes useful to relieve engorgement of the breasts, although breast pumps usually make this unnecessary. Pumping can increase milk production and relieve sore nipples.

Formula feeding
Although breast-feeding is considered superior to formula feeding, many infants receive and thrive well on formula from birth, although this may be associated with excessive weight gain and higher incidence of infections and allergies. Guidelines for successful formula feeding include:
➤ The infant should be hungry, warm, dry and fully awake.
➤ The bottle should be held above the horizontal so that milk, and not air, flows through the teat.
➤ Milk warmed to body temperature is usually given, although no harmful effects have been found from feeding at room temperature or cooler.

COMMON NEONATAL PROBLEMS
Birth marks
➤ **Milia** are multiple pearly white or pale yellow papules or cysts which are scattered on the face, especially on the nose. They disappear within a few weeks of life. No treatment is required.
➤ **Salmon patch** is by far the most common vascular lesion in neonates: a midline or symmetrical pink macule over one or both upper lids.
➤ **Mongolian spots** are present at birth in > 80% of Black and Asian children and in 5–10% of Caucasian infants. They may be solitary over the sacral area but can be multiple over the legs and shoulders. Mongolian spots (bluish, present at birth) should not be confused with bruises.
➤ **Erythema toxicum neonatorum** is seen in about half of healthy newborns and is often mistaken for staphylococcal pustules. The child appears well and the rash is asymptomatic.
➤ **Café-au-lait spots.** Single or a couple of lesions of café-au-lait, 1–3 cm in length, occur in about 20% of all healthy children. In neurofibromatosis there should be 6 or more café-au-lait spots > 0.5 cm in diameter in pre-pubertal children and > 1.5 cm in diameter (patch) in post-pubertal individuals before the diagnosis can be made.
➤ **Haemangiomas** (strawberry naevi) (Fig 1.5– *see* Plate section) are found in about 10% of all children. They are usually not present at birth; they appear in the first few weeks of life, enlarge during early infancy and usually regress at age 5 years. Lesions > 5 cm in diameter may be associated with Kasabach–Merritt syndrome, which is characterised by a vascular lesion (haemangioma), thrombocytopenia and chronic

consumption coagulopathy as platelets are consumed and destroyed within the haemangioma.

Referral is indicated if there is:

➤ visual, airway or ear canal obstruction

➤ extensive growth

➤ proptosis

➤ severe disfigurement such as facial disfigurement

➤ recurrent bleeding, infection, ulceration.

BIRTH TRAUMA

➤ **Moulding** of the head is frequent, particularly if the head has been engaged for a long time.

➤ **Cranial caput succedaneum** consists of subcutaneous and extra-periosteal oedema of the soft tissues of the scalp with no limitation to the sutures.

➤ **Cephalohaematoma** is sub-periosteal haemorrhage which is always confined by one cranial bone. Most cephalohaematomas disappear within 2 weeks to 2 months of life. A few remain for years as a bony protuberance. There may be an underlying skull fracture. They require usually no treatment; massive cephalohaematoma may require blood transfusion and phototherapy. Aspiration is contraindicated.

🏳 RED FLAG

- Cranial meningocele is rare but can occasionally be mistaken for cephalo-haematoma. It is differentiated by pulsation, increased pressure on crying, and bony defect on skull X-ray.

Intracranial haemorrhage (ICH) is common in pre-term infants, particularly those with a birthweight < 1500 g, occurring in 20–40% of babies with low birth weight. ICH may lead to post-haemorrhagic hydrocephalus. Checking the skull sutures and head circumference (HC) is recommended each time the baby is seen in the clinic. Infants may present with poor feeding, excessive somnolence, apnoea, temperature instability and seizures. Findings include hypotonia and bulging anterior fontanelle.

➤ **Fracture of the clavicle** is a common injury in babies delivered with shoulder dys-tocia. The infant may be asymptomatic or display pseudo-paralysis on the affected side. Palpable bony crepitations and irregularity at the site of the fracture are the physical findings.

➤ **Brachial palsy.** Injury to the 5th and 6th cervical spinal nerves (Erb's palsy) causes adduction and internal rotation of the arm with extension of the elbow and flexion of the wrist. Injury to the 7th and 8th cervical and 1st thoracic spinal nerves (Klumpke's palsy) is rare and leads to weakness of the hand and absence of the grasp reflex.

INFECTION

Sticky eyes are a very common finding and the majority of eye discharges are benign. Ophthalmia neonatorum is a severe form of conjunctivitis occurring within the first month of life. It is a potentially blinding condition. The main differential diagnoses include:

➤ **Viral conjunctivitis.** Onset is acute, 1–14 days, unilateral or bilateral with serous discharge. The condition is usually benign and self-limiting except with herpes simplex virus (HSV), which usually occurs as a result of intrapartum transmission and may also cause keratitis, cataracts and retinopathy.

➤ **Chlamydia** is the most common cause of ophthalmia neonatorum in the UK. The infection usually appears 5–14 days after birth, with a purulent discharge which varies from mild to severe and is associated with a swelling of the eyelids.

➤ **Gonococcal infection** presents in the first few days of life with a rapidly progressive profuse purulent discharge and lid oedema. The cornea is rapidly affected. Urgent treatment with systemic antibiotics is needed.

➤ The above infections need to be differentiated from the far more common **obstruction of the nasolacrimal duct**. This resolves spontaneously in over 95% of infants over the next few months. Diagnosis is made by:

  ➢ A history of initial watery discharge, often followed by sticky and crusty discharge, sometimes copious and thick

  ➢ The discharge being reproduced by pressure over the lacrimal sac

  ➢ The eye is not red and the child is otherwise well.

RED FLAGS

There is an indication for referral if:

- The discharge is thick and/or purulent and/or rapid-onset, as these often suggest bacterial infection (*Chlamydia*, *Gonorrhoea*, staphylococcal infection or *Pseudomonas*).
- The conjunctivitis is associated with skin vesicles. Vesicles of HSV infection typically appear in the second week of neonatal life on the presenting part of the body.
- Both eyes are affected without prior history of watery eyes.
- There is suspicion of maternal sexually transmitted disease (STD). The mother may be asymptomatic.
- The child is unwell or distressed.
- The inflammation affects the bulbar conjunctiva (over the sclera).
- If signs of nasolacrimal blockage do not resolve by 1 year of age, referral for possible probing is indicated.

➤ **Omphalitis**, spreading erythema around the umbilicus with purulent umbilical discharge, is a serious neonatal infection which may spread to adjacent tissue causing peritonitis, hepatic vein thrombosis and hepatic abscess. Immediate referral to hospital is required for parenteral antibiotics.

Congenital infections

➤ **Cytomegaloviruses** (CMVs) are members of the herpesvirus family. About 1 : 100 babies is born with CMV infection, but only about 10% have clinical symptoms including petechiae, deafness, hepatosplenomegaly, chorioretinitis and microcephaly causing later neurodisability.

➤ **Rubella** (*see* Chapter 4).

➤ **HIV** infection usually arises as a result of vertical transmission from an HIV-infected mother to her child, mostly during parturition. Without treatment, the rate of mother-to-baby transmission is approximately 25–30%. This rate is significantly reduced with prophylactic retroviral therapy (Zidovudine or AZT). The majority of infected children are asymptomatic at birth, but symptoms may develop within the first month of life, including persistent thrush, lymphadenopathy, hepatosplenomegaly, recurrent or persistent diarrhoea and failure to thrive.

➤ **Parvovirus** is known to cause fetal infection resulting in non-immune hydrops fetalis. The virus can cause severe anaemia and myocarditis. It can also cause neonatal infection, manifested by rash, anaemia, hepatosplenomegaly and cardiomegaly.

Perinatal infections
(*See* Chapter 4.)
➤ Herpes simplex virus
➤ Varicella zoster virus
➤ Hepatitis
➤ Sepsis and meningitis.

Clinical signs of congenital infection
These clinical findings of systemic infection may often be non-specific and subtle (Box 1.3).

BOX 1.3 Non-specific signs of infection

- Respiratory distress
- Instability of body temperature
- Gastrointestinal: poor feeding, vomiting, abdominal distension
- Diminished activity or lethargy
- Seizures

RESPIRATORY DISORDERS
➤ **Respiratory distress syndrome (RDS).** The primary cause is inadequate surfactant leading to diffuse alveolar atelectasis, oedema and cell injury. Risk factors for developing RDS are mainly prematurity and, to a lesser extent, maternal diabetes and maternal infection. Clinical signs include tachypnoea > 60 breaths/min, subcostal retractions, grunting, flaring of nasal alae and cyanosis.

➤ **Meconium aspiration.** The passage of meconium in utero may cause hypoxia. Gasping by the fetus or newly born infant can cause aspiration of the amniotic fluid which contains meconium. Meconium aspiration can cause RDS by obstructing airways and interfering with gas exchange.

➤ **Transient tachypnoea of the newborn (TTN).** This is a mild and self-limiting respiratory distress characterised (in contrast to RDS) by:
  ➤ Tachypnoea usually without subcostal recession
  ➤ Babies are usually born at term
  ➤ Babies frequently are born by caesarean section.

PRACTICE POINTS
- Referral of babies with RDS is required.
- If symptoms and signs of TTN are mild, the baby may be kept at home under observation provided the condition is stable and improving, the baby is feeding well and there are no parental concerns.

METABOLIC DISEASE

➤ **Hypoglycaemia** is defined as a blood glucose level < 1.7 mmol/L. A level < 2.3 mmol/L should be a cause for concern. Prematurity, intrauterine growth retardation, asphyxia and infection are the main causes. Symptoms include lethargy, jitteriness, apnoea, seizures and poor feeding. Many infants are asymptomatic.

➤ **Hypocalcaemia** is defined as a total calcium of < 2.1 mmol/L in children and < 2.0 mmol/L in term neonates. Causes for early hypocalcaemia (during the first 3 days of life) include prematurity, infant of diabetic mother, and birth asphyxia. Late-onset hypocalcaemia usually presents at the end of the first week of life and is caused by hypoparathyroidism, magnesium or vitamin D deficiency, and others. Symptoms are similar to those of hypoglycaemia.

CONGENITAL HEART DISEASE (CHD)

The birth prevalence of CHD is around 1%. The most common presentations of CHD are murmur, cyanosis, respiratory distress and poor feeding. Important diagnostic clues of the presence of CHD in young infants are given in Box 1.4.

Early detection is important:

➤ Missed or delayed diagnosis of CHD distresses parents, even if the delay does not cause any harm to the baby.

➤ Early diagnosis may prevent the occurrence of irreversible changes (e.g. pulmonary hypertension with left to right shunt), rapid deterioration with worsening prognosis and the development of endocarditis.

BOX 1.4 Important diagnostic clues for CHD

- Normal findings in the neonate do not guarantee that serious CHD does not exist. On the other hand, the presence of an innocent murmur is very common, occurring in at least 50% of children. The most common problem in auscultation of the heart is the difficulty in distinguishing innocent from pathological murmurs (*see* Chapter 10)
- It is important to check the femoral and dorsalis pedis pulses as part of the clinical examination. However, they are often not easily detectable and may occasionally be palpable even in the presence of coarctation
- In a baby who tires rapidly and sweats during feeding, CHD must be excluded
- In an infant with respiratory distress, VSD could be the cause. There may be no murmur at birth but this appears by the age of 6 weeks

NEONATAL JAUNDICE

Jaundice (apparent if total bilirubin > 35 μmol/L) is very common during the neonatal period. Jaundice appearing after 3 or 4 days of life suggests an infection, e.g. urinary tract infection or sepsis. Jaundice after the first week of life suggests breast-milk jaundice, biliary atresia, infection or metabolic disorders, e.g. galactosaemia or hypothyroidism (Box 1.5). After the neonatal period, viral hepatitis remains the most common cause of jaundice worldwide.

Physiology

➤ Physiological jaundice occurs in most neonates during the first few days of life. It is not a disease, is not present in the first 24 hours and is always an indirect hyperbilirubinaemia.

➤ Breast-milk jaundice is nothing other than physiological jaundice, which may persist for weeks. Mothers should be encouraged to continue breast-feeding.

➤ An infant with yellow skin but normal white sclera usually has carotenaemia.

➤ There is no evidence that a well full-term baby without haemolysis will experience ill-effects from a bilirubin level < 400 μmol/L.

➤ Conjugated bilirubin is water-soluble, not fat-soluble, and therefore does not damage the brain tissue to cause kernicterus. It is, however, associated with serious diseases such as congenital hepatitis and biliary atresia. Unconjugated bilirubin is fat-soluble and may enter the brain tissue, causing kernicterus.

BOX 1.5 List of causes of neonatal jaundice

- Physiological jaundice
- Haemolytic (e.g. Rh or ABO incompatibility)
- Breast-milk jaundice
- Polycythaemia
- Parenteral hyperalimentation
- Congenital spherocytosis
- Infection (e.g. congenital hepatitis such as cytomegalovirus)
- Biliary atresia
- Metabolic (e.g. galactosaemia)
- Hypothyroidism
- Crigler–Najjar syndrome

Recommended investigations

All babies with significant and/or prolonged jaundice need serum bilirubin estimation, which is usually performed by the community midwife. Guidelines for referring cases for further evaluation are provided in Box 1.6. First-line investigations are listed in Box 1.7.

BOX 1.6 Guidelines for referring babies with neonatal jaundice

- > 300 μmol/L of total bilirubin in a breast-fed term infant and > 270 μmol/L in formula-fed term infant
- Serum bilirubin level increasing by > 85 μmol/L per day
- > 34 μmol/L of direct bilirubin
- Persistent jaundice after 8 days in a term infant or 14 days in a premature infant
- Clinical jaundice prior to 36 hours of age
- Any hyperbilirubinaemia in an unwell or distressed child
- Any hyperbilirubinaemia with anaemia

BOX 1.7 Baseline tests for jaundice

(Usually performed in hospital.)
- Urine: Dipsticks to exclude UTI
- Full blood count (FBC): haemoglobin (Hb) low in haemolysis; leukocytosis in infection; reticulocytosis in haemolysis
- Liver function tests (LFTs): direct hyperbilirubinaemia indicates hepatocellular disease such as hepatitis; indirect hyperbilirubinaemia with otherwise normal LFTs is very suggestive of Gilbert syndrome; raised transaminase and alkaline phosphatise may indicate biliary obstruction. A positive direct Coombs' test supports ABO and Rhesus (Rh) incompatibility
- Blood group and Rh-status of the mother and infant

ANAEMIA

Erythropoiesis declines rapidly with the rise of arterial oxygen saturation (AOS) at birth to 95%, and remains low for 6–10 weeks. This causes a decline of haemoglobin (Hb) to 90–110 g/L in full-term infants and 70–90 g/L in premature infants. The low Hb level is the best stimulus for erythropoiesis and should not be suppressed by blood transfusion unless the child is symptomatic.

Anaemia is defined as an Hb level of less than 110 g/L. Causes of anaemia in neonates are given in Box 1.8. First-line tests are given in Box 1.9.

BOX 1.8 Main causes of anaemia in neonates and early infancy

- Blood loss (twin-to-twin transfusion, fetomaternal bleeding, placenta previa, massive cephalohaematoma
- Haemolytic anaemia:
  > ABO, Rh or minor blood group incompatibility (e.g. c, E, Kell, Duffy)
  > Maternal disease (e.g. lupus, autoimmune or haemolytic disease)
  > Red blood cell membrane defects (e.g. spherocytosis)
  > Metabolic defects (e.g. G6PD deficiency)
  > Haemoglobinopathies
- Infection
- Physiological anaemia
- Iron-deficiency anaemia (IDA)
- Red cell aplasia (Diamond–Blackfan syndrome)

BOX 1.9 Baseline tests for suspected anaemia

(Usually performed in hospital.)
- Full blood count (FBC): haemoglobin (Hb) < 110 g/L indicates anaemia, low mean corpuscular volume (MCV) (< 70 fL) and mean corpuscular haemoglobin (MCH) (< 26 pg) suggests microcytic, hypochromic anaemia. (Remember that capillary blood samples are 3.7 ± 2.7% higher than venous haematocrit. Warming the foot reduces the difference to around 2%)

- Reticulocyte count (elevated in haemolysis and chronic blood loss)
- Serum ferritin low in iron-deficiency anaemia, normal or high in haemolytic anaemia
- Coombs' test
- Liver function tests (LFTs): hyperbilirubinaemia: suggestive of acute or chronic haemolysis
- Reticulocyte count high in haemolytic anaemia, and response to iron treatment

PRACTICE POINTS

- Anaemia of prematurity is very common. It is usually normocytic and normochromic and does not respond to iron therapy.
- The time of umbilical cord clamping remains controversial (Box 1.10).
- Mild anaemia is usually asymptomatic; pallor and clinical symptoms first occur when the Hb falls below 70–80 g/L.
- By far the most common cause of anaemia is nutritional IDA, which can be easily diagnosed by low Hb, MCV, MCH, and ferritin level. IDA is rare in neonates.
- Premature infants are often comfortable with an Hb of 60.5–70.5 g/L. The level itself is not an indication for transfusion unless the infant is symptomatic (e.g. tachypnoeic) or has an infection.
- Iron supplement (2 mg/kg per day as fortified formula or therapeutic iron) should be given to all premature infants for the first year of life. This prophylaxis should start after the baby is 8 weeks old to prevent late anaemia of prematurity.
- Resist the wish of the parents to add tonics, vitamins or trace metals to iron therapy. There is no evidence to support their use. Vitamin D is recommended for all infants with a dose of 400 IU (10 mcg) per day PO.
- Treatment with oral iron should be given to all children with Hb < 110 g/L for 4–6 weeks. Hb needs to be checked to ensure recovery of the anaemia.

BOX 1.10 Early versus late clamping of the cord

- Early cord clamping (within the first minute after birth) is advocated on the grounds that it can prevent polycythaemia (haematocrit > 60%) and decreases the risk of postpartum haemorrhage
- Delaying clamping of the cord for at least 2–3 minutes does not appear to increase the risk of postpartum haemorrhage and leads to improved iron status, particularly in infants where access to good nutrition is poor, although this increases the risk of jaundice (Cochrane search: Pregnancy and Childbirth Groups Trials register, December 2007)

RED FLAGS

- All babies with anaemia (even mild) should be investigated; its presence may indicate a serious underlying disorder.
- Iron preparations are an important cause of accidental overdose. Ensure that parents keep the medicine away from children. Parents should also be told about common side-effects of iron therapy.

BLEEDING (PURPURA)

Core messages

➤ Purpura indicates extravasation of blood into the skin or mucosal membranes. It may be due to vasculopathy, thrombocytopathy, coagulopathy, or a combination of these mechanisms. It may represent a benign condition or a serious underlying disorder (Box 1.11). Depending on their size, purpuric lesions are either petechiae (pinpoint haemorrhages < 1 cm, usually < 2 mm, in diameter) or ecchymoses (> 1 cm in diameter).

➤ In contrast to exanthem and telangiectasia, purpura does not blanch on pressure. Once purpura is suspected or diagnosed, baseline tests are needed to confirm it (Box 1.12).

➤ In neonates, petechiae are commonly observed on the presenting part during delivery, particularly if the delivery was traumatic.

BOX 1.11 Causes of bleeding/purpura

- Infection (intrauterine or acquired)
- Hypoxia (DIC)
- Drugs
- Vitamin K deficiency
- Thrombocytopenia
- Infection, e.g. meningococcal septicaemia (MCS)
- Child abuse
- Thrombocytopenia, absent radius (TAR)
- Kasabach–Merritt syndrome (thrombocytopenia with haemangioma)
- Liver disease
- Histiocytosis
- Hereditary coagulation defects (haemophilia A and B)
- Vascular purpuras, e.g. Von Willebrand's disease
- Ehlers–Danlos syndrome
- Wiskott–Aldrich syndrome

BOX 1.12 Baseline tests for a child with purpura

(Usually performed in hospital.)

- Full blood count (FBC): to confirm thrombocytopenia; leukocytosis in bacterial infection
- Blood culture, urea & electrolytes (U&E), calcium, blood glucose
- LFT for underlying renal and liver disease
- Coagulation screen: bleeding and clotting time, partial thromboplastin time (PTT) (screen for factor VIII; haemophilia) and prothrombin time (PT) (for factors VII, V, X), clotting factors such as VIII, IX if PT and/or PTT abnormal

PRACTICE POINTS

- In a neonate with petechiae, maternal history for presence of idiopathic thrombocytopenic purpura (ITP), systemic lupus erythematosus (SLE), drugs, and infections during pregnancy should be sought. History is more important than extensive tests.
- The crucial factor in diagnosing and managing an infant with bleeding is determining whether he/she is well or ill (Table 1.3).

TABLE 1.3 Main causes of bleeding in neonates

	Diagnosis	Platelets	PT	PTT
Healthy-appearing	Immune thrombocytopenia	↓	–	–
	Haemorrhagic disease of newborn (vitamin K deficiency)	–	↑	↑
	Hereditary clotting factor deficiency (e.g. haemophilia)	–	–	↑
Ill-appearing	Disseminated intravascular coagulopathy (DIC)	↓	↑	↑
	Infection	↓	–	–
	Liver disease	–	↑	↑

1. PT = prothrombin time; PTT = partial thromboplastin time.

Haemorrhagic disease of the newborn occurs in 1 in 200–400 neonates who did not receive vitamin K prophylaxis. Vitamin K 1.0 mg IM is offered to all neonates.

➤ In 1992 a link was suggested between IM administration of vitamin K at birth and an increased risk of cancer in children. Although this was not confirmed by other studies, parents are given the option to instead administer 3 doses of oral vitamin K, usually at birth, at 7–10 days and at 28 days.

➤ Modern formulae contain sufficient vitamin K, but babies who are breast-fed should receive prophylaxis.

➤ Administration of the last dose is often missed and should be specifically asked about at the 6-week check.

RED FLAGS

- Of all diseases with purpura, those caused by sepsis or meningococcal septicaemia are the most serious and require urgent management in hospital.
- Any acutely ill child with purpura should receive immediate management, including benzylpenicillin injection 75 mg/kg before urgent transfer to hospital.

Whenever there are unexplained bruises, non-accidental injury (NAI) should always be considered. Lesions are suspicious when they are found in areas of the body not normally subjected to injury (trunk, buttocks and cheeks). Additional clues for NAI should be sought: inflicted cigarette burns, retinal haemorrhages, intra-oral injury; and a skeletal examination performed. Radiological skeletal survey may be indicated

APPENDIX
Definitions of terms

Embryo	< 9 weeks' gestation
Fetus	9 weeks' gestation to delivery
Miscarriage	Spontaneous loss of pregnancy < 24 weeks' gestation
Stillbirth	Birth of baby > 24 weeks' gestation with no signs of life. It is either intrauterine death (IUD) or intrapartum death during labour
Abortion	The termination of pregnancy by the removal or expulsion of a fetus or embryo from the uterus, either spontaneous or induced
Multiple pregnancy:	
– monozygotic (identical twins)	A single ovum fertilised by a single sperm which splits into two embryos. About a quarter of twins are identical
– dizygotic (non-identical twins)	Ovulation of two ova fertilised by two sperms
Term	37–42 weeks
Pre-term	< 37 weeks
Post-term	> 42 weeks
Low birthweight	$\leq 2500\,g$
Small for gestational age (SGA)	Also known as intrauterine growth retardation (IUGR), a birthweight < 10th centile for the gestational age. Babies may be:
	Asymmetrical – weight on a lower centile than head circumference
	Symmetrical – weight and head circumference on the same centile
Large for gestational age	Birthweight > 90th centile for gestational age
Perinatal mortality rate	Number of stillbirths + deaths within 7 days per 1000 deliveries

Growth, development and disability

NUTRITIONAL REQUIREMENTS

Children need enough calories to grow and develop. Daily requirement of calories for children at different ages is shown in Table 2.1. This is about 80–120 kcal/kg during the first year of life, with subsequent decrease of calories per kg bodyweight except during puberty when rapid growth requires increased caloric consumption. Energy expenditure is utilised:

➤ 12% for daily growth (Table 2.2)
➤ 25% for physical activity
➤ 13% for thermic effect and faecal loss
➤ 50% for basal metabolism.

The principal source of fluid is from milk during the early years of life (Table 2.3).

TABLE 2.1 Calorie requirements in different ages

Age (years)	Calories per day (kcal)	
	Boys	Girls
1–3	1,230	1,165
4–6	1,715	1,545
7–10	1,970	1,740
11–14	2,220	1,845
15–18	2,755	2,110
Adults	2,550	1,940

TABLE 2.2 Approximate growth increase during the first few years of life

	Weight	Length	Head circumference
At birth (term baby)	2.7–4.6 kg	47–55 cm	33–37 cm
0–3 months	25–30 g/day	3.5 cm/month	2 cm/month
3–6 months	20–25 g/day	2.0 cm/month	1 cm/month
6–12 months	12–15 g/day	1.2–1.5 cm/month	0.5 cm/month
1–3 years	8 g/day	0.8–1.0 cm/month	0.25 cm/month
4–6 years	6 g/day	4–5 cm/year	1 cm/year

TABLE 2.3 Daily fluid intake requirements at different ages

Age	mL/kg/day
0–6 months	150
7–12 months	120
1 year	120–135
2 years	115–125
4 years	100–110
10 years	70–85
14 years	50–60
18 years	40–50

GROWTH MONITORING

Routine measurement of weight, height and head circumference is widely accepted among professionals for monitoring growth. There is, however, no clear consensus on how often growth should be measured. Benefits of growth monitoring include:
➤ Assessing the overall nutritional status
➤ Detecting impaired growth caused for example by child neglect or abuse
➤ Detecting overweight children at an early stage
➤ Detecting other growth disorders such as:
  ➢ Rapid growth, e.g. precocious puberty
  ➢ Constitutional growth delay
  ➢ Endocrine or chromosomal disorders, e.g. Turner's syndrome and growth hormone deficiency
  ➢ Chronic diseases, e.g. coeliac or Crohn's disease
  ➢ Syndromes, e.g. Noonan's syndrome or bone dysplasia.

Measurement of weight
➤ Weight is a useful guide to the child's nutritional status.
➤ Infants should be weighed naked or with a nappy at most, subtracting the weight of the nappy afterwards. Older children should be weighed with underwear on.
➤ During the first year of life, a child's weight and height may cross 1 centile line. After the age of 1 year, growth measurements in most healthy children tend to stay within the same centile until the onset of puberty unless a growth disorder such as obesity or growth failure intervenes.

Measurement of height
➤ Any child older than 2 years should be measured for height standing up. In children younger than 2 years of age, recumbent length is significantly greater than standing height.
➤ Length is no longer routinely measured, but should be measured at the 6-week check if the infant was small for dates, failing to thrive or has dysmorphic features.
➤ Early identification of short stature associated with hormonal deficiencies is important because early treatment improves the outcome for adult height.
➤ The World Health Organization (WHO) 9-centile growth charts should be used, showing the 0.4 and the 99.6 centiles. Only one child in 250 lies above or below these

centile lines. A child below the 0.4 centile has a significant probability of having an organic cause for short stature. The current growth charts can be downloaded from: www.rcpch.ac.uk/growthcharts.
➤ Children with achondroplasia have a normal sitting height but a markedly reduced standing height.

Measurement of head circumference (HC)

➤ HC should be recorded carefully following birth and at 6–8 weeks of age.
➤ A large head, known as benign familial macrocephaly, is by far the most common cause of large HC in a healthy child, often exceeding 2 standard deviations or more above the mean. The presence of a large head in one of the parents, usually the father, should establish the diagnosis.
➤ If HC measurements are crossing centiles upwards, other conditions (e.g. hydrocephalus, subdural effusion and haematoma) should be considered. These conditions are associated with increased intracranial pressure (ICP), which clinically presents with tense fontanelle, suture separation, prominent scalp veins, downward gaze and irritability.
➤ If there are no accompanying symptoms or signs of ICP, two HC measurements over a 4-week period are sufficient. There is no justification for further repeated measurements because these cause excessive anxiety. GPs must either decide that this enlargement is normal or refer the child urgently.
➤ A small HC often suggests a benign familial small head with no additional problem. The rate of growth is normal and one of the parents is likely to have a smaller than average HC.
➤ Other causes of small HC include premature fusion of the suture, which is clinically diagnosed by a palpable elevated bony ridge along the length of the fused suture and abnormal head shape depending on which particular sutures have closed prematurely (*see* Chapter 1).

GROWTH DISORDERS

Failure to thrive (FTT) and weight loss

➤ Although there is no agreement about a definition of FTT, a child whose weight is below the 0.4 centile or has weight loss that has crossed 2 centiles is considered as FTT. Box 2.1 lists causes of FTT.
➤ Children with FTT have poorer cognitive, neurological and psychomotor development. Associated problems include immunodeficiency and increased susceptibility to infections.

BOX 2.1 Common causes of FTT

- Small-for-dates (after the age of 3 years)
- Psychosocial (e.g. emotional deprivation)
- Eating disorder (e.g. anorexia nervosa)
- Chronic infection (e.g. HIV, parasitic)
- Malnutrition
- Malabsorption (e.g. coeliac disease)
- Inborn errors of metabolism
- Depression, anxiety
- Inflammatory bowel disease
- Malignancy
- Endocrine (e.g. hyperthyroidism)

➤ FFT is divided into two main categories: organic and non-organic causes. In children, in contrast to adults, psychosocial causes are far more common than organic causes. If the history and physical examination do not suggest a specific underlying organic disease in a child who fails to thrive, psychosocial causes are likely and laboratory and imaging are unlikely to provide the answer. Table 2.4 provides distinguishing features of the two categories.

TABLE 2.4 Distinguishing features between organic and psychosocial causes of FTT

	Organic causes	Psychosocial causes
History usually	Diagnostic	Diagnostic
Acute history	Likely	Unlikely
Abnormal examination	Often positive	Usually negative
Child's behaviour	Likely normal	Likely abnormal
Family interaction	Likely normal	Likely abnormal
Laboratory data and imaging	Positive results	Usually negative

Recommended investigations
➤ Urine dipsticks for possible infection and proteinuria
➤ Full blood count (FBC): looking for anaemia suggesting malnutrition, infection or malabsorption
➤ Inflammatory markers (C-reactive protein (CSR) or erythrocyte sedimentation rate (ESR)): elevated in infections
➤ Thyroid function tests (TFTs) will confirm hyperthyroidism
➤ Coeliac screening tests
➤ Liver function tests (LFTs) and bone profile

PRACTICE POINTS

- In pre-term infants: when plotting growth parameters, the weeks of prematurity should be subtracted from the postnatal age. For example, if a child is seen at a chronological age of 15 months but was born 3 months early, the corrected age is 12 months. This correction should be done up to the age of 2 years.
- Small-for-gestational-age (SGA) babies (weight < 10 centile for gestational age) whose poor growth dated from the 1st trimester are symmetrically affected with low weight, height and HC. They often remain underweight for a few years and should not be categorised as FTT. Those with SGA from the 3rd trimester are only underweight with their height and HC unaffected. They are more likely to catch up on growth.
- High-quality child care and a loving home favourably influence a child's development and growth, while poor-quality care adversely affects development and growth.
- Neglect, either physical or emotional, is the most common cause of underweight in infancy and may account for > 50% of cases of FTT.
- Children at high risk of abuse are often those with excessive crying during infancy, physical handicap, chronic illness, or behavioural or learning difficulties.

- Neglected children returning to their parents without any medical or social intervention may face serious re-injury (in about 25%) or death (in about 5%).
- Depressive disorder occurs in about 50% of adolescents. They may show either a decrease or an increase in weight.
- Weight loss in adolescent girls is likely to be due to eating disorder. Diagnosis can be difficult in the early stages. Asking about attitude (e.g. by using a self-administered test of four simple questions) towards eating and weight can screen for 'eating disorder risk' (*see* Chapter 3).

Excessive weight gain (obesity)

➤ The number of obese children (Table 2.5) has tripled over the past 20 years.

➤ Obesity is linked to adult obesity, with the potential risk of increased mortality, cardiovascular disease, hypertension, type 2 diabetes, back pain, osteoarthritis, hyperlipidaemia, cholelithiasis, some cancers and sleep apnoea. It reduces the life expectancy by an average of 9 years.

➤ Obese children often do not eat more than their peers. Genetic factors and reduced energy output (long hours sitting in front of the TV or computer) are more important causal factors.

➤ Obesity usually results from increases in the number of fat cells (adipocytes), occurring during the gestational months and the first year of life. Any early obesity may persist.

➤ Other causes of obesity (Box 2.2), including hormonal and endocrine, are rare in clinical practice but are often considered by parents to be the reason for the obesity.

TABLE 2.5 Weight definition of healthy and overweight children

Classification	Body mass index (BMI) (kg/m^2)
Healthy weight	18.5–24.9
Overweight	25–29.9
Obesity I	30–34.9
Obesity II	35–39.9
Obesity III	40 or more

Recommended investigations

➤ Urine: proteinuria in case of oedema caused by renal disease
➤ TFTs: for hypothyroidism
➤ Electrolytes and urea (U&E) in blood: deranged in Cushing's syndrome
➤ Blood glucose for diabetes and Beckwith–Wiedemann syndrome
➤ Calcium and parathyroid hormone for hypoparathyroidism
➤ Serum cortisol levels for Cushing's syndrome
➤ Bone age: normal in simple obesity, delayed in endocrine causes
➤ Pelvic ultrasound scan: will confirm ovarian cysts in PCOS, or abnormalities of adrenals in Cushing's syndrome
➤ CT scan or MRI for suspected cases of Cushing's syndrome

BOX 2.2 Possible causes of obesity

- Simple obesity
- Infant of diabetic mother
- Polycystic ovarian syndrome (PCOS)
- Endocrine (e.g. Cushing's syndrome, hypothyroidism)
- Drugs (e.g. steroids, pizotifen, anticonvulsants)
- Insulinoma
- Oedema (renal or cardiac)
- Beckwith–Wiedemann syndrome
- Cerebral gigantism (Sotos syndrome)
- Laurence–Moon–Biedl syndrome (polydactyly, learning disability, retinitis pigmentosa)

PRACTICE POINTS

- Obesity due to a syndrome or endocrine causes is rare. Table 2.6 provides differential diagnosis between simple and endocrine/syndrome causes of obesity.
- BMI gives no indication of body fat distribution, while waist circumference (midway between the 10th rib and the top of the iliac crest) is a marker for central body fat accumulation and is more accurate than BMI. Normal ranges for waist circumference are shown in Table 2.7.
- Clinical intervention should be considered for children with a BMI $\geq$ 91st centile and assessment for co-morbidities if $\geq$ 98th centile.
- Much time is wasted by giving unwanted advice about food. The child with obesity is aware of that and is often upset by hearing that he or she is eating too much; dietary restriction is in any case notoriously unsuccessful in treating the condition. Box 2.3 shows evidence-based treatment of obesity.
- The main cause of childhood obesity is not overeating, but genetic factors and decreased energy output. The latter can be estimated indirectly by the total hours spent in front of the TV and computer per day.
- Non-insulin-dependent diabetes mellitus (NIDDM or type 2 diabetes), elevated levels of low-density lipoproteins (LDLs) and low levels of high-density lipoproteins (HDLs) occur in association with obesity and are risk factors for cardiovascular disease and stroke.
- The finding of supernumerary digits with obesity raises the likelihood of Laurence–Moon–Biedl syndrome (obesity, polydactyly, retinitis pigmentosa and progressive nephropathy).
- An uncommon but important physical sign in an obese child: when the hand is fisted it may show short fourth and fifth knuckles; a sign seen in pseudohypoparathyroidism and in girls with Turner's syndrome.
- Blood pressure should be recorded in any child with obesity. It may be elevated in those with Cushing's syndrome and Turner's syndrome.

TABLE 2.6 Differential diagnosis between simple and endocrine obesity

	Simple obesity	Endocrine obesity
History	Long duration	Shorter duration
Family history (obesity)	Often positive	Usually not positive
Height	Average or above	Short
Findings in physical examination	Otherwise normal	Usually abnormal
Fat distribution	Diffuse	More localised (e.g. truncal)
Bone age	Normal or advanced	Delayed
Sexual development	Appropriate for age	Delayed
Striae	Pink, appear at puberty	Often violaceous, appear early

TABLE 2.7 Normal ranges of waist circumference (cm)[1]

Age (years)	Boys			Girls		
	10th centile	50th centile	90th centile	10th centile	50th centile	90th centile
2	43.2	47.1	50.8	43.8	47.1	52.2
5	48.4	53.2	61.0	48.5	53.0	61.4
10	57.0	63.3	78.0	56.3	62.8	76.6
15	65.6	73.5	95.0	64.2	72.6	91.9

MANAGEMENT OF OBESITY

Drug and surgical treatment

➤ Drug treatment is generally not used for children younger than 12 years except in life-threatening co-morbidities, e.g. sleep apnoea.

➤ For children aged 12 years or older, treatment with Orlistat (the drug prevents the absorption of fat by inhibiting the enzyme lipase) is indicated only:
  ➤ If physical co-morbidities such as sleep apnoea or orthopaedic or severe psychological problems are present
  ➤ For a trial for 6–12 months with regular review to assess effectiveness, side-effects and adherence.

➤ Orlistat should be prescribed for obesity in children only by a multidisciplinary team with expertise in:
  ➤ drug monitoring
  ➤ psychological support
  ➤ behaviour intervention such as increased activity
  ➤ nutrition and how to improve diet.

➤ Surgical intervention (e.g. gastric banding) may be considered only in exceptional circumstances and after the patient has:
  ➤ received intensive management in a specialised obesity service
  ➤ been found to be generally fit for surgery and anaesthesia
  ➤ been found committed to the need for a long-term follow-up.

BOX 2.3 Management of obesity in children

Activity

- Encourage regular physical activity daily (even if they do not lose weight) such as cycling and swimming
- Children may need to change their daily routine habits such as taking the stairs instead of lift, walking and cycling to school and shops
- Maintain good glycaemic control and reduce the risk of type 2 diabetes and cardiovascular events
- Diabetic children are at risk of hypoglycaemia during or after exercise. Ensure that:
  1. Pre-exercise blood glucose is in the target range to avoid hypoglycaemia. High levels of BS > 14 mmol or the presence of ketones are unsafe
  2. The child wears an identification, e.g. medicalert bracelet
  3. The child has an extra snack prior to activity, e.g. 15–30 g carbohydrate 15–30 min pre-exercise
  4. The child has some fast-sugar food on hand at all times

Diet

Children with type 1 diabetes should:

- See a trained dietitian who can advise on a balanced diet with carbohydrates, protein and fat
- Know that there are no forbidden foods, including sugar. Carbohydrate restriction is not recommended. Better glycaemic control is established by providing 40–55% of the total caloric intake as carbohydrate
- Opt for fruits, whole-grain foods such as whole-grain bread, beans, brown rice, pasta and starchy vegetables, low-fat dairy products, lean meat as foundation of diet
- Be encouraged to lose weight if appropriate
- Eat regular meals in a pleasant, sociable environment without distraction such as TV watching. Parents should eat the same food as their children whenever possible
- Get children involved in meal preparation

NORMAL DEVELOPMENT
Developmental assessment

The goal of developmental assessment is to answer the following questions:

➤ Is the child's development in the 'normal range' and comparable to that of his/her peers?
➤ Are the key areas of development – gross motor, fine motor, language and personal/social – developing at the same rate?
➤ Has the child's development been progressing at a steady rate or has there been evidence of regression?

The Denver Developmental screening test is the most widely used test to screen for developmental abnormality. In summary:

➤ Primary care teams, in particular health visitors, need a good knowledge of normal child development and this should be updated regularly. GPs are no longer routinely involved in child surveillance except at the 6-week check.
➤ Routine surveillance is now focused on high-risk children, including those who were treated in special care units, where concerns were raised at the 6-week check and if there are parental concerns.

➤ The test generates pass–fail ratings in four categories of development (gross motor, fine motor, personal/social, and language) for children from birth to 6 years (summarised for the age group 0–36 months in Table 2.8).

➤ One or two screening questions in each key area of development are usually sufficient to assess development.

➤ Language and personal/social skills should be assessed first because gross and fine motor milestones can be observed during physical examination.

TABLE 2.8 Summary of developmental milestones

Age in months	Gross motor	Fine motor	Personal/social	Language
0–1	Knees under the abdomen. In ventral suspension, head below the body level	Hands fisted	Regards human face with interest	Responds to sounds (bell) if active or crying, startles if quiet
2	Prone: lifts head to 45°, knees no longer under the abdomen. In ventral suspension, head held erect	Hands open most of the time	Smiles in response	Coos, vocalises with vowel sounds (ah, uh)
3	Lifts head to 45° for sustained period. In ventral suspension, head up above the level of body	Hands open, holds placed object actively	Anticipates feeding, smiles spontaneously	Chuckles
4	Bears weight briefly on extended legs, rolls front to back	Reach and grasp begin, puts toys to mouth	Excited when toys presented, smiles and vocalises at self in mirror	Laughs loudly, increased vocalisation
6	When pulled to sit, no head lag, assists by lifting head, sits leaning forward on arms	Transfers objects from one hand to another, reaches for toy with one-hand approach	Takes solids well, bites and chews, pats at mirror image	Increasing babble, expresses with sounds
9	Sits indefinitely, pulls to stand	Explores pellet with index finger	Imitates waving, straightens arm through sleeve	Non-specific 'Mama' and 'Dada'
12	Stands independently well, walks a few steps	Helps turn book pages, imitates scribbling	Throws toys away in play	One word besides 'Mama' and 'Dada'
15	Gets to standing without support, walks well	Tower of 2 or 3 cubes	Starts to handle spoon and cup	4 or 5 words
18	Walks carrying objects, runs stiffly	Tower of 3–4 cubes, turns 2–3 book pages	Feeds self with spoon, handles regular cup	Follows simple commands, points to 1–4 body parts
21	Runs well, walks up and down stairs holding rail, kicks a large ball	Tower of 5–6 cubes, completes 3-piece form board	Uses fork, helps with simple household tasks	20–50 words, combines 2 words

Age in months	Gross motor	Fine motor	Personal/social	Language
24	Jumps with both feet off floor	Tower of 6–7 cubes, threads shoelace through holes	Feeds self with little spilling	At least 50 words, 3-word sentences
30	Stands briefly on one foot, alternates feet going upstairs	Tower of 8–10 cubes, turns single book pages	Accomplishes toileting, puts on shoes	Names many familiar objects, names many body parts
36	Pedals tricycle, alternates feet going upstairs	Tower of at least 10 cubes, holds crayon in fingers, tries to cut with scissors	Toilet training, dresses with supervision	Recites nursery rhyme, gives first and last name

Primitive reflexes

(*See* Chapter 1)

These reflexes do not usually persist (except the parachute reflex), and their persistence is a sign of abnormal development (Table 2.9).

TABLE 2.9 Some primitive reflexes, with age of disappearance

Reflex	Usual occurrence and disappearance
Rooting	From birth until 4 months of age
Placing	From birth until about 6 weeks of age
Moro	From birth until about 3 months of age
Palmar grasp	From birth until 3 months of age
Atonic neck	From 2 months until 6 months of age
Parachute	From 9 months of age and persists

Performing developmental assessment

➤ Child's performance must be interpreted against the background of the history. Testing provides a general impression of whether the child is performing within the expected age range.
➤ It is best to start assessment with the child on the parent's lap or in a seat that provides good support and allows both arms to be free.
➤ Test for fine motor and problem-solving tasks (tower building with blocks or colouring should be the initial steps, as these are engaging to children).
➤ Language testing is done once the child is cooperating well.
➤ Gross motor and physical examination should be done last to avoid losing the child's cooperation.

The following items for performing the assessment (4 months to 6 years) are needed:
➤ Table of age-appropriate milestones (summary in Table 2.8), as there is no need to memorise the long lists of milestones

➤ Useful materials are commercially available which include:
  ➢ a plastic spoon
  ➢ non-transparent cup
  ➢ safety scissors
  ➢ a book with simple pictures of common household items
  ➢ at least 10 identical 1-inch blocks for tower building
  ➢ a form board puzzle with removable geometric blocks
  ➢ pellets for fine motor assessment
  ➢ shoelace
  ➢ paper and pencils for drawing a circle (imitates vertical stroke and circle scribble aged 2 years), cross (4 years), square (5 years), triangle (5 years), diamond (6 years).

Developmental delay

Identification of a child with developmental delay is usually achieved through:
➤ Routine neonatal and 8-week examinations
➤ Specialist follow-up of high-risk babies
➤ Parental or professional concerns.

Developmental delay may be due to non-specific genetic factors, specific conditions or environmental factors. Behavioural and developmental problems often go hand in hand. These problems include:

➤ **Significant emotional, psychological or behavioural problems.** These are common at some stage of development and affect as many as 20% of children, but they are not sufficiently severe to be regarded as psychiatric disorders. However, when these problems become frequent or severe, or inappropriate for the child's age, they become a source of considerable misery and distress to the child and/or the parents and may interfere with the child's development. Examples include temper tantrum, aggressive behaviour, eating or sleeping disorders (refusing food or not settling at night), disobedience, school phobia, overactivity and enuresis and encopresis. Rates of these problems are higher in inner cities, socially deprived families and children with learning difficulties including delayed language development.

➤ **Delayed language development.** There are wide variations among healthy children in the rate of language acquisition. Genetic influences and socio-economical factors play important roles in determining the rate of language development. Delayed language development is best defined as 2 standard deviations below the mean, e.g. fewer than 10 words at the age of 24–26 months. This can be caused by:
  ➢ Normal variation (other causes below should be excluded)
  ➢ Hearing impairments (sensorineural or middle ear disease)
  ➢ Aphasia
  ➢ Neurological diseases, e.g. cerebral palsy
  ➢ Classical autism.

➤ **Delay in walking** can be caused by:
  ➢ Normal variation
  ➢ Prematurity
  ➢ Associated bottom shuffling
  ➢ Neuromuscular diseases, e.g. Duchenne muscular dystrophy.

RED FLAGS

- Any child who walks later than at 18 months should have creatinine phosphokinase (CPK) check to exclude Duchenne muscular dystrophy (DMD). About 50% of children with DMD walk later than at 18 months.
- It is essential to distinguish the child who has always been delayed in development from the one who began normally and subsequently slowed or regressed. The latter may indicate neurodegenerative diseases, autism or seizures.
- Warning signs:
  - No smile by 8 weeks of age
  - Not sitting by 9 months of age
  - No single word by 18 months of age
  - No sentences by 30 months of age.

DISABILITY[2]

Disability indicates any restriction or lack of ability to perform an activity which is considered normal for the child's age. The WHO defines learning disability as 'a state of arrest or incomplete development of mind'. Disability includes:

➤ Motor involvement such as cerebral palsy or Duchenne muscular dystrophy
➤ Delayed speech and language acquisition
➤ Learning difficulty or disability –
  ➣ global learning difficulty denotes the presence of lower than normal intelligence
  ➣ specific learning difficulty denotes an impairment in one particular skill or function (Table 2.10).

TABLE 2.10 Summary of specific learning difficulties

Specific disability in:	Brief description of the difficulties
Reading (dyslexia)	Understanding the relationship between words and letters, misspelling words
	Reading with fluency and speed
Mathematics (dyscalculia)	Solving maths problems, understanding time and using money
Fine motor (dyspraxia)	Hand–eye coordination, balance
Writing (dysgraphia)	Handwriting, spelling, organising ideas, accurately copying words or letters
Language (dysphasia)	Producing or understanding spoken words

A GP can refer a child with suspected developmental delay to:

➤ a Child Development Team, which includes specialists such as community paediatricians, nurses, psychologists and speech therapists (sometimes the team includes a child psychiatrist)
➤ a Community Learning Disability Team, available in some areas.

All educational authorities have a Parent Partnership Scheme to advise parents on education provision.

FURTHER READING

1. Fernandez JR, Redden DT, Pietrobelli A, et al. Waist circumference percentiles in national samples of African-American, European-American, and Mexican-American children and adolescents. J Pediatr 2004; 145: 439–44.

2. Sources of further information:
   - The young mind. An essential guide to mental health for young adults, parents and teachers. Bantam Press, 2009
   - Contact a Family offers information and advice for parents of children with any special needs or disability
   - MENCAP – leading UK charity for people with a learning disability
   - Every Disabled Child Matters website, which campaigns for rights and justice for every disabled child
   - UK government websites for citizens which contain useful information regarding special educational needs:
   - www.childrendisabilities.info
   - www.councilfordisabledchildren.org.uk

CHAPTER 3

Behavioural problems and mental health

TEMPER TANTRUM

Core messages

➤ Temper tantrums include excessive screaming, kicking, hitting and breath-holding. Their frequency and intensity vary considerably.

➤ The vast majority of temper tantrums can be regarded as a normal part of development and most parents can expect some forms of temper tantrum from the age of 1½ years up to the age of 4 years.

➤ Between 1½ and 2 years of age, children are usually very egocentric, want to be independent and self-controlled and resist domination by parents. If an adult stands in their way and they cannot reach their goals, they become frustrated and a temper tantrum is triggered. By the age of 3 years, temper tantrums often become less frequent and intense as children learn to use language to express themselves.

➤ Situations that commonly trigger tantrums include bedtime, bath and playtimes, getting dressed and shopping.

MANAGEMENT TIPS (PROMOTING POSITIVE BEHAVIOUR)

● Parents should not *ask* children to do something when they must do it anyway, e.g. do not ask '"When would you like to eat (or sleep)?' but rather say 'It is now lunchtime (or bedtime)'.

● Children need to know how their parents want them to behave. Parents should give praise and attention for ordinary good behaviour. Instant approval is much more effective than bribery.

● Parents should spare a little time each day to share an activity or game with their children, and to let them feel their parents are enjoying this shared activity.

● Parents should allow their children to feel important and grow in self-confidence by giving them little tasks suitable for their developmental ability.

● Parents should remain calm and hang on to a sense of humour, and not punish or argue with the child. Parents must manage their own behaviour before expecting their child to manage his or hers. Yelling back or spanking will only make the situation worse.

● Parents should not give in to a child having tantrums; that attitude will only increase their frequency.

- Temper tantrums may be ignored if they are attention-seeking.
- After the child has calmed down from a tantrum, parents can teach him/her skills to help avoid temper tantrums in the future, e.g. how to try to express feelings without hitting or screaming, how to learn better ways to get what he/she wants and how to interact successfully with his/her peers.
- If despite the use of these interventions the temper tantrums are worsening in terms of frequency, intensity and duration, a **referral** may be considered, particularly if:
  - there is evidence of self-injury or physical assaults on others
  - there are signs of withdrawal or frustration
  - there is suspicion of neglect or abuse.

RED FLAGS

- When a child presents with temper tantrums, primary-care physicians should check the child for possible co-morbid conditions which may cause or contribute to such behaviour, e.g. hearing or visual impairment, language and learning difficulties.
- Severe temper tantrums are sometimes an early symptom of autism, occurring particularly when the child is interrupted from performing routines or rituals.

BREATH-HOLDING ATTACKS (CYANOTIC AND PALLID ATTACKS)
Core messages
➤ This common condition affects about 5% of children, and is characterised by an episodic apnoea, often leading to changes in postural tone and consciousness and may end in seizure. Peak age is 6–18 months. The attacks are unusual before 6 months and after the age of 5 years. Family history is positive in 25% of cases.
➤ About one-third of affected children have 2–5 attacks a day; another third have one attack per month and the remaining third have attacks either more or less frequently than these two ranges.
➤ Attacks usually are triggered by anger, frustration or pain. The child will recover within 1–2 minutes. There is no prolonged post-ictal-phase drowsiness or confusion as occurs in seizures. The child is well between the attacks.
➤ The more common cyanotic attacks have a stereotypical course: pain → crying → apnoea (lasting about 10 seconds) → cyanosis (or pallor in the pallid form) → loss of consciousness → possible seizure, which is usually very brief.
➤ It is important to differentiate between the cyanotic and pallid forms, because the pallid form may be associated with cardiac rhythm abnormalities (Box 3.1).
➤ Combination attacks (both cyanotic and pallid forms) occur in about 20% of the total cases.

BOX 3.1 Differentiating between cyanotic and pallid forms of breath-holding attacks

- Cyanotic attacks are far more common than the pallid form
- Cyanotic attacks are triggered by anger or frustration; the pallid attacks are usually triggered by a painful event
- Crying is the rule in the cyanotic type and very brief or absent in the pallid form
- Following loss of consciousness, cyanotic attacks may be associated with clonic jerks and bradycardia. Pallid attacks may be associated with tonic seizure; bradycardia and/or cardiac asystole. Seizure may occasionally need to be differentiated from epilepsy (Box 3.2)

BOX 3.2 Differentiating between breath-holding attacks and epileptic seizures

- Excluding febrile seizures, epileptic seizures are uncommon and 10 times less common (0.5%) than breath-holding (5%)
- Epilepsy occurs at any age; breath-holding attacks usually occur between 6 and 18 months of age
- Cyanosis in breath-holding occurs first, before the onset of subsequent seizure, while cyanosis occurs late and after the onset of epileptic seizure
- Breath-holding attacks are nearly always stereotyped (*see* text above); epileptic seizures are unpredictable in the way they manifest
- Recovery is fast in breath-holding (1–2 minutes) while the recovery in epileptic seizure usually takes much longer
- There is no post-ictal phase in breath-holding, in contrast to epileptic seizures
- EEG is normal in breath-holding, and usually abnormal in epilepsy

MANAGEMENT TIPS

- The first step of management is to establish the diagnosis.
- Reassurance that the child will grow out of it is the cornerstone of management.
- Distract the child whilst in pain and avoid the situations which lead to breath-holding.
- CPR is usually unnecessary and unhelpful. When the child is unconscious or fitting, he/she should be placed on its side in the recovery position.
- Some parents find splashing cold water on the face helpful in terminating the duration of the attacks. There is little evidence to support this.
- Extra attention or worry, or bending to the child's will, may reinforce the attacks.
- ECG, haemoglobin (Hb) and ferritin are usually indicated in the pallid form (*see* Red Flags below) and Hb and ferritin in cyanotic attacks. EEG may be requested if the diagnosis is unclear and history may suggest epilepsy.
- There is no definitive treatment available. There is evidence that iron is beneficial if the ferritin level is found to be low. Iron may also be prescribed even in the absence of iron-deficiency anaemia if the attacks are frequent and/or severe.
- **Referral** should be considered if the history is unclear, or the attacks are frequent and/or severe.

🏳 **RED FLAGS**

- It is essential to exclude seizure in any child presenting with breath-holding (Box 3.2). If the diagnosis is in doubt, referral should be made.
- An ECG is an essential investigation in pallid attacks to exclude prolonged QT-syndrome which is a potentially life-threatening but treatable form of cardiac arrhythmia.
- Pallid attacks can in some cases be induced by ocular compression (oculocardiac reflex). This should not be attempted in primary care.
- Some children with pallid attacks are treated with atropine by specialists. This medication should not be given in very hot weather (e.g. holidays abroad) because of the risk of hyperthermia.

HEAD BANGING AND ROCKING

Core messages

➤ Head banging and rocking, also termed rhythmic movement disorder, is a common stereotyped repetitive behaviour usually seen in children around naptime and bedtime.

➤ The head movements are commonly seen in healthy children aged 6–9 months, and usually resolve by 18 months of age. In 3% of cases they persist beyond the age of 2 years.

➤ Head banging and rocking may also be due to attention-seeking, self-stimulation and self-comfort. This behaviour is more common in children with developmental delay or learning difficulty.

➤ The condition typically occurs with the child lying face down, banging the head into a pillow or mattress. In the upright position, the head is banged against the wall or bedside furniture.

BOX 3.3 Management tips for children with head banging and rocking

- Children need to be carefully examined to ensure they are healthy with normal development. The head should be examined to exclude any injury
- Parents can be reassured if the child:
  - ❭ is healthy and has a normal development
  - ❭ is showing this behaviour only at bedtime and naptime
  - ❭ has no associated sleep disorder such as sleep apnoea or night terrors
- Parents can be advised:
  - ❭ to give plenty of attention to the child during the day and ignore the head movements at night
  - ❭ to try soothing routines, e.g. warm bath, before putting the child to sleep
  - ❭ to not put the child to sleep until he or she is tired and ready to go to sleep, rather than making bedtime a battle of wills
  - ❭ that padding of the bed is often unnecessary as there is a small risk of trapping the head
  - ❭ that the child's bed or crib should be moved away from the wall or furniture as this can cause injury and worsen the noise

➤ The head movements are considered abnormal if they are very frequent, occur outside bedtime and naptime, interfere with sleep or have caused head injury. Management is shown in Box 3.3.

TEETH GRINDING (BRUXISM)

➤ This unconscious habit usually occurs during sleep. In adults the habit is often caused by stress. In children it may be caused by:
  ➢ Improper teeth alignment
  ➢ Stress, anger, frustration
  ➢ Unknown causes.
➤ Management depends on the cause. Dentists may correct any non-alignment of teeth if this condition exists. They may prescribe a plastic mouth guard to be worn at night. If stress is suspected as the cause, parents should help the child relax by reading his or her favourite book before bedtime. A warm bath before sleep may help.
➤ Teeth grinding is usually harmless. Severe grinding may cause damage to the teeth enamel. Because teeth grinding usually occurs in sleep, the habit is very difficult to stop.

THUMB SUCKING AND NAIL BITING

➤ Thumb sucking is observed in utero as early as 29 weeks' gestation. In infancy, as many as 25–50% suck their thumbs. This incidence declines to 15–20% in children aged 5–6 years.
➤ Nail biting is found in as many as 45–60% of school age children to adolescents.
➤ In at least some children, the habit may be considered as a form of self-stimulation or self-comfort. Occasionally the habit is caused by stress or tension.
➤ Both habits (thumb sucking and nail biting) may cause some complications, including dental problems, deformities of the thumb or nails, and paronychia.
➤ Averse-tasting substances are often used in young children and may occasionally help.

SELF-STIMULATION (MASTURBATION) IN PRE-PUBERTAL CHILDREN
Core messages

➤ It is virtually impossible to eliminate masturbation, which is almost universal at puberty in response to the normal sexual drive.
➤ In pre-pubertal children it can often be regarded as normal behaviour, in particular in infants and toddlers as part of normal development and body exploration. Stimulation of the genitalia is usually done for pleasure and self-comfort.
➤ Self-stimulation occurs as repetitive and stereotyped episodes of tonic posturing associated with body rocking. The child may sit on the edge of a chair performing these movements for a few minutes but without actual manual stimulation of the genitalia. During the act the child is noted to be dazed, flushed and fully preoccupied. The child may grunt, and breathes irregularly. The act is often repeated several times a day.

MANAGEMENT PLAN

- Reassure parents that the habit does not pose any health risk or physical injury. Parents have to understand that their child has learned about it and he or she enjoys it.
- Reassure parents that the habit does not mean that the child will be promiscuous or a sex maniac.
- The habit usually ceases by 3 years of age.
- A reasonable approach by the parents is to allow the act to be carried out in the bedroom or bathroom.
- Self-stimulation only becomes a problem if parents overreact by punishing the child or stopping him or her by force, or making it appear 'dirty' or 'wicked'. These actions may cause emotional harm to the child.
- Some acts may be caused by boredom or inattention. The child may therefore be distracted by the parents spending more time together with the child and increasing activity, including physical activity.
- Occasionally this behaviour is associated with abnormality of the genitalia, such as nappy rash. Therefore, with appropriate consent, inspection of this area is important.
- **Referral** may be considered if:
  - The child continues doing it in public, particularly if this is done deliberately
  - The parents suspect that the child is demonstrating abnormally sexualised behaviour
  - Despite adequate steps taken by parents, the frequency of the act increases
  - There is evidence of child abuse.

TICS

Core messages

➤ This is a very common condition affecting about 20% of school-age children at some time during their childhood.

➤ Tics consist of sudden, involuntary, repetitive movements of muscles (motor tics) or sounds (vocal or phonic tics).

➤ Simple motor tics involve one muscle group, such as eye blinks, neck twisting or shoulder shrugging. Complex motor tics involve more than one muscle group, such as jumping or squatting.

➤ Tourette syndrome is a lifelong inherited neuropsychiatric disease with a prevalence of approximately 1 : 2000. It is characterised by:

➣ Motor tics, mainly affecting eyelids, face and shoulders

➣ Uncontrollable vocal tics, e.g. throat clearing, sniffling and coprolalia (obscene words)

➣ Obsessive-compulsive disorder (OCD)

➣ Attention-deficit hyperactivity disorder (ADHD).

MANAGEMENT OF TICS

- Avoid calling attention to the tics.
- Avoid telling your child to stop or control the tics.
- Avoid allowing the child to become over-excited, e.g. by video or computer games.
- There is usually no cure or effective medication for tics. Explanation, reassurance and education are the most important part of management.
- The goal of management is often to achieve optimum functioning rather than eliminating symptoms.
- Medications, such as haloperidol, clomipramine and clonidine, should be considered when the motor tics or vocalisations interfere significantly with social life or school functions.
- Clomipramine is effective in over 50% of patients with Tourette syndrome and OCD. These drugs are normally initiated in secondary care.
- **Referral** should be considered for:
  - ○ Persistent tics for several months
  - ○ Tics causing distress to the child or family
  - ○ Tics interfering with school function, social or family life
  - ○ Suspected Tourette syndrome.

RED FLAGS

- In severe cases of tics, including Tourette syndrome, co-morbidities are common and should be searched for, such as ADHD, OCD, learning and sleep difficulties.
- A child with tics or Tourette syndrome with co-morbidity of ADHD should not receive psychostimulant medications such as methylphenidate because they make the conditions worse. Some reports implicate methylphenidate in unmasking Tourette syndrome, but it is unlikely to cause it.

ANOREXIA NERVOSA

Core messages

➤ Anorexia nervosa is a serious mental illness with a high incidence of co-morbidities and mortality. It mainly affects girls, with a prevalence of 1%. Typical age used to be 13–17 years – this peak age has decreased in recent years and the age of onset can be as low as 9 years.

➤ In contrast to post-pubertal adolescents and adults, pre-pubertal children are at high risk of:
  ➢ Rapid weight loss due to low energy stores
  ➢ Rapid dehydration which may affect activity and wellbeing
  ➢ Stunting of growth, including height.

Anorexia nervosa is also an eating disorder characterised by:
➤ Fear of gaining weight, which continues as the weight loss progresses
➤ Denial of hunger, preoccupation with food preparation, obsession with calories and fat content and dieting despite weight loss and being underweight

➤ Refusal to maintain bodyweight within the normal range
➤ Weight loss, often rapid
➤ Purging, often using laxatives, e.g. ipecac
➤ Distorted self-image
➤ In females, loss of menstrual cycle for at least 3 months
➤ Frequent and strenuous exercise
➤ Excoriation.

Clinical findings are mostly the results of malnutrition and include:
➤ Weight well below the 3rd centile for age
➤ Cardiac arrhythmia or signs of congestive cardiac failure
➤ Bradycardia, low blood pressure and low body temperature
➤ Excoriation on the dorsum of the hand as a result of induced vomiting
➤ Sleep disturbance
➤ FBC often showing anaemia and leucopenia
➤ Reduced bone density (osteopenia).

Screening for eating disorders[1]

This can be done using the SCOFF questionnaire:
1. Do you make yourself **Sick** because you feel uncomfortably full?
2. Do you worry you have lost **Control** over how much you eat?
3. Have you recently lost more than **One** stone in a 3-month period?
4. Do you believe yourself to be **Fat** when others say you are too thin?
5. Would you say that **Food** dominates your life?

Interpretation of the test
➤ An answer 'No' to every question excludes an eating disorder.
➤ An answer 'Yes' to one question with the rest answered as 'No' should exclude an eating disorder but suggest that the individual may have some issues with food or body image.
➤ An answer of 'Yes' to at least two questions indicates the likelihood of anorexia nervosa or bulimia. Further assessment is required, including medical assessment if this has not already been done.

Recommended investigations

➤ Full blood count with CRP or ESR
➤ Blood glucose
➤ U&E, magnesium and phosphate
➤ Liver function tests
➤ Plasma protein with fractions (albumin and globulin)
➤ Thyroid function tests
➤ ECG for pulse rate, QT interval and possible arrhythmia

Management

➤ The **nutritional management** (Box 3.4) of patients with anorexia nervosa forms an essential part of treatment.

BOX 3.4 Recommendation on assessment and management of anorexia nervosa

- Assess the degree of dehydration. Weight and height should be measured and plotted on a growth chart. Dry mouth mucosa is the first sign of dehydration. Loss of skin elasticity (turgor loss) is a late sign
- Assess weight loss (BMI) and muscle wasting. The thigh muscles are affected first; cheek muscles are the last. This can be assessed using the squat and sit-up tests (Box 3.5)
- Examine the skin for breakdown and purpuric rash
- Examine the mouth, looking for glossitis and loss of taste sense (caused by iron or zinc deficiency), bleeding of gums and fissure of the lips (caused by riboflavin (vitamin B_2) or vitamin C deficiency)
- Inspect the teeth, as recurrent induced vomiting can erode teeth enamel leading to pain and caries
- Examine the circulation: systolic and diastolic blood pressure, postural hypotension and pulse rate
- Measure body temperature. Low body temperature is often present, and improves rapidly with improved nutrition
- Feed slowly. The amount of food given should be small at first, and be increased gradually
- Monitor weight. A weekly weight gain of 0.5–1.0 kg is optimal and an intake of 2200–2500 kcal (9211–10467 kJ) will achieve this in most patients

Based on guidelines by the Royal College of Psychiatry.[2,3]

BOX 3.5 Squat and sit-up tests

Squat test
- Patient squats down and is asked to stand up without using the arms as levers. Outcomes:
  - ❭ Able to get up without using hands at all
  - ❭ Unable to get up without using arms for balance
  - ❭ Unable to get up without using arms as leverage

Sit-up test

- Patient lies flat on a firm surface and has to sit up without using his/her arms. Outcomes:
  - ❭ Able to sit up without using the hands at all
  - ❭ Unable to sit up without using arms as leverage
  - ❭ Unable to sit up at all

Further management includes:
➤ All children with features suggestive of anorexia nervosa should be referred to the local eating disorders service or CAMHS (Child and Adolescent Mental Health Services) for multidisciplinary assessment, which include psychotherapy, behaviour-modification therapy and dietary rehabilitation. Admission to a rehab clinic is also possible.[4] Recovery occurs in about 70%. The mortality rate is around 10%. Death is usually due to cardiac arrhythmia or electrolyte disturbance.

🔖 **RED FLAGS**

- The diagnosis of anorexia nervosa should not be made without excluding organic diseases causing severe loss of appetite, such as endocrine disorders (e.g. hypopituitarism), occult malignancy, tuberculosis (TB) or gastrointestinal disorders (Crohn's or coeliac disease).
- Patients may develop peripheral oedema in the early stage of re-feeding. This has to be distinguished from cardiac failure by the absence of other signs of cardiac failure.
- With height reduction, weight loss will be underestimated if assessment is based on BMI alone.

AUTISM SPECTRUM DISORDERS (PERVASIVE DEVELOPMENTAL DISORDERS)

Core messages

➤ Autism is a lifelong disorder which has shown an increased prevalence. At least 1% of children are affected.

➤ The term *autistic spectrum disorders* encompasses three subtypes: autistic disorder, pervasive developmental disorder (PDD) and Asperger's syndrome. They are caused by a dysfunction of the CNS leading to disordered development.

➤ Global developmental delay in children with autism occurs in approximately 70–80%, of which 15–20% are severely delayed. Over 10% have average or above-average intelligence (Asperger's syndrome).

➤ About one-third of patients develop seizures in early childhood or adolescence.

➤ The symptoms and signs of autism are summarised in Box 3.6.

Diagnosis

➤ Although most children with autism are diagnosed aged 2–3 years, early diagnosis may be suspected if the following features are present:
  ➤ Reduced or absent interaction with others, paying attention instead to (for example) a toy
  ➤ Reduced or absent ability to imitate (which may explain difficulty with acquired language later)
  ➤ Reduced or absent non-verbal communication skill.

➤ Asperger's syndrome is a specific pervasive developmental disorder in children without developmental or speech delay who have deficient sociability and a narrow range of interest.

Primary-care physicians are required to take a history and perform physical examination looking specifically for conditions which may be mistaken for autism:
➤ Fragile X-syndrome, which has been found in about 10% of autistic children
➤ Neurofibromatosis and tuberous sclerosis
➤ Maltreatment of or injury to child
➤ Dysmorphic disorders
➤ Degenerative CNS diseases
➤ Specific language delay
➤ Intellectual disability or global developmental delay

BOX 3.6 Symptoms and signs of possible autism

Impairment in social interaction
- Impairment in non-verbal behaviours such as eye-to-eye gaze, facial expression and body postures
- Failure to develop peer relationships appropriate to developmental level
- Lack of spontaneous seeking to share enjoyment, interests or achievements with others
- Reduced or absent responsive social smiling
- Rejection of cuddle initiated by parent or carer

Impairment in communication
- Language delay or total lack of the development of spoken language (e.g. no single words by the age of 16 months or fewer than 10 words by the age of 2 yrs)
- Regression in speech
- In individuals with adequate speech, marked impairment in the ability to initiate or sustain a conversation with others
- Stereotyped and repetitive use of words
- Lack of varied social play

Repetitive or obsessive behaviour
- Engagement in repetitive movements such as rocking and twirling, hand flapping or rolling
- Self-abusive behaviour such as biting, head banging, or eye poking
- Reduced or absent responsiveness to other people's facial expression or feeling
- Pre-occupation with certain objects, ritualised and repetitive play, coping badly with changes to routine

---

➤ ADHD
➤ Mood or anxiety disorder
➤ OCD
➤ Visual or hearing impairment.

Autism should not be ruled out because of:
➤ Good eye contact, smiling and showing affection to other family members
➤ Report of normal language milestones
➤ A previous assessment that concluded that there was no autism.

Referring children to a paediatrician, paediatric neurologist or the autism team for multidisciplinary assessment should be done if there is:
➤ Concern about possible autism on the basis of reported or observed or signs and/or symptoms of autism
➤ Parental concern that their child has autism
➤ Any child with static or regression in language or motor skills.

The multidisciplinary team includes:
➤ Community paediatrician and/or child and adolescent psychiatrist

➤ Speech and language therapist
➤ Clinical and/or educational psychologist
➤ Occupational therapist whenever possible.

Management

The **foundations of therapy** remain educational and behavioural interventions which address:

➤ Communication
➤ Maladaptive behaviour
➤ Social and play skills
➤ Daily living skills
➤ Academic achievement.

Drug therapy plays a minor role in management. The atypical antipsychotic drug Risperidone may have a beneficial effect on general core symptoms such as maladaptive behavioural symptoms and irritability. Methylphenidate is regarded as ineffective unless ADHD co-exists.

Autism support groups

➤ The National Autistic Society
www.autism.org.uk
email: nas@nas.org.uk.
Tel: +44 (0) 20 7833 2299

➤ Autism Advice & Info UK
email: oassis@cambiangroup.com
Tel: 0800 1973907

ATTENTION-DEFICIT HYPERACTIVITY DISORDER (ADHD)

Core messages

➤ ADHD is a common heterogeneous behavioural syndrome affecting 3–9% of school-age children and young people. It is characterised by the core symptoms of:
  ➢ Hyperactivity
  ➢ Impulsivity
  ➢ Inattention
  In addition, these symptoms should be persistent for > 3 months and present in more than one environment.
➤ Three subtypes of ADHD are recognised: combined, predominately inattentive and predominately hyperactive–impulsive.
➤ Common co-morbidities include oppositional defiant disorder (negativistic, disobedient and hostile behaviour) and disorders of conduct, mood, learning, motor control, communication and anxiety.
➤ It is essential that information be obtained directly from teachers about children with behaviour problems at school.
➤ Research suggests that children with ADHD have lack of activity in the frontal lobe processes.
➤ When a child presents with symptoms suggestive of ADHD, primary-care practitioners should:
  ➢ Not make the initial diagnosis or start drug treatment (Box 3.7)
  ➢ Determine the severity of the problems and how these affect the child and the family

➤ Request a report from school confirming that the behaviour reported by the parents also occurs in the school environment

➤ Consider a period of watchful waiting for up to 10 weeks

➤ Offer a referral to secondary care (child psychiatrist, paediatrician, specialist in ADHD or CAMHS, depending on local service provision) for assessment if the symptoms persist with at least moderate impairment.

BOX 3.7 Management of ADHD

- Management usually requires a comprehensive approach which includes health professionals, school and parent support, parent/child education, behaviour management and medications if needed
- Healthcare professionals should stress the value of a good nutrition and regular exercise. Colouring and additives should not be eliminated from the diet unless these appear to influence their behaviour
- Teachers who have received training about ADHD and its management should provide behavioural intervention in the classroom
- Following diagnosis of ADHD, parents should receive written information about diagnosis and assessment, self-help and support groups. Parents should be offered a group-based parent-training/education programme. A behavioural modification plan should be considered at home and includes:
  > Involving the child in setting up the plan
  > Identify the behaviour parents want to see (e.g. make the bed every day, completing home work) and behaviour they want to decrease or eliminate (e.g. refusing to get out of bed in the morning, interrupting when others are speaking)
  > Devise an appropriate system for good behaviour using rewards or privileges such as seeing a movie, buying a small item like toys, having friends come over)
- Medications
  > CNS stimulant treatment should always form part of a comprehensive treatment plan that includes psychological, behavioural and educational programmes
  > In school-age children with severe ADHD, drug treatment is the first-line treatment. Children with moderate ADHD can be treated with stimulants when psychological interventions have been unsuccessful or are unavailable
  > Before medications are prescribed, doctors should take a detailed history (including a family history of cardiac disease, any exercise syncope or undue dyspnoea, mental health and social status), and perform physical examination including measurements of weight, height, pulse and BP
  > Parents should be advised of the common side-effects of the drug such as reduced appetite, weight loss and insomnia
  > Medications available are:
  > Methylphenidate for ADHD without significant co-morbidity (modified-release preparation is available as a single dose in the morning)
  > Methylphenidate or Atomoxetine for ADHD with co-morbid conduct disorder
  > Dexamfetamine for refractory cases of ADHD ((initiated by specialist)

RED FLAGS

- The diagnosis of ADHD must exclude any possible medical conditions that have similar presentation, such as hearing or visual impairment, sleep disorders and substance abuse.
- Children with ADHD who are treated with psychostimulants should be closely monitored for the onset of tics.

ADHD support group

➤ National Attention Deficit Disorder Information and Support Service, ADDISS
www.addiss.co.uk
email: info@addiss.co.uk
Tel: 020 8952 2800

CONDUCT DISORDERS

Core messages

➤ Conduct disorders are defined as repetitive and persistent patterns of behaviour that violate the basic rights of others or major age-appropriate societal norms or rules. They refer to conduct disorder and oppositional defiant disorder (ODD).

➤ They include stealing, lying, truancy, delinquency, repeat disobedience and aggressive behaviour.

➤ The onset of conduct disorders can occur in children < 10 years of age (childhood-onset) or aged 10 years and greater (adolescent-onset).

➤ ODD is characterised by persistently hostile or defiant behaviour outside the normal range but without aggression or anti-social behaviour. The prognosis is particularly poor in childhood-onset disorder because of its likely persistence.

➤ Conduct disorders often occur as part of co-morbidities with other disorders such as ADHD and substance use or abuse.

➤ Co-morbidities include ADHD, depression, learning disability, substance misuse and (rarely) psychosis and autism.

➤ Risk factors for conduct disorders include marital discord, abused parents, social isolation, poverty and overcrowding, substance misuse.

Diagnosis

Diagnosis is based on the presence of at least three of the following criteria exhibited in the past 12 months, with at least one criterion present in the last 6 months:

➤ Bullying, threats or intimidation towards others
➤ Initiating physical fights
➤ Use of a weapon that can cause serious physical harm to others
➤ Being physically cruel to people
➤ Being physically cruel to animals
➤ Deliberately setting fires
➤ Stealing while confronting a victim (e.g. mugging or purse-snatching)
➤ Being a rapist
➤ Destroying other property
➤ Breaking into someone else's house or building
➤ Often lying to obtain goods or favours.

Conduct disorders may cause major problems, including:
➤ Affecting the child's development
➤ Interference with learning and prospects of employment
➤ Isolation and difficulty in making friends
➤ Feelings of unworthiness and depression
➤ Disruption of family life, leaving home
➤ Early unprotected sexual activity with the risk of STD, teenage pregnancies.

Management

Management may include the following steps:
➤ Provision of considerable attention from parents, who should agree how to handle their child's behaviour
➤ Behavioural management involving parents and the rest of the family
➤ Relationship-enhancing strategies such as children and parents spending time and playing together
➤ Discipline at school and home should be fair and consistent. Children should be encouraged to live within social rules and the law
➤ Children may need to be praised and rewarded if they improve their behaviour
➤ NICE guidelines[7] recommend group-based parent-training/education programmes in the management of children with conduct disorders. Individual-based programmes are only recommended where the family's needs are too complex for group-based programmes. These programmes have been found to achieve substantial and sustained changes in behaviour.

ANXIETY DISORDERS

Core messages

➤ Anxiety is one of the most common mental conditions in children. Approximately 12–20% of children are affected.
➤ Anxiety disorders include generalised anxiety disorder, separation anxiety, phobias (such as school phobia), obsessive compulsive disorder (OCD) and post-traumatic stress disorder (PTSD).
➤ Anxiety is regarded as a part of normal development during childhood, related to genetic causes, maternal anxiety and environmental factors including trauma reaction and anxiety response to abuse of the child.
➤ Anxiety may disrupt family functioning, and can impede the child's development, school performance and social interactions.
➤ School phobia affects some 1–2% of children. Common co-morbidities include anxiety or depression, or both.
➤ Young children (< 7–8 years) often have school phobia as a result of separation fear from the main carer. Older children are more likely to be anxious about school performance.
➤ OCD is an anxiety disorder characterised by intrusive thoughts that produce apprehension, fear or worry leading to repetitive behaviours. Its incidence in adults is about 2%, and one-third to one-half of them report the onset of their disorder in childhood.

Management of anxiety

➤ Therapy for anxiety may begin with interviews designed to provide children with an opportunity to express their feelings, including feeling of sadness, helplessness and fear.

➤ The most effective therapy for children with anxiety is cognitive behavioural therapy (CBT), which helps patients modify the way they think, feel and behave.

➤ The best way that CBT is administered is through play (CBPT), where children learn to gain power over their thoughts and to manage their anxious emotions in enjoyable and developmentally appropriate ways.

➤ In some cases medications can be helpful, including fluoxetine or clomipramine for OCD, and benzodiazepines or tricyclic antidepressants for panic disorder.

DEPRESSION

Core messages

➤ Children with a high genetic risk (parental depression) may develop depression in association with the following adverse environmental factors:
  ➢ Own or parental substance misuse
  ➢ Bullying at school
  ➢ Bereavement, parental divorce or separation or marital conflicts
  ➢ Associated disability or chronic illness.

➤ Assessment of severity of depression in primary care is as follows (based on NICE guidelines).[8]
  Key questions: at least one of the following key symptoms is present on most days, most of the time, for at least 2 weeks:
  ➢ Persistent sadness or low mood
  ➢ Loss of interest and/or pleasure
  ➢ Fatigue or low energy.

➤ If any key symptoms are present, the following **associated questions** should be asked about:
  ➢ Poor or increased sleep
  ➢ Poor concentration or indecisiveness
  ➢ Low self-confidence
  ➢ Poor or increased appetite
  ➢ Suicidal thoughts or acts
  ➢ Agitation or slowing of movement
  ➢ Guilt or self-blame.

MANAGEMENT

➤ A psychogenic cause of anxiety or depression should only be considered after excluding organic causes, including endocrine causes, e.g. thyroid diseases, chronic illness causing chronic aches and fatigue, and systemic lupus erythematosus (SLE). Bullying and child abuse should also be considered.

➤ For all children and young people with **mild depression**:
  ➢ Those who do not want intervention should be re-assessed within 2 weeks. If they fail to attend their follow-up appointments, they should be contacted.
  ➢ After up to 4 weeks of watchful waiting, children with continuing mild depression

should be offered a non-directive supportive therapy, group CBT or guided self-help. If this is ineffective within 2–3 months, referral to CAMHS should be carried out.

➤ Antidepressants should not be initiated in primary care because of the possible increased risk of suicide during the first few weeks of therapy.

➤ Factors that favour watchful waiting include:
  ● Four or fewer of the symptoms listed above
  ● No past or family history of depression
  ● Social support available
  ● Symptoms are intermittent or of less than 2 weeks' duration
  ● Patient is not actively suicidal
  ● No, or mild, associated disability.

➤ All children with **moderate to severe depression** should be assessed by CAMHS, particularly if they voice suicidal ideas. They should be offered, as a first-line treatment, a specific psychological therapy (CBT, interpersonal or short-term family therapy). Antidepressants should not be offered except in combination with psychological therapy. When drug treatment is considered necessary, attention should be given to the following:

  ➤ Antidepressants may be considered in children with moderate or severe depression and in cases refractory to psychological treatment.

  ➤ Antidepressant drugs have significant risks when given to children with depression. Children should be monitored for suicidal behaviour and self-harm, particularly at the beginning of treatment.

  ➤ There is no evidence that tricyclic antidepressants are effective for treating children with depression.

  ➤ The selective serotonin re-uptake inhibitors (SSRIs) should be considered first. Fluoxetine is probably the only antidepressant for which benefits outweigh the risks. Recommended starting dose should be 10 mg daily. This dose can be increased to 20 mg after a week.

  ➤ Hyponatraemia has been associated with all types of antidepressants, particularly with SSRIs.

  ➤ If treatment with fluoxetine is unsuccessful or not tolerated, second-line treatment may be considered with sertraline or citalopram.

SELF-HARM

➤ This is defined as 'non-fatal, self-poisoning or self-injury irrespective of the apparent purpose of the act'.[9] Most of these acts involve a behaviour (e.g. cutting the wrists), ingestion of a substance in excess of the prescribed or therapeutic dose, ingestion of recreational or illicit drugs or ingestion of a non-ingestible object.

➤ In a school survey, 13% of young people aged 15 or 16 reported having self-harmed at some time in their lives. In children aged 5–15 years, 1.3% have tried to harm themselves. Risk factors of self-harm are shown in Box 3.8. Self-harm is less common in the Asian community.

BOX 3.8 Risk factors associated with self-harm

- Families of low socio-economic status
- Lack of family or social support, child–parent conflicts
- Mental or physical maltreatment, sexual abuse
- Loss of friend's or family member's relationship
- Females living in single-parent families
- Smoking, alcohol drinking
- Substance abuse
- Chronic physical illness, e.g. disability
- Mental illness, e.g. depression, psychosis
- Stressful events, e.g. bullying at school

Management guidelines in primary care

➤ The management of self-harm consists of
  ➣ assessment
  ➣ referral
  ➣ treatment.
➤ Children and young people who have self-harmed should normally be admitted overnight to a paediatric ward, and assessed fully the following day before discharge.
➤ If a person who has self-harmed has to wait for treatment, he or she should be offered an environment that is safe and supportive and minimises any distress. For many patients this may be a separate, quiet room, with supervision and regular contact with a named member of staff to ensure safety.
➤ In any assessment or treatment of self-harm in children, special attention should be paid to the issues of confidentiality, the young person's consent (if Fraser-competent), and parental consent.
➤ Drugs should be prescribed in small quantities or under supervision of another family member to minimise the risk of drug overdose.
➤ All people who have self-harmed should be offered an assessment of needs, which should be comprehensive and include evaluation of the social, psychological and motivational factors specific to the act of self-harm, current suicidal intent and hopelessness as well as full mental health and social needs assessment.
➤ All children and young people who have self-harmed must be assessed for the risk of repetition of self-harm and of suicide, including the identification of mental illness.

SUBSTANCE ABUSE

Core messages

➤ The UK's rates of recorded illegal drug misuse are among the highest in the Western world. In particular, the UK has comparatively high rates of heroin and crack cocaine misuse. Degrees of severity of substance abuse are shown in Table 3.1.
➤ About one-third of all cases of hepatitis B, over 90% of cases of hepatitis C, and 5.6% of HIV infections in England are associated with injecting drugs.[10]
➤ Substance abuse is defined as a maladaptive pattern of substance use leading to clinically significant impairment or distress as manifested by one of the following, occurring within a 12-month period:
  ➣ Recurrent substance use resulting in a failure to fulfil major role obligations at work, school or home (e.g. repeated absences or poor work performance)
  ➣ Recurrent substance use in hazardous situations, e.g. driving a car

➤ Recurrent substance-related legal problems (e.g. arrest for conduct disorder)
➤ Continued substance use despite persistent or recurrent social or interpersonal problems caused or exacerbated by the effects of the substance (e.g. physical fights).

Box 3.9 shows risk factors leading to substance abuse.

TABLE 3.1 Assessment of severity of substance abuse

	Mild	Severe
Age of starting use	> 15 years	< 15 years
Family history of use	No	Yes
Type of drug use	Marijuana	Heroin
Administration of drug	Oral, inhalation	IV
Circumstance of use	Group setting	Alone
Frequency of use	Occasional, weekends	Daily
Pre-morbid personality	Happy	Depressed
Family support	Present	Absent
School performance	Good	Poor
Recognition of school achievement	Present	Absent
Co-morbidities	No	Present

BOX 3.9 Some of the risks causing or contributing to substance abuse

Behavioural/social
- Interruption of a child's normal development
- Domestic violence, physical and sexual abuse
- Mental illnesses (depression, anxiety, suicidal attempts)
- Legal problems (arrests, imprisonment)
- Unemployment

Health
- Substance-related CNS disorders, e.g. psychosis
- Stress-related gastrointestinal disease
- Malnutrition
- Hepatitis B, hepatitis C and HIV from IV drug misuse

Education
- Poor school performance
- Expulsion from school
- Isolation, low self-esteem

MANAGEMENT
➤ Except in Northern Ireland, there is no longer a legal requirement for doctors in the UK to notify the authorities of suspected drug abuse.
➤ Clinicians have a responsibility to assess risk to children, e.g. neglect or abuse. This may require referral to social services with the patient's knowledge but not necessarily with the patient's consent.

➤ Management goals include:
  ➢ Reducing health and social problems
  ➢ Attaining controlled, non-dependent and non-problematic drug use
  ➢ Abstinence from all drugs, including the main problem drugs
  ➢ Harm reduction (e.g. oral rather than IV, needle exchange, etc).
➤ Treatment is given for acute episodes of illness.
➤ Identification screening for hepatitis A and B (and immunisation if negative)
➤ Counselling and advice about testing for a blood-born virus infection, especially hepatitis B and C, is provided.
➤ Advice is given on:
  ➢ Safer injection
  ➢ Referral to a local drug misuse service
  ➢ Contraception, including safer-sex advice.
➤ The NICE guidelines (2007)[11] identifies a number of formal psychosocial treatments as having a high-quality evidence base. Psychosocial interventions are the mainstay of treatment.

REFERENCES/NOTES

1. www.disordered-eating.co.uk
2. Guidelines for the nutritional management of anorexia nervosa. Report by the Royal College of Psychiatry, 2005. www.rcpsych.ac.uk/files/pdfversion/cr130.pdf
3. MARSIPAN: Management of really sick patients under 18 with anorexia nervosa. Report from the Junior Marsipan Group, January 2012. www.rcpsych.ac.uk/files/pdfversion/CR162.pdf
4. Patients also receive help and advice from BEAT, the Eating Disorders Association. www.b-eat.co.uk
5. NICE guidelines, 2011. CG128: Autism spectrum disorders in children and young people: recognition, referral and diagnosis. http://guidance.nice.org.uk/CG128/Guidance
6. NICE Guidelines, 2008. CG72: Diagnosis and management of ADHD in children and young people. www.nice.org.uk/CG072
7. NICE Guidelines, 2013. CG158. Antisocial behaviour and conduct disorders in children and young people. http://guidance.nice.org.uk/CG158
8. NICE guidelines. CG28: Depression in children and young people: identification, and management in primary care, community and secondary care. www.nice.org.uk/CG028
9. Nice guidelines, 2004. CG 16: Self-harm: the short-term physical and psychological management and secondary prevention of self-harm in primary and secondary care. www.nice.org.uk
10. Department of Health. Drug misuse and dependence: UK Guidelines on clinical management. www.nta.nhs.uk/guidelines-clinical-management.aspx
11. NICE guidelines, 2007. CG51: Drug misuse: psychosocial interventions. http://publications.nice.org.uk/drug-misuse-psychosocial-interventions-cg51

CHAPTER 4

Common infectious diseases

INTRODUCTION

Childhood infectious diseases are a common presentation in general practice. Rather than providing an exhaustive list of causes, this chapter aims to cover common and important infectious diseases. There are excellent books available that deal with this subject in more detail for the interested reader.[1,2]

UNEXPLAINED FEVER (FEVER WITHOUT FOCUS)

Core messages

➤ Fever without focus (FWF) is defined as an acute febrile illness without an apparent source, which lasts for less than 1 week and where the history and physical examination fails to find a cause. In contrast to FWF, pyrexia of unknown origin (to be discussed later) lasts longer than 1 week.

➤ About 20% of all febrile episodes demonstrate no localising signs on presentation.

➤ The most common cause of FWF is a viral infection, mostly occurring during the first few years of life. Such an infection should be considered only after excluding urinary tract infection (second most-common cause) and bacteraemia (Box 4.1).

➤ Bacteraemia indicates the presence of bacteria in blood, while septicaemia suggests tissue invasion by the bacteria, causing tissue hypoperfusion and organ dysfunction. Neonates, young and ill-looking children and those with immunodeficiency or sickle-cell anaemia more often have septicaemia rather than bacteraemia. For these groups there should be a low threshold for admission to hospital.

➤ Clinicians facing a case of FWF must decide who can be safely managed at home and who require admission or investigation.

BOX 4.1 Causes of fever without focus

Viral infection	Urinary tract infection	Occult bacteraemia
Post-vaccination	Occult abscess	Drug fever
Connective tissue/	Brucellosis	Sinusitis
autoimmune diseases	Malaria	

Recommended investigations

➤ Urine: dipsticks – positive nitrite is highly sensitive for urinary tract infection (UTI).

➤ If a child with FWF is admitted to hospital, tests should include full blood count (FBC), blood culture, (particularly for highly febrile children with a temperature

> 39°C, age > 3 months or any ill child), anti-nuclear antibodies for connective tissue autoimmune disease, and abdominal ultrasound scan looking for any hidden abscess.

PRACTICE POINTS

- Viral infections are the main causes of childhood febrile illnesses in 90–95% of cases and in 40–60% in FWF. It is essential to identify a bacterial cause in the minority of children who may need antibiotics.
- Children with a viral infection often appear well with good eye contact, have reasonable levels of activity and are usually eating and drinking satisfactorily.
- Roseola infantum (caused by human herpesvirus HH-6) is the most common febrile exanthem in children < 3 years, occurring in about 30% of children. Onset of fever is abrupt (sometimes triggering a febrile seizure) and characteristically continuous, often with temperatures as high as 40–41°C and without a focus. The temperature usually drops abruptly on the third or fourth day of fever onset, coinciding with the appearance of a rash. Characteristically, the child becomes well and afebrile when the rash erupts.
- Children aged 3–24 months have the highest incidence of bacteraemia. For these children, GPs should have a low threshold for seeing and examining them rather than giving advice over the phone.
- While the risk of bacteraemia is negligible with temperatures of 38–39°C, a strong correlation exists between the incidence of bacteraemia and higher temperatures: it is 7% with temperatures of 40–40.5°C, 13% with temperatures of 40.5–41.0°C, and 26% with a temperature higher than 41.0°C.
- Although bacteraemia occurs more often as a primary isolated disease, meningitis is associated with positive blood culture in 50–80% of cases, pneumonia in about 10%, and otitis media in 1.5%.
- Abnormal findings in children with bacteraemia are usually absent, ill-appearance being the only manifestation of the disease. Occasionally children with bacteraemia may still look well.

RED FLAGS

- Children < 3 months of age, those with immune deficiency (e.g. HIV or on chemotherapy), sickle-cell anaemia (SCA), cystic fibrosis (CF), asplenia or with body temperature > 41°C should be considered as having bacterial infections until proved otherwise. Antibiotic treatment and/or admission is essential.
- Examination of a child with FWF is not complete without urine dipstick examination for infection.
- Normal body temperature does not preclude serious bacterial infection. It is important to safety-net, providing carers with clear instructions as to what signs of deterioration to look for and when to bring the child back for review.

RECURRENT FEBRILE INFECTIONS

Core messages

➤ Recurrent infections are a source of great concern to parents, and a common reason to bring children for medical advice (Box 4.2).

➤ It has been estimated that normal young children may have as many as 12–16 infections per year if he or she attends nursery, nine infections per year if a sibling attends school, and six or eight per year if the child and a sibling are not at school. Fortunately, these infections decline as the child grows older.

BOX 4.2 Common causes of recurrent fevers

● Viral infections, common in those visiting daycare centres
● Immunodeficiency, including neutropenia and asplenia, immunoglobulin A (IgA) deficiency, DiGeorge syndrome (thymic hypoplasia)
● Sickle-cell anaemia (SCA)
● Underlying chronic disease (e.g. cystic fibrosis)
● Neurodisability (e.g. causing aspiration)
● Left-to-right cardiac shunt
● Periodic fevers (other than malaria)

Recommended investigations

➤ Urine: for dipstick testing and if necessary for culture
➤ FBC: looking for neutrophil and lymphocyte counts
➤ Serum immunoglobulins
➤ Chest X-ray or ultrasound scan to assess the presence and size of the thymus.

PRACTICE POINTS

● Children with mainly viral recurrent infections which are common in children attending daycare centres (at least 50% of cases with recurrent infections) are unlikely to have an immunodeficiency. These children often receive unnecessarily frequent courses of antibiotics, contributing to the development of antibiotic resistance.
● Primary immunodeficiency diseases (B- and T-cell diseases) are rare except for selective IgA deficiency which has a prevalence of 1 : 333. Normal absolute neutrophil and lymphocyte counts alone eliminate most causes of immunodeficiency.
● Chemotherapy-induced neutropenia remains one of the most common causes of neutropenia, which is predisposing to serious and recurrent febrile diseases.
● Cyclic neutropenia is an autosomal dominant disease, which is easily diagnosed by recognising the periodicity of symptoms in association with isolated neutropenia every 3 weeks. During the phase of neutropenia, patients often suffer from stomatitis, oral ulcers, fever and lymphadenopathy. When asymptomatic, the neutrophil count is usually normal.

- Other causes of recurrent fever are:
  - Periodic fever (PF) and relapsing fever, which are characterised by episodes of fever recurring at regular or irregular intervals. Each episode is followed by 1 to several days, weeks or months of normal temperature. Examples of PF are seen in malaria, brucellosis and familial Mediterranean fever. Relapsing fever is caused by numerous species of *Borrelia* and transmitted by lice (louse-borne) or ticks (tick-borne).
  - PFAPA (periodic fever, aphthous stomatitis, pharyngitis, and adenitis)
  - FCUS (familial cold urticaria syndrome)
  - MWS (Muckle–Wells syndrome)
  - TRAPS (TNF-receptor associated periodic syndrome)
  - HIDS (hyperimmunoglobulinaemia D syndrome) is also characterised by recurrent episodes of fever, but they are rare compared with familial Mediterranean fever.

PYREXIA OF UNKNOWN ORIGIN (PUO)

Core messages

➤ The term PUO is applied when fever (body temperature > 38.0°C) without localising signs persists for 1 week or longer with no apparent cause.

➤ The patient's history should include a search for animal exposure, ingestion of raw milk, travel abroad, prior use of antibiotics, and exposure to infections. Causes of PUO are listed in Table 4.1.

➤ Physical examination should include checking for tenderness over the sinuses, bones and muscles and palpation of lymph nodes; eye examination looking in particular for uveitis as an early clue for rheumatoid arthritis; bulbar conjunctivitis for leptospirosis, choroid tubercles for tuberculosis (TB).

➤ The prognosis of PUO is better in children than in adults, mainly because of the higher incidence of infection and lower incidence of malignancy. Death may occur in less than 5% of patients, primarily due to neoplastic cases.

TABLE 4.1 Principal causes of PUO

Cause	Reason for misdiagnosis
Infection (60–70%)	
Localised	
• Sinusitis	Symptoms not obvious of sinuses, e.g. headaches
• Endocarditis	Previously unsuspected of having a cardiac defect
• Occult abscess	Absence of localised clinical signs
Systemic	
• Viral (e.g. Epstein–Barr virus)	Absence of clinical signs, and fever as the only sign
• Tuberculosis	Extrapulmonary, tuberculin test negative
• Kawasaki disease	Incomplete or atypical presentation
• Brucellosis	Diagnostic tests for *Brucella* not performed

Cause	Reason for misdiagnosis
Collagen (about 20%)	
Juvenile rheumatoid arthritis	Pre-arthritic manifestation
Systemic lupus erythematosus	Atypical manifestations or absence of clinical signs
Neoplasms (5%)	
Leukaemia	Atypical presentation; blood tests negative
Lymphoma	Unusual localisation, absence of lymphadenopathy
Neuroblastoma	Disseminated
Miscellaneous (5–10%)	
Drug fever	Diagnosis not considered, suspected drug not stopped
Factitious fever	Diagnosis not considered, temperature measured by patient and not by clinician
Undiagnosed (5%)	

Recommended investigations

(Apart from urine, stool and possibly FBC, other tests are usually performed in hospital.)

➤ Urine (microscopy and culture)
➤ Stool (microscopy and culture)
➤ FBC, C-reactive protein (CRP), erythrocyte sedimentation rate (ESR), blood film
➤ Blood culture
➤ Liver function tests
➤ Anti-nuclear antibody
➤ Serology for brucellosis, toxoplasmosis, cytomegalovirus, mononucleosis
➤ X-ray of chest/sinuses
➤ Tuberculin test
➤ Ultrasound scan of the abdomen.

MANAGEMENT OF FEVER

Core messages

➤ Antipyretics do not influence the clinical course of the disease or the number of days of subsequent fever, or prevent febrile seizures.
➤ The main effect of antipyretics is to relieve the child's discomfort and thereby the parents' anxiety.
➤ There is no evidence that fever, in contrast to hyperthermia, is injurious to tissue. Fever per se is self-limiting and rarely serious provided that the cause is known and fluid loss is replaced. If there is morbidity or mortality, it is due to the underlying disease. The associated fever may well be protective.
➤ Bacterial growth rates and viral replication rates are significantly reduced at elevated temperatures. Fever enhances immunological processes, including mobility of poly-morphonuclear cells, activity of interleukin-1, T-helper cells and cytolytic T-cells, as well as B-cell activity and possibly immunoglobulin synthesis.

PRACTICE POINTS

- Accurate body temperature measurement is essential (Box 4.3).
- Detection of signs of dehydration is outlined in Table 4.2.
- Paracetamol is the most commonly used antipyretic and analgesic drug. A therapeutic dose is 10–15 mg/kg every 4–6 hours. Recurrence of fever is expected in 3–4 hours. Clearance is reduced in neonates; 8- to 12-hourly dosing is recommended.
- Ibuprofen suspension is available for children who are at least 6 months old. Its anti-inflammatory and analgesic properties provide additional therapeutic advantages over paracetamol. Rectal ibuprofen is available. Ibuprofen is used:
  ○ As an antipyretic in a dose of 5 mg/kg for at least 3–4 hours. A dose of 10 mg/kg is more potent and has longer-lasting fever suppression than paracetamol.
  ○ For analgesic and anti-inflammatory effects, e.g. in juvenile idiopathic arthritis. A dose of 20–40 mg/kg/day has a greater therapeutic effect.
- Combining antipyretics – paracetamol is frequently used in an alternating manner with ibuprofen for the treatment of febrile children. The practice is common but has no scientific basis (Box 4.4).
- Physical measures (fan, tepid sponging) for fever are unnecessary and unpleasant for the child; their use is discouraged. Offering extra fluids, keeping the room cool and dressing the child lightly are beneficial.

BOX 4.3 Evidence-based measurements of body temperature[3]

- Axillary temperature measurement is inaccurate
- Oral temperature measurement is not recommended in children aged < 5 years
- Infrared ear thermometry – the technique is fast and easy to use without risk of cross-infection and is not influenced by environmental temperature

---

TABLE 4.2 Assessment of dehydration

Dehydration is assessed by looking for the following features:	
Overall appearance	Poor
Fontanelle	Sunken
Mouth	Dry
Eyes	Sunken, absence of tears
Skin	Cold limbs, skin turgor
Heart and circulation	Weak pulse, prolonged CRT*
Respiration	Abnormal pattern

* CRT = capillary refill time; prolonged if > 2–3 seconds.

BOX 4.4 Reasons for not recommending combined antipyretics

- There is presently no scientific evidence in support of this practice, including lack of evidence of its safety
- There is no evidence that greater antipyretic effect influences the underlying disease or duration of fever
- The practice may increase the risk of incorrect dosing
- The practice may suggest to the parents that fever is a grave situation. It may increase their fever phobia

---

MANAGEMENT

Table 4.3 outlines a procedure for assessment and management of febrile children < 5 years old.

TABLE 4.3 Assessment scale of febrile children < 5 years of age

	Signs not suggestive of a serious illness (e.g. viral infection)	Signs suggestive of a serious illness (e.g. serious bacterial illness)	Life-threatening signs (requiring emergency admission, Box 4.5)
Colour	• Normal pink colour of skin, lips and tongue	• Pallor reported by parents	• Very pale, mottled or blue or ashen
Response/ activity	• Normal response to social cues, play • Content/smiles • Alert or awakens quickly • Strong normal cry	• Not responding normally to social cues • Wakes only with prolonged stimulation • Decreased activity • No smile	• Ill appearing • Unrousable or if roused does not stay awake • Weak/high pitched/ continuous cry, moaning
Respiration	• Normal	• Nasal flaring age • Tachypnoea, RR > 50 bpm age 6–12 months or > 40 aged > 12 months • Grunting • O_2-saturation< 95% in air • Crackles on chest auscultation	• Irregular breathing, intermittent apnoea • Tachypnoea, RR > 60 bpm (at any age) • Moderate to severe chest indrawing • O_2-saturation <92% in air
Hydration	• Normal skin and eyes • Moist mucous membranes • Normal urine output	• Dry mucous membranes • Reduced urine output	• Reduced skin turgor • Sunken eyes • Anuria
Other	• Feeding well	• Fever ≥ 5 days • Swelling of a limb or joint • No weight bearing or not using an extremity • Not feeding or takes little fluid	• Bile-stain vomiting • Non-blanching rash • Bulging fontanelle • Neck stiffness • Focal neurological signs • Focal seizures

RR= respiratory rate; bpm= breath per minute

TABLE 4.4 Managing feverish children under 5 years in primary

No serious signs of illness	Serious signs of illness	High risk
• Manage at home with appropriate advice on warning symptoms and how to access further healthcare • Follow up if fever persists 48–72 h or if clinical course changes • Paracetamol or ibuprofen as required • Test urine for UTI if no obvious focus for the fever • No routine blood tests • Antibiotics are usually not indicated	• Refer to paediatric care if clinically indicated • Verbal or written information on warning symptoms and how to access further health care. The safety net is information on the symptoms indicating a deterioration of the child's condition which requires urgent review in primary care or referral to hospital • Clean catch urine to exclude UTI, particularly if no focus for the fever is present • FBC, CRP and blood culture • Chest X-ray if fever > 39°C and WBC > 20 000 • Antibiotics before transfer for suspected meningitis or meningococcal septicaemia	• Refer urgently to hospital

Indications for admission (Box 4.5)

BOX 4.5 Indications for hospital admission or sending home

Febrile children should be considered for hospital admission for:
- Neonates (less than 28 days), and infants < 3 months
- Those who appear toxic or ill-looking (*see* signs of a serious illness in Table 4.3)
- Those with a history of prolonged fever > 5 days
- Suspected serious bacterial infection (SBI)
- Those with bloody diarrhoea, increased abdominal tenderness
- Any child with skin petechiae
- An infant with fever > 40°C (particularly > 40°C without a focus)
- A child with his/her first febrile seizure (FS)
- Child with tachypnoea, grunting, rash, headaches, or vomiting
- Parents appear unreliable and follow-up is not assured
- Cases with immunodeficiency or sickle-cell disease
- Child with high white blood cell (WBC) count > 20 000, or high C-reactive protein
- Any young child with urinalysis suggestive of urinary tract infection

Febrile children may be sent home provided that:
- They appear well and playful
- A urine sample has been sent for culture or urine dipsticks are negative for nitrate and WBC
- A follow-up appointment is set within 24–48 hours if fever persists
- Parents are informed to return if condition worsens

KAWASAKI DISEASE (KD)

Core messages

➤ Kawasaki disease is an acute inflammatory disease that principally affects infants and young children, with a peak incidence at 1–2 years of age.

➤ The disease is a form of vasculitis of unknown origin.

➤ Diagnostic criteria are shown in Box 4.6.

BOX 4.6 Diagnostic criteria of Kawasaki disease

Fever persisting for at least 5 days plus at least 4 of the following:
1. Bilateral, painless conjunctival inflammation without exudates
2. Changes of the oropharynx mucosa, cracking lips, strawberry tongue
3. Acute unilateral non-purulent cervical lymphadenopathy > 1.5 cm
4. Polymorphous rash, primarily truncal
5. Changes of peripheral extremities: oedema/erythema/peeling

---

➤ The most serious features are those affecting the cardiovascular system:
  ➢ Myocarditis occurs in about 25% of cases. Presentation includes tachycardia, gallop rhythm, and non-specific ST–T wave changes on the ECG
  ➢ Pericardial effusion occurring towards the second week
  ➢ Coronary artery aneurysm. Dilation occurs in 15–20% of cases and can be detected as early as 6 days after the appearance of fever. Aneurysms may also occur in other arteries, such as renal, axillary and iliac arteries
  ➢ Fatality may occur in about 2% and is usually the consequence of myocardial infarction secondary to thrombosis in the coronary artery aneurysms.

➤ **Laboratory findings** include:
  ➢ Leucocytosis with increased neutrophils, mild to moderate normocytic normochromic anaemia, almost universally increased ESR and CRP and thrombocytosis
  ➢ Other findings are: raised aspartate and alanine aminotransferase, increased anti-streptolysin 0 (ASO) titre, immunoglobulins IgG, IgA and IgM, and pyuria and proteinuria
  ➢ Echocardiography is usually performed 14, 21 and 60 days after onset.

Management

➤ Referral of all those suspected to have KD is essential. Patients should receive:
  ➢ Aspirin for its anti-thrombotic effect. If the patient cannot take aspirin, dipyridamole (persantin) is recommended.
  ➢ Intravenous immune gamma globulin (IVIG) plus aspirin, which reduces the incidence of coronary artery disease.

➤ Fever usually resolves within 1–2 days after initiation of aspirin and gamma globulin treatment.

VIRAL EXANTHEMS

Exanthem (from Greek, 'a break out') is defined as a widespread skin eruption usually occurring as a symptom of an acute viral disease (*see* Table 4.5).

TABLE 4.5 Some clinical characteristics of viral exanthem

Diseases	Incubation time (days)	Infectious period (days)	Characteristics of the exanthem
Measles	8–12	4 before and 4 after the onset of the rash	The exanthem appears at the peak of symptoms, first behind the ears and then spreads to the face, neck, trunk and extremities. The rash begins to clear on the third day
Varicella	10–21	2 before the onset of the rash until all vesicles have crusted, or 5–7 days after the start of the rash	Macules rapidly progressing to papules and to vesicles on the face and scalp (may appear first on the back and trunk), which spread to the trunk and extremities. After 7 days the vesicles begin to crust and children are no longer infectious
Rubella	14–21	1–2 days before the rash, and 3 days after	The rash usually starts behind the ears before spreading around the head and neck, trunk and legs. The rash fades after 3 days and usually the child is no longer infectious
Erythema infectiosum	4–20	1–2 days before onset of the rash and probably not infectious after the rash appears	Starts on the face with a 'slapped cheeks' appearance, resembling scarlet fever. The rash spreads to the trunk and extremities in 1–4 days after onset of the facial rash. It disappears after 2–4 days
Roseola infantum	5–15 (mean about 10)	1–2 days before onset of fever and 1–2 days after the fever subsides	The rash is pink or red and appears predominately on the neck and trunk, lasting 24–36 hours. Characteristically, the child becomes well and afebrile when the rash erupts.

MEASLES

Core messages

➤ Measles is a notifiable disease in the UK.

➤ Figure 4.1 shows the rapid decline in measles notifications since the introduction of measles vaccination; deaths have declined likewise.

➤ Clinical course:

➢ The pre-exanthem stage begins like a common cold, with abrupt fever (from 39 to 40.5°C), sneezing, dry cough and conjunctivitis. About 24 hours prior to the appearance of exanthem, Koplik's spots can be detected in about 80% of cases as tiny, about 1 mm, whitish spots in the buccal mucosa opposite the lower molars.

➢ Rash.

➢ Pharyngitis, cervical lymphadenopathy and occasionally a mild splenomegaly.

➤ The infectivity decreases considerably with the onset of the rash.

➤ Measles–mumps–rubella (MMR) vaccination is given at 12–13 months and again at 3–5 years of age.

➤ Confirmation of the diagnosis by buccal swab is usually arranged by the Health Protection Agency.

➤ Gamma globulin (0.25 mg/kg) within 5 days of exposure to measles virus prevents the disease, and is indicated for certain susceptible individuals including:
  ➢ immunocompromised patients
  ➢ pregnant non-immune women
  ➢ children < 1 year of age.
➤ Oral vitamin A (400 000 U) can decrease mortality in children in developing countries.
➤ **Recommended investigations:** The diagnosis is mainly clinical and investigations are not usually required. FBC often shows leucopenia and lymphopenia.

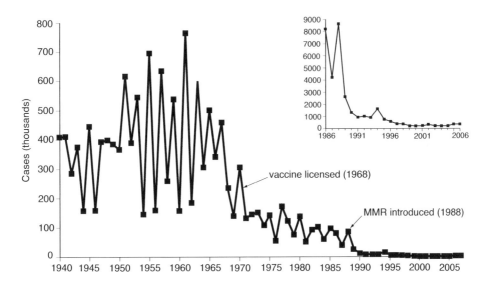

FIGURE 4.1 Measles cases in England and Wales, 1940–2007. There was an increase in the number of confirmed cases of measles in 2009 and a major outbreak in Wales in 2013.

VARICELLA
(Fig 4.2– *see* Plate section)

Core messages
➤ Varicella is highly infectious via the respiratory route.
➤ Varicella is not notifiable in England, Wales and Scotland, but is so in Northern Ireland.
➤ Varicella is usually a benign disease. Complications include pneumonia in about 1% (affecting primarily adults and newborn infants), secondary staphylococcal skin infection, thrombocytopenic purpura, cerebellar ataxia and encephalitis.
➤ At least 90% of older children and adults are varicella zoster virus (VZV) IgG-seropositive, indicating prior infection.
➤ In patients with impaired cellular immunity, and those receiving cytotoxic drugs, varicella is often severe and may be fatal. Severe varicella occurs in children with leukaemia and lymphoma, and the mortality is about 20%. Children with hypogammaglobulinaemia recover normally from varicella.

➤ When maternal varicella develops within 4 days of delivery, neonates develop severe varicella within 5–10 days postpartum (Box 4.7).

BOX 4.7 Congenital varicella infections

- Infection with varicella during pregnancy may produce **congenital varicella syndrome** (e.g. skin scarring and loss, microcephaly, cataracts, limb malformation). The risk of infection is highest if the infection occurs within the first 20 weeks of pregnancy
- Delivery within 1 week before or after the onset of maternal varicella infection may cause **severe infection** within 5–10 days postpartum. The disease is associated with a mortality of around 20% due to disseminated chickenpox, usually with severe pneumonitis. The disease requires varicella zoster immunoglobulin (VZIG) and aciclovir
- If there was an interval of ≥ 1 week between maternal varicella and parturition, neonates receive sufficient protective transplacental antibody to the virus
- For these reasons, pregnant women with unknown immunity to VZV should have their VZV IgG status checked

---

Management

➤ The majority of patients require no special treatment. Itching can be relieved by simple soothing lotions such as calamine and oral antihistamine. Fever is managed with paracetamol. Aspirin should not be administered because of the risk of Reye's syndrome.

➤ Patients with severe varicella or with complications should receive aciclovir. This antiviral drug reduces the duration of fever.

➤ Zoster (shingles) can be treated with oral aciclovir within 72 hours of onset of symptoms. This can reduce the duration of viral shedding and post-herpetic neuralgia.

➤ Varicella zoster immunoglobulin (VZIG) is recommended for those who test sero-negative within 10 days (ideally within 7 days) of exposure to VZV. The duration of protection is 3 weeks. VZV vaccination information is shown in Box 4.8.

BOX 4.8 Information and guidelines on varicella zoster virus (VZV) vaccination

- Two varicella vaccines have been licensed in the UK since 2003 for use in susceptible individuals: Varilrix (Glaxo SmithKline) and Varivax (Aventis Pasteur MSD). Both vaccines contain live attenuated VZV
- Two doses of vaccine are given 4–8 weeks apart, and provide 75% protection against varicella and over 90% protection against severe infection. Immunity may wane over time, causing a mild varicella if exposed to VZV
- At present, varicella vaccine is not offered routinely but it may be given to:
  > Close contacts of chickenpox sufferers who are at high risk of complications from varicella or zoster
  > High-risk children within 3 days of exposure to chickenpox. Varivax (and not Varilrix) is licensed for post-exposure prophylaxis

---

RUBELLA (GERMAN MEASLES)

Core messages

➤ The incubation time of rubella is 14–21 days. The infection is usually mild, and children usually present with sore throat, rash (distinctive light-red or pink), lymphadenopathy (prominent in the posterior cervical and suboccipital areas) and low-grade fever (rarely exceeding 38.0–38.5°C) for several days. The infectious period is 1–2 days before the rash appears.

➤ In older children, particularly in females after puberty, the infection is more severe and prolonged. There are usually painful and visibly enlarged lymph nodes, involving post-auricular, occipital and posterior cervical nodes, with polyarthralgia or arthritis.

➤ Infection with rubella virus is particularly important to diagnose because of possible fetal–maternal transmission causing congenital rubella syndrome (Table 4.6).

➤ Prevention of maternal rubella used to be through routine vaccination of all girls aged 11–14 years and women of child-bearing age. The use of the MMR vaccine has been very successful in preventing congenital and acquired rubella. Outbreaks still occur in developing countries where vaccination is not widespread.

➤ Contraindications to MMR vaccination are shown in Box 4.9.

TABLE 4.6 Congenital rubella syndrome

This syndrome may occur if a mother is infected within the first 20 weeks of pregnancy, particularly during the early weeks. It manifests as:

Eye disease	Cataract, retinopathy, glaucoma
Auditory	Sensorineural deafness
Heart	Pulmonary stenosis, patent ductus arteriosus
Hepatic	Hepatitis
Neurological	Microcephaly, neurodisability
Blood	Thrombocytopenic purpura, anaemia

BOX 4.9 Contraindications to measles–mumps–rubella (MMR) vaccine

● Women who are pregnant or trying to conceive (women should be advised to avoid conception within 28 days after vaccination)

● Immunocompromised individuals including those who are receiving chemotherapy or high doses of steroids, with the exception of HIV-infected patients who have no signs of AIDS

● People receiving blood products such as immunoglobulin. In this case, MMR administration should be deferred for 3 months

● Children who are unwell with acute illness. Symptoms such as mild cough or runny nose due to upper respiratory tract infection may still receive the MMR

MUMPS

Core messages

➤ Mumps is a paramyxovirus infection which begins with swelling and tenderness of one or both parotid glands. About 30–40% of infections are subclinical.

➤ Following an incubation period of 16–18 days, the parotid swelling peaks in 2–3 days and subsides within 3–7 days. Swelling of the submandibular glands occurs frequently, either accompanying the parotid swelling or alone in about 10% of cases.
➤ The infectious period starts 1 day before the parotid swelling and ends 3 days after the swelling has subsided.
➤ Common complications include:
   ➢ Meningoencephalitis occurs in more than 50% of cases, but only 10% of cases are clinically apparent
   ➢ Orchitis usually occurs within 8 days of the onset of parotitis, mainly in post-pubertal boys. The affected testis is tender and swollen. Infertility is rare even with bilateral orchitis. Oophoritis may present as pelvic pain and tenderness, mainly in post-pubertal females
   ➢ Other less-common complications are pancreatitis, arthritis, neural deafness, myocarditis and thyroiditis.
➤ Diagnostic IgM antibodies are detectable within the first few days of infection.
➤ There has been a dramatic reduction in mumps cases since the introduction of MMR vaccination in 1988. Mumps is a notifiable disease.

ERYTHEMA INFECTIOSUM (SLAPPED CHEEKS)
Core messages
(Figure 4.3– *see* Plate section)
➤ Erythema infectiosum, or 5th disease, is an acute benign, communicable disease caused by parvovirus B19. It usually affects children aged 5–15 years.
➤ The rash is diagnostic, with bright red cheeks often followed by a lacy rash spreading onto the trunk. There may be mild flu-like prodromal symptoms. Complications from parvovirus are uncommon and are shown in Table 4.7.

TABLE 4.7 Complications of parvovirus infection in pregnancy

Arthritis	Often symmetrical, affecting the wrists, hands, knees and ankles. It usually resolves within a few days. In some cases it may persist for 2 months or longer, causing diagnostic difficulty to differentiate it from juvenile idiopathic arthritis. Arthritis is seen mainly in female adults
Aplastic anaemia	A transient anaemia affecting particularly those with chronic haemolytic anaemia such as thalassaemia, sickle-cell anaemia and spherocytosis
Fetal hydrops	As well as miscarriage and fetal loss in non-immune pregnant women
CNS infection	Rarely meningitis, encephalitis or neuropathy

ROSEOLA INFANTUM (RI) (EXANTHEMA SUBITUM)
Core messages
➤ RI is caused by human herpesvirus 6 (HHV-6), identified in 1988, and less commonly by HHV-7. The virus is recognised as a major cause of febrile illness with viraemia and a high temperature (mean 39.7°C), sometimes with rash.
➤ RI is the most common febrile exanthem in children under the age of 3 years. Approximately 30% of children develop this disease, most commonly aged 6–24 months.
➤ Children may develop a short period of irritability and malaise before the onset of

fever, which is abrupt (sometimes triggering a febrile seizure in 10–15% of cases) and characteristically continuous, with temperatures often as high as 40–41°C. Fever usually persists for 3–4 days in about 75% of cases and for 5–6 days in the remaining 25%. The temperature usually drops by crisis over a period of a few hours, coinciding with the appearance of the rash.
➤ There may be mild pharyngitis, suboccipital or posterior cervical lymphadenopathy.
➤ Laboratory findings commonly show leukocytosis of 12 000–20 000 with a slight increase in neutrophils.

BACTERIAL DISEASES
Meningococcal disease (MCD)
Core messages
➤ Neck stiffness or meningism refers to an abnormal position of the neck or restricted range of movement, usually associated with pain during passive and active movement.
➤ Meningism is extremely important and requires immediate evaluation because of the possibility of infection (Box 4.10). Non-infectious causes include torticollis (wry neck), sleeping in an awkward position and dystonic drug reaction. In contrast to children with non-infectious meningism, those with an infectious cause usually look ill and have a fever.

BOX 4.10 Differential diagnosis of neck stiffness (meningism)

Infection
- Meningitis
- Pneumonia (particularly upper-lobe pneumonia)
- Viral upper respiratory tract infection with cervical lymphadenitis

Non-infection
- Muscular torticollis (mainly in infancy)
- Neck trauma
- Sandifer syndrome (gastro-oesophageal reflux)
- Congenital abnormalities of the cervical spine
- Dystonic drug reaction
- Hysteria

Meningococcal disease (MCD)
The NICE guidelines[4] on MCD include:
➤ Encouraging the parent/patient to trust their instincts and seek medical help again if the illness worsens, even if this is shortly after the patient was seen.
➤ Information should be provided about symptoms of serious illness, including how to identify a non-blanching rash, e.g. tumbler test (pressing a tumbler firmly against the skin to see if the rash blanches; Fig 4.5 – *see* Plate section).
➤ A review within 4–6 hours may be necessary.
➤ Ensure that the parent/patient understands how to get medical help after normal working hours.
➤ Temperature, heart rate, respiratory rate (RR), and capillary refill time (CRT) should routinely be measured and recorded in all feverish children < 5 years of age (NICE guidelines on feverish illness). A child with RR > 60 breaths/min requires urgent

referral to a paediatric specialist. Normal values of these vital signs are shown in Table 4.8.

TABLE 4.8 Normal values of vital signs

Age (years)	Pulse (beats/min)	RR (breaths/min)	BP (systolic) (beats/min)
< 1	110–160	30–40	70–90
1–2	100–150	25–35	80–95
2–5	95–140	25–30	80–100
5–12	80–120	20–25	90–110
> 12	60–100	15–20	100–120

Source: Advanced Paediatric Life Support Manual. Resuscitation Council 2010. www.resus.org.uk/pages/pals.pdf

Clinical features

➤ MCD has two main clinical presentations: meningitis and septicaemia, which may occur together.
➤ Septicaemia is more common, progressing more rapidly and more dangerously than meningitis. It is most likely to be fatal when it occurs without meningitis.
➤ Patients with septicaemia may present with very different symptoms from those with meningitis (Box 4.11).
➤ Meningococcal disease is a notifiable disease. There is a legal duty to notify the case to the local Consultant and Communicable Disease Control (CCDC), Consultant in Public Health Medicine (CPHM) or the on-call Public Health Specialist.

BOX 4.11 MCD should be considered in patients with the following symptoms and signs

Septicaemia
- Limb/joint pain
- Cold hands and feet and prolonged capillary refill time
- Pale/mottled/blue skin
- Tachycardia
- Tachypnoea/laboured breathing
- Rigors
- Oliguria, thirst
- Rash anywhere on the body
- Abdominal pain
- Impaired consciousness/confusion

Meningitis
- Severe headache
- Neck stiffness (not always present in young children)
- Photophobia (not always present in young children
- Frequent vomiting
- Confusion/impaired consciousness
- Seizure (late sign)
- Focal neurological deficit (e.g. cranial nerve involvement)

In babies
- Poor feeding
- Irritability or lethargy
- Tense fontanelle
- Abnormal muscle tone (increased or decreased)
- Vacant look, staring

Clinical assessment
(*See* Box 4.12.)
(Fig 4.4 – *see* Plate section)
(Fig 4.5 – *see* Plate section)

BOX 4.12 Rapid assessment in children with suspected MCD

Assessment of skin rash (*see* Fig 4.4 and Fig 4.5)
- About 60% of children with MCD have a rash when seen by their GP. Assessment is best done in good light, searching the entire body for small petechiae especially in a febrile child

Level of consciousness can be assessed using AVPU:
- **A**lert
- **R**esponds to **P**ain
- **R**esponds to **V**oice
- **U**nresponsive

Assessing the CRT:
- Press for 5 seconds on the big toe, finger or sternum
- Count the seconds it takes for the skin to return to normal
- If the CRT > 2 seconds the possibility of MCD should be considered, particularly in association with tachycardia and tachypnoea

Assessment of neck stiffness:
- Whether patient has the ability to 'kiss' his/her knees
- The ease of passive neck flexion

Treatment guidelines
➤ If meningeal infection is suspected, the patient should be transferred to hospital by the quickest possible means of transport, usually 999 ambulance, and IM antibiotics administered prior to transfer.
➤ For suspected meningitis without a rash, NICE recommends urgent transfer without giving antibiotics, mainly to enable administration of dexamethasone within 4 hours of the first dose of antibiotics, and because the disease progresses more slowly than septicaemia.
➤ If urgent transfer to hospital is not possible (e.g. in remote locations or if adverse weather conditions), then antibiotics should be administered in primary care (Box 4.13).
➤ Antibiotics can be administered IV or IM. IM should be given as proximally as possible into a part of a limb that is still warm.

BOX 4.13 Penicillin dosage for suspected meningococcal disease

- Adults and children aged 10 years or older: 1200 mg
- Children 1–9 years: 600 mg
- Infants: 300 mg

Follow-up care for survivors

➤ GPs should be alert to possible late-onset sensory, neurological, orthopaedic and psychosocial effects of MCD, as some sequalae may not become evident until years after the illness. These include:

  ➤ Hearing loss – hearing assessment should be carried out as soon as possible

  ➤ Neurodisability including learning, motor and neuro-developmental deficit and epilepsy

  ➤ Psychological and behavioural problems including post-traumatic stress disorder.

➤ Parents should be given information on self-help groups, including:

  ➤ Meningitis 24-hour helpline: 080 8800 3344 offers support, including home visits to patients and their families whether currently ill, recovering or bereaved. www.meningitis.org

  ➤ The Meningitis Research Foundation, www.meningitis.org

  ➤ The National Meningitis Trust, www.meningitis-trust.org 24-hour helpline: 0808 80 10 388

RED FLAGS

- According to a recent national study,[5] at least 50% of children presenting to a GP with MCD were sent home on their first visit; these children were more likely to die.
- The first symptoms reported by parents of children with meningitis and septicaemia are 'viral-like symptoms'. This prodromal phase usually lasts 4 hours in young children and as long as 8 hours in adolescents.
- Early signs of MCD are circulatory shutdown including pale or mottled skin and cold hands or feet, limb pain and tachycardia, occurring at a median time of **8 hours from onset of illness**.
- Other signs are drowsiness, rapid or laboured respiration, sometimes diarrhoea. Thirst may occur in older children.
- In the early stages the rash may be blanching and maculopapular, but it nearly always develops into a non-blanching, red or brownish petechial rash, appearing at a median time of **8–9 hours after onset**. Examining the whole body is important.
- Although the majority of children seen in primary care with petechial rash will not have MCD, a child with a non-blanching rash should be urgently referred to hospital.
- In MCD a non-blanching rash should not be mistaken for a viral rash, trauma or abuse; or joint pain for arthralgia or arthritis; or impaired consciousness for drug or alcohol intoxication.
- The rash can be more difficult to see on dark skin, but it is often visible on the soles of the feet, palms of the hands, conjunctivae or palate.

Scarlet fever

Core messages

➤ Tonsillitis is nowadays usually caused by viruses. Isolation of streptococci from a throat culture does not necessarily indicate that the infection is caused by these organisms. Therefore administration of antibiotics to these patients may not be indicated and may contribute to antibiotic resistance.

➤ Scarlet fever is caused by certain strains of haemolytic streptococci in the throat producing an erythrogenic toxin. Scarlet fever may follow infection of wounds, burns or streptococcal skin infection. It mostly affects children aged 5–15 years. The incubation time is 2–4 days. The disease is notifiable in the UK.

➤ Onset is usually sudden with fever (temperature usually ranges from 39 to 40.5°C), sore throat (tonsillitis often with petechiae on the palate), vomiting and headaches.

➤ A rash appears typically on the 2nd day of illness and is characterised by an erythematous punctiform eruption that blanches on pressure and spares the area around the mouth (circumoral pallor). It appears typically on the neck and chest, later on the trunk and legs. The rash is more prominent in skin creases, with confluent petechiae.

➤ Initially the tongue has a thick white coating, which develops in a few days into typical strawberry tongue. Tonsillitis may show exudates with cervical lymphadenopathy.

➤ From 6–10 days after the eruption, peeling (desquamation) begins and usually lasts several weeks.

➤ Apart from the rash and the tongue, there is essentially no difference between streptococcal tonsillitis, viral tonsillitis (including EBV infectious mononucleosis) and scarlet fever. Normal throat culture for streptococci and anti-streptolysin O (ASO) titres favour viral aetiology. Scarlet fever can be differentiated from Kawasaki disease by an older age at onset, absence of conjunctival involvement and rapid response to penicillin (Box 4.14).

➤ Complications include peri-tonsillar or retropharyngeal abscess, acute rheumatic fever, glomerulonephritis, meningitis, otitis media osteomyelitis and arthritis.

BOX 4.14 Antibiotic therapy for children with scarlet fever

● Oral penicillin (Phenoxymethylpenicillin=penicillin V): 125 mg–500 mg (depending on the child's age) 4 times daily for 10 days
● Oral erythromycin 250–500 mg (depending on the child's age) 4 times daily for 10 days (for those allergic to penicillin)
● It is unnecessary to treat asymptomatic children with positive throat culture for group A streptococci
● Children should not return to school or daycare until they have completed 24 hours of antibiotic therapy

---

Tuberculosis (TB)

Core messages

➤ The incidence of TB has declined progressively in the past few decades. However, it is still a cause of significant illness and mortality. After 4 decades of steady decline, the annual case rate levelled off in 1985 and has increased in some areas since then.

➤ Children usually acquire the infection from adults who have active disease and are expectorating tubercle bacilli. Children themselves are usually non-contagious, therefore every effort should be made to identify the adult source to enable eradication of the source bacilli.

➤ In older children, **primary infection** is asymptomatic in most cases. Radiologically, a parenchymal lesion is usually not visible, but hilar adenitis is prominent and may cause compression of the adjacent soft bronchus, causing wheezing and non-productive cough. With increased compression, or following perforation of an infected lymph node into the bronchus, segmental atelectasis may ensue.

➤ Other presentations are erythema nodosum, phlyctenular conjunctivitis, and TB pneumonia. Pneumonia resembles radiologically bacterial pneumonia with high fever, cough and dyspnoea.

➤ **Miliary TB** in children usually presents with no specific symptoms and signs. Fever is present in about 75% of cases, with anorexia, weight loss, night sweats and dyspnoea. Ophthalmoscopy may detect typical choroidal tubercles in the retina. Almost one-third of the children with active TB may have extrapulmonary manifestations, such as adenitis (frequently as a non-tender, firm-to-tender, or firm cervical lymphadenitis), or TB meningitis (see section on meningitis above).

➤ **Neonatal TB** occurs through vertical transmission of infection from mother to infant via the placenta or amniotic fluid. Neonates present with feeding difficulty, failure to thrive, jaundice, respiratory distress or hepatosplenomegaly. Fever is usually absent. Chest X-ray shows bronchopneumonia. The disease often runs a fulminant course with rapid multiplication of tubercle bacilli and minimal giant cell formation.

➤ Diagnosis of TB is as shown in Box 4.15.

BOX 4.15 The diagnosis of TB

● **History of contact** with an infectious case
● **Symptoms:** persistent, unremitting cough, persistent fever and fatigue, night sweating, chest pain and weight loss
● **Identification of the mycobacteria** (positive in about 30–40% of cases) from sputum, gastric fluid, pleural fluid, CSF or other tissues, or by PCR. Acid-fast smear is positive in 10–20% of cases
● **X-ray findings**, often in the form of "unresolved pneumonia", with enlarged mediastinal lymphadenopathy.
● **Positive tuberculin test** (Fig 4.6)

Mantoux test: use 0.1 mL of 1:1000 tuberculin PPD (100 U/mL)
Reaction for detection of induration after 48–72 hours

< 5 mm	5–10 mm	> 10 mm (more definite if > 15mm)
↓	↓	↓
Negative	Previous BCG	Infection

↓
Treat as TB infection if:
• Known contact
• From high prevalence area
• Abnormal chest X-ray
• Symptoms present

FIGURE 4.6 Diagnosis of tuberculosis by the outcomes of a Mantoux test

PRACTICE POINTS

- BCG (Bacille Calmette-Guérin) vaccination has been shown to give 70–80% protection against TB. The BCG vaccine is no longer given as part of the routine childhood vaccination schedule, but only to those children considered at risk of developing TB (Box 4.16).
- HIV infection may occur in association with TB, which often presents as unresolving pneumonia. The infection carries a high mortality rate despite adequate anti-TB and anti-HIV therapy.
- Patients receiving anti-TB drugs may develop hypersensitivity to these drugs (usually appearing between the third and fifth day of treatment). This should be considered in any patient with persistent fever after initiation of therapy. Such a drug reaction should be suspected if the fever becomes higher than it was prior to therapy.
- Drugs used for treatment of TB are shown in Table 4.9. A 6-month regimen for drug-susceptible TB with INH, rifampicin and pyrazinamide for the first 2 months followed by INH and rifampicin for the remaining 4 months is recommended. If drug resistance is possible, initial treatment should include ethambutol, streptomycin, amikacin or ciprofloxacin until a drug susceptibility result becomes available (*See* Table 4.9). Shorter regimens using four drugs in the initial phase are increasingly being adopted.

BOX 4.16 Indications for BCG vaccination

BCG vaccination is offered to:
- All infants living in areas of the UK where the annual incidence of TB is ≥ 40/100 000
- All infants with a parent or grandparent who was born in a country where the annual incidence of TB is ≥ 40/100 000
- Previously unvaccinated children aged 1–5 years with a parent or grandparent who was born in a country where the annual incidence of TB is ≥ 40/100 000
- Previously unvaccinated tuberculin-negative children aged from 6 to under 16 years of age with a parent or grandparent who was born in a country where the annual incidence of TB is ≥ 40/100 000
- Previously unvaccinated tuberculin-negative individuals under 16 years of age who are contacts of cases of respiratory TB
- Previously unvaccinated, tuberculin-negative individuals under 16 years of age who were born in or have lived at least 3 months in a country with an annual TB incidence of ≥ 40/100 000

TABLE 4.9 The main drugs used to treat children with TB (6-month therapy)

Isoniazid (INH)	10 mg/kg	maximum 300 mg
Rifampicin	15 mg/kg	maximum 600 mg
Pyrazinamide	35 mg/kg	
Ethambutol	20 mg/kg	

Malaria

Core nessages

➤ Malaria is caused by protozoal infection transmitted by *Anopheles* mosquitoes. The four species of protozoa that commonly infect humans are *Plasmodium vivax, P. ovale* (benign tertian malaria), *P. falciparum* (malignant tertian malaria), and *P. malariae* (benign quartan malaria).

➤ The number of malaria cases and deaths is estimated at 200–300 million and 2–3 million respectively. Over 50% of childhood deaths in many parts of Africa are attributed to malaria.

➤ Most cases of malaria imported to the UK are *P. falciparum* (about three-quarters of cases) and *P. vivax*, with 1500–2000 cases each year (total number of cases of all forms).

➤ Typical symptoms include paroxysm of fever (see below), lethargy, headache, cough, anorexia, vomiting, diarrhoea, and abdominal pain. Physical examination reveals splenomegaly (detected in almost 100% of cases) and hepatomegaly.

The presenting symptoms of *falciparum* infection are an irregular pattern of fever, severe headache, irritability, delirium, coma, hyperpyrexia, convulsion and meningism. Infection is most likely to occur within 3 months of return from malaria-endemic areas, especially if anti-malarial prophylaxis has been inadequate or not taken.

➤ A typical tertian paroxysm (*P. vivax* and *P. ovale*) is characterised by fever with rigor, which often triggers febrile seizures. The next stage is marked by high fever, up to a temperature of 41°C. In tertian infection the paroxysm recurs at 48-hour intervals, while in quartan infection the paroxysm recurs at 72-hour intervals. The third stage is characterised by a drop in body temperature to normal, with sweating.

➤ Malaria can present as pyrexia of unknown origin only, without other associated signs such as anaemia or splenomegaly

Complications include:

➤ Nephrotic syndrome may occur with *P. malariae* infection.

➤ Blackwater fever, a state of acute intravascular haemolysis accompanied by haemoglobulinuria, may occur as a complication of *P. falciparum*.

➤ Human parvovirus B19 infection may occur, adding to the severity of anaemia. This virus is highly erythrotropic, infecting erythroid progenitor cells.

Diagnosis

➤ Diagnosis is easy when children present with typical paroxysms of fever. Children may, however, present with misleading symptoms such as sore throat, myalgia and gastrointestinal and respiratory symptoms.

➤ Definitive diagnosis is made via Giemsa-stained blood smear (thick and thin smears), which should be arranged urgently if the diagnosis is suspected.

➤ Rapid diagnosis tests (RDTs) based on detection of parasite antigens or enzymes are commonly used in addition to the blood slides.

➤ Laboratory findings include anaemia, with Hb concentration of 50–110 g/L, and leukopenia. Thrombocytopenia, hyponatraemia and hypoglycaemia may also occur.

Management

➤ Hospitalisation for any child with suspected or confirmed malaria is always indicated to assess the severity and extent of the infection.
➤ Treatment consists of:
  ➢ Oral 3-day course of chloroquine, which remains the treatment of choice for benign malarias
  ➢ Oral quinine is for uncomplicated *falciparum* malaria, usually combined with doxycycline
  ➢ Atovaquone + proguanil (Malarone) or co-artemether (Riamet; artemether + lumefantrine) are also effective against *P. falciparum*
  ➢ For parasites persisting in the liver after treatment of *P. vivax* or *P. ovale* infection, primaquine is effective
  ➢ Severe cases of *P. falciparum* are treated with IV quinine.

Prophylaxis of malaria

➤ Malarone Paediatric tablets should be started 1–2 days before entering a malaria-endemic area and continued for 1 week after leaving:
  ➢ 1 tablet daily for 3 days for a bodyweight of 11–21 kg
  ➢ 2 tablets once daily for 3 days for a bodyweight of 21–31 kg
  ➢ 3 tablets once daily for 3 days for a bodyweight of 31–40 kg
  ➢ 4 tablets once daily for 3 days for a body weight over 40 kg.
➤ Travellers should be warned about the importance of avoiding mosquito bites, of taking prophylaxis regularly and seeking medical assessment urgently if a child becomes ill within 1 year and especially within 3 months of return from the malaria-endemic area.
➤ Proguanil is usually used with chloroquine (only occasionally alone) for the prophylaxis of malaria. The drug(s) should be used 1 week before entering a malaria-endemic area and continued for 4 weeks after leaving.

⌂ RED FLAGS

- Some drugs used for prophylaxis and treatment of malaria, in particular primaquine, should not be administered before checking for glucose-6-phosphate dehydrogenase (G6PD) deficiency status. This drug can cause severe haemolysis in case of deficiency.
- Children with malaria may present with atypical symptoms. Diagnosis should always be considered in a feverish or unwell child who has visited any malaria-endemic areas.
- *Falciparum* infection is a medical emergency requiring immediate admission to the hospital, as death can occur within 24 hours of onset.

Brucellosis

Core messages

➤ Brucellosis is primarily a zoonotic infection caused by small, non-motile, Gram-negative coccobacilli of the genus *Brucella*.
➤ There are four important species pathogenic to humans: *B. melitensis* (Malta fever,

found primarily in goats and sheep), *B. abortus* (abortus fever, in cattle), *B. suis* (swine) and *B. canis* (dogs).

➤ The infection is transmitted to humans through direct contact with infected animals or their products, and through consumption of infected milk, milk products or meat. More than half a million cases per year occur worldwide.

➤ Clinically, brucellosis is characterised by the following features:
  ➢ Symptoms and signs include fever, arthritis, arthralgia, backache, anorexia and weight loss, tender hepatosplenomegaly and lymphadenopathy. These symptoms and signs are more severe with *B. melitensis*.
  ➢ Fever occurs in almost every patient (90–100 % of cases), often insidiously over the course of several days. Fever may also manifest as periodic fever, with symptoms lasting a few days or weeks followed by symptom-free intervals that last weeks and months, or as pyrexia of unknown origin (PUO).

➤ **Complications** include spondylitis, osteomyelitis, granulomatous reaction of the eye, meningitis or meningo-encephalitis. *Brucella* endocarditis is rare and may be responsible for the majority of deaths due to the disease.

Laboratory findings
➤ FBC, looking for anaemia, leucopenia, lymphopenia
➤ Liver function tests: raised liver enzymes
➤ The diagnosis is established by positive culture of *Brucella* organisms from blood or bone-marrow aspirate, or positive serological tests (agglutination titre of > 1 : 80).

Management
Antibiotics for 6 weeks are the cornerstone of management:
➤ In children older than 8 years, a combination of doxycycline 100 mg BD with rifampicin 600–900 mg PO. Gentamicin, streptomycin and ciprofloxacin in combination with doxycycline have also been found to be effective.
➤ In children below 8 years of age, a combination of rifampicin and trimethoprim-sulfamethoxazole (Septrin) is effective.
➤ Rifampicin has also been used successfully in combination with streptomycin in the treatment of *Brucella* endocarditis.

Lyme disease
Core messages
➤ Lyme disease (LD) is a multisystem inflammatory disease caused by the spirochete *Borrelia burgdorferi*. It is transmitted by infected ticks (Fig 4.7 – *see* Plate section). There may currently be around 3000 cases of Lyme disease in the UK each year.
➤ LD has been divided into three stages:
  ➢ The first stage occurs 3–30 days after the tick bite and is characterised by an annular skin rash (erythema migrans – Fig 4.8 – *see* Plate section), which develops at the site of the bite. Associated features include flu-like symptoms such as fatigue, myalgia and low-grade fever, which occurs in about 50% of children. Antibiotics at this stage may prevent subsequent stages.
  ➢ The second stage follows 2–12 weeks after the tick bite and is characterised by disseminated infection causing:
    ● carditis (most commonly presenting as atrioventricular block or myocarditis)

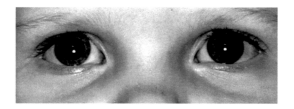

FIGURE 1.3 Normal right eye with abnormal red reflex in the left eye. Possible causes include congenital cataract or retinoblastoma. Urgent referral is indicated

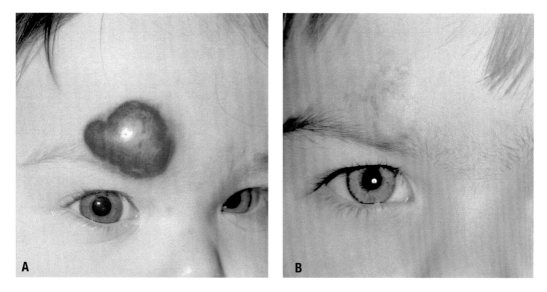

FIGURE 1.5 Strawberry naevus at the age of 1 year (A) and at the age 5 years (B)

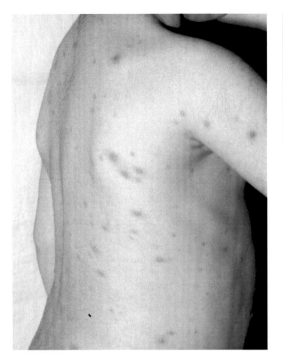

FIGURE 4.2 Varicella on the trunk showing pink macules, which change rapidly into papules, vesicles, pustules and then crusts

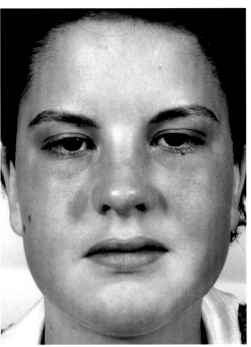

FIGURE 4.3 Erythema infectiosum

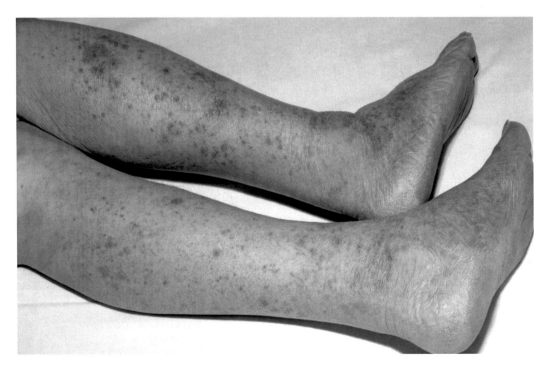

FIGURE 4.4 Purpuric skin rash of meningococcal septicaemia

FIGURE 4.5
Tumbler test: skin
is non-blanching
with glass pressed
against it

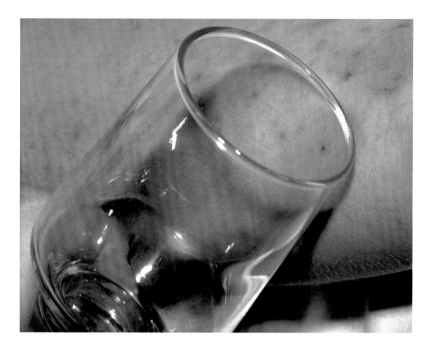

FIGURE 4.7 Ticks
before (left) and
after feeding (right)

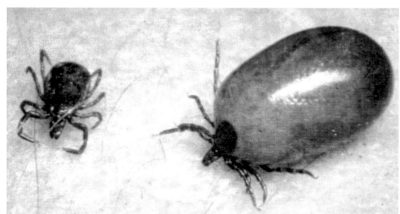

FIGURE 4.8 Large
erythema migrans

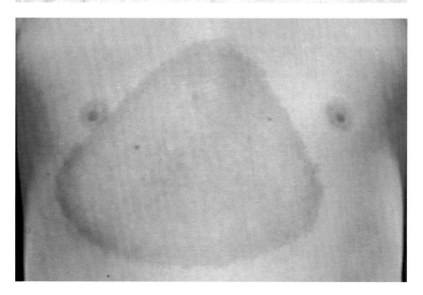

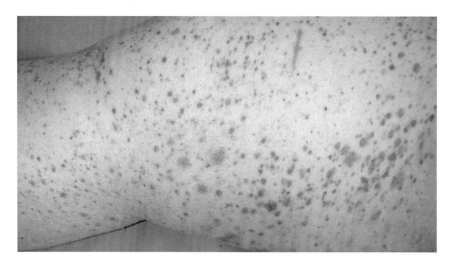

FIGURE 6.1 Extensive purpuric lesions on the leg

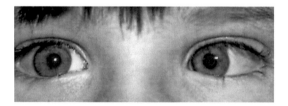

FIGURE 13.3 Abnormal positioning of a light reflex in the left eye, indicating squint. There is also anisocoria (unequal size of the pupils), which is a common finding affecting 20% of the population. Acquired squint that is not congenital could be the first presentation of retinoblastoma

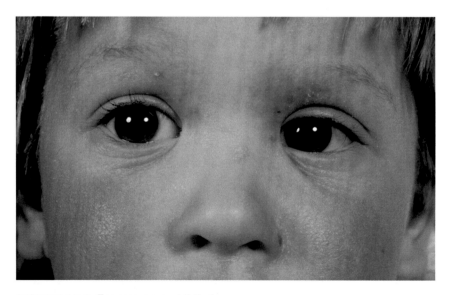

FIGURE 17.1 Eczema on a child's face

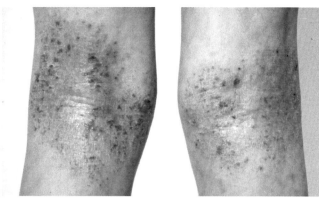

FIGURE 17.2 Eczema involving the popliteal fossae

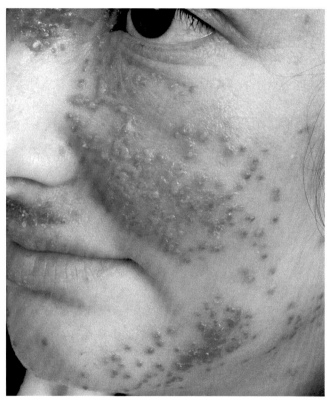

FIGURE 17.3 Eczema herpeticum

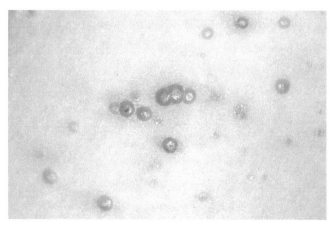

FIGURE 17.4 Molluscum contagiosum

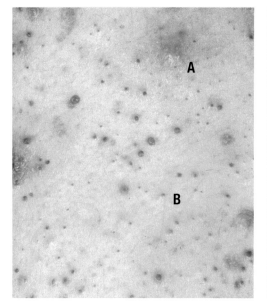

FIGURE 17.5 Acne. A: upper right: pustule B: comedones (blackheads)

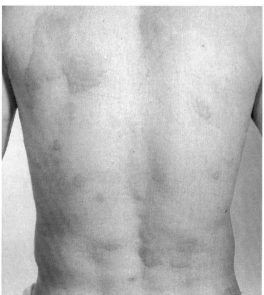

FIGURE 17.6 Urticaria with large wheals

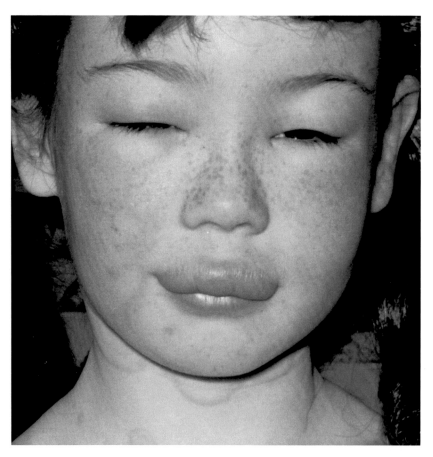

FIGURE 17.7
Angioedema
involving eyelids
and upper lip

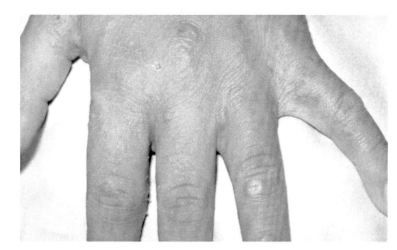

FIGURE 17.8 Scabies, showing burrows in the webs between the fingers

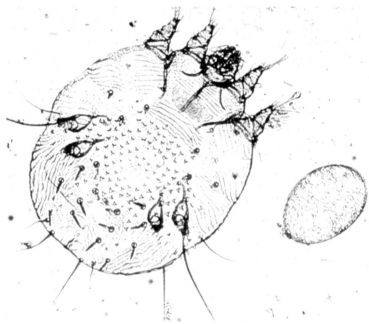

FIGURE 17.9 Scabies mite and egg

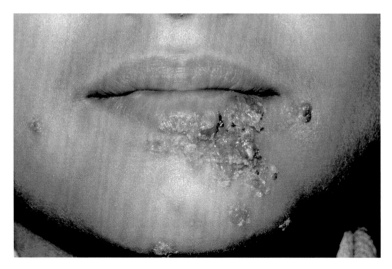

FIGURE 17.10 Impetigo with typical honey-coloured crusts on the chin

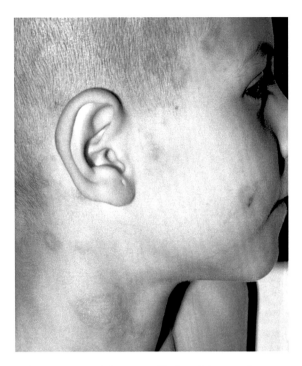

FIGURE 17.11 Tinea capitis involving scalp, face and neck. This photo unusually shows tinea capitis involving multiple sites

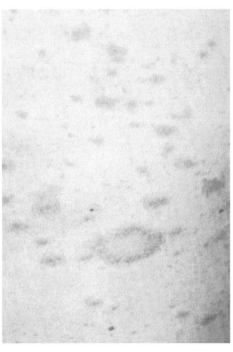

FIGURE 17.13 Pityriasis rosea on the trunk with a herald patch

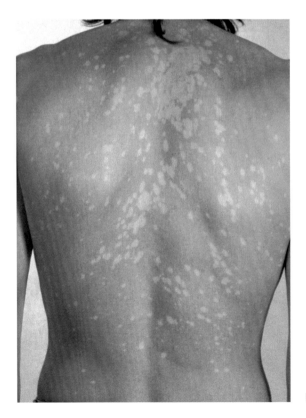

FIGURE 17.14 Pityriasis versicolor

- aseptic meningitis with neck stiffness and severe headaches
- cranial neuritis most commonly presenting as Bell palsy
- intermittent arthritis.

➤ The third stage is characterised by oligoarticular arthritis and acrodermatitis chronica atrophicans, occurring between 6 weeks and 2 years after the tick bite in 50–80% of patients.

Diagnosis of Lyme disease (LD) depends on:

➤ Characteristic, clinical features, in particular the appearance of erythema migrans

➤ Specific IgM antibodies against *B. burgdorferi* appearing 3–4 weeks after the infection and peaking after 6–8 weeks. Specific IgG antibodies usually become detectable in the second month after the onset of infection.

Treatment

➤ Uncomplicated cases of LD are treated with oral penicillin (125–500 mg daily) or amoxicillin (125–250 mg) divided into 3 doses for 21 days.

➤ For children older than 12 years, doxycycline twice daily for 21 days or tetracycline for the same duration is effective. For arthritis, antibiotic therapy should continue for 4 weeks and often includes a third-generation cephalosporin. For meningitis, penicillin G/cephalosporin is given intravenously for 2–3 weeks.

RED FLAGS

- Symptoms in the 3rd stage may often be mistaken for fibromyalgia or chronic fatigue syndrome.
- Negative enzyme linked immunosorbent assay (ELISA) antibody testing does not exclude LD.

REFERENCES

1. Feigin and Cherry's Textbook of Pediatric Infectious Diseases (2 volume set). 6th edition. Publisher: Saunders 2009.
2. Principles and Practice of Pediatric Infectious Diseases. By S S Long, LK Pickering, CG Prober. Elsevier, Churchill, Livingstone 2012.
3. El-Radhi AS, Barry W. Thermometry in paediatric practice. Arch Dis Child 2006; 91: 351–356.
4. Meningococcal meningitis and septicaemia. Diagnosis and treatment in general practice (2011). NICE guideline CG102, SIGN: meningococcal disease guideline 102, and NICE guideline CG47. www.sign.ac.uk/guidelines/fulltext/102/ and www.nice.org.uk
5. Thompson MJ, Minis N, Perera R, et al. Clinical recognition of meningococcal disease in children and adolescents. Lancet 2006; 367: 397–403.

CHAPTER 5

Allergy

PREVALENCE

➤ In Western countries, almost 30% of the population develops one or more allergic diseases, ranging from mild transient eczema or hay fever to severe life-threatening asthma or systemic anaphylaxis. Table 5.1 shows an overall prevalence of allergy in these countries.

➤ There has been an increasing prevalence of allergic diseases during the last few decades. Many environmental factors appear to be responsible for this increase, including:

  ➢ Increased exposure to allergens

  ➢ The modern lifestyle with its insulated homes, high indoor humidity, and wall-to-wall fitted-carpets that contribute to house dust mite proliferation

  ➢ Changing dietary habits, with greater consumption of processed food and less natural food

  ➢ The hygiene theory: infection suppresses those immunological reactions responsible for allergic responses. With the decline of the prevalence of infection, the prevalence of allergy has increased. In support of this theory is the lower prevalence of atopy among children of large families or those attending daycare nurseries compared with those of small families or those not attending nurseries. Also, children who experienced numerous febrile episodes during the first year of life have a lower incidence of allergy than those with fewer febrile episodes.

TABLE 5.1 Prevalence of various allergic diseases in Western countries

Prevalence	Average cases reported (%)
Asthma	20–30
Seasonal allergic rhinitis	20
Perennial allergic rhinitis	11–15
Atopic dermatitis	10–15
Food allergy	6–8
Cow's milk allergy	2–3
Egg allergy	2

DIAGNOSIS OF ALLERGY

History and physical examination

A detailed allergy-focused history exploring exposure to potential allergens is essential and is often diagnostic. Symptoms are either caused by immunoglobulin E (IgE)-mediated or non-IgE-mediated reactions (*see* Table 5.3, in the section below on food allergy). Allergy history should include:

➤ Immediate family history of atopy (asthma, hay fever and atopic dermatitis or urticaria)

➤ Seasonal respiratory and/or nasal symptoms which may suggest seasonal allergens such as pollens

➤ Perennial symptoms, occurring particularly at the end of the summer, suggesting allergy to house dust mites

➤ Symptoms occurring shortly after acquisition of a pet and relief when the child is away from the house, which suggest allergy to animal dander

➤ Symptoms of asthma occurring in a damp musty basement, suggesting allergy to inhaled fungal spores

➤ Symptoms produced by dusting or carpet cleaning, suggest allergy to house dust mites

➤ Symptoms occurring after moving to a new house or during trips, suggesting environmental causes of allergy.

Physical examination often contributes to the diagnosis, e.g.:

➤ Mouth-breathing and frequent, habitual wiping of a runny nose with the palm of the hand suggest allergic rhinitis.

➤ The presence of seasonal conjunctivitis with watering and peri-orbital oedema makes the diagnosis of allergic conjunctivitis most likely.

➤ Examination of the skin may reveal patches of atopic dermatitis, which is often associated with allergic rhinitis and asthma.

➤ Chest examination may reveal tachypnoea, wheezing and subcostal recession.

Laboratory tests

(*See* Table 5.2.)

➤ **Total IgE.** Normal values of IgE increase with age and vary in different populations. The mean concentration of IgE in atopic individuals is often higher than in non-topic people. However, a large number of atopic patients have normal IgE levels. This suggests that low levels of IgE may be more useful in excluding atopic diseases than elevated levels are in confirming their presence. Furthermore, many non-allergic conditions are associated with increased levels of IgE (Box 5.1).

➤ **Skin prick testing (SPT)** is currently the most common way of demonstrating skin sensitivity to an allergen. Infants and young children show less-pronounced reactions compared with older children and adults. A summary of common allergens used in SPT is shown in Box 5.2. Intradermal tests are less often used, but they are several thousand times more sensitive than epidermal testing. They are indicated if the allergy extracts used for SPT are not strong enough to give a reaction.

➤ **The RAST (radioallergosorbent) test** determines antigen-specific IgE concentrations in serum using an allergen extract which is a mixture of numerous protein allergens. Although there is a good correlation between RAST and skin prick results, the RAST is on the whole less sensitive than SPT by about 70–80%. Tests can be specified for either foods or inhalants, or both.

➤ **Direct challenge** (to be carried out in hospital). Many specialists believe that the challenge test is the gold standard for diagnosis of allergy, particularly food allergy. It is performed by introducing the suspected allergen (usually food, an extract or aerosol of the material) to the mucous membranes of the affected organ, e.g. the mouth or bronchus. Challenge testing is indicated if there is a need for definitive diagnosis or if the history is equivocal and symptoms improve during an elimination diet.

TABLE 5.2 Summary of diagnostic testing for allergy

Diagnostic tool	Details
Skin prick tests (SPTs)*	Most commonly used method to test for allergy; it has higher specificity than blood tests
Blood:	
• IgE	The finding of a normal level is more important in excluding allergy than a high level is in confirming allergy, i.e. high sensitivity and low specificity
RAST	Sensitivity is no more than 70–80%, which is lower than SPT
Direct challenge*	Useful, particularly for milk allergy (resuscitation measures should be available)

* Not usually performed in a primary-care setting.

BOX 5.1 Non-allergic diseases with increased IgE

Infection
• Systemic candidiasis
• Mononucleosis

Neoplasm
• Hodgkin's lymphoma

Parasites
• Ascariasis

Pulmonary
• Cystic fibrosis
• Haemosiderosis

Skin disorders
• Erythema nodosum

Immunodeficiency
• IgA deficiency
• Hyperimmunoglobulinaemia

Vascular–rheumatic
• Kawasaki disease
• Rheumatoid arthritis

Others
• Liver disease

BOX 5.2 Common allergens tested for by skin prick testing (SPT)

Aeroallergens
• Pollens – grass mix, tree mix, weed mix, birch
• Mites – house dust mites (*Dermatophagoides pteronyssinus*)
• Animals – cat, dog, horse
• Moulds – mould spores

Stinging insects
• Bees, wasps

Food
• Cow's milk, eggs, fish, peanuts, shellfish, wheat

FOOD ALLERGY

Core messages

➤ Food allergy is defined as an adverse immunological-mediated (IgE-mediated) or non-IgE-mediated response to food protein. IgE-mediated reaction is rapid and may occur within a few minutes. Non-IgE-mediated reaction is cell-mediated and occurs over hours or days. Symptoms differ in each reaction (Table 5.3).

➤ There has been a dramatic increase in the prevalence of allergy, including food allergy, in the last 20 years. As many as 8% of young children and 2% of adults in Westernised countries have an allergy, and the prevalence is rising. Hospital admissions in the UK for allergies have increased 500% since 1990.[1]

➤ Food intolerance manifests with gastrointestinal symptoms (vomiting, nausea, crampy abdominal pain, bloating, discomfort and diarrhoea). Food allergy should be distinguished from *food intolerance* which is usually caused by deficiency of intestinal enzymes. The classical example is milk intolerance due to deficiency of the enzyme lactase rather than being mediated by IgE.

Almost any food is capable of inducing allergy, most commonly cow's milk, fish, shellfish, eggs, peanuts, sesame, soy, wheat and kiwifruit. Allergy to cow's milk and eggs has been estimated to have a prevalence of 2–4% in the infant population (UK). Fortunately, the prevalence of most food allergy declines with age, and some 80% of children are no longer allergic by the age of 4 years.

TABLE 5.3 Summary of signs and symptoms of possible food allergy[1]

IgE-mediated	Non-IgE-mediated
Skin	**Skin**
• Pruritis	• Pruritis
• Erythema	• Erythema
• Acute urticaria	• Atopic eczema
• Acute angioedema (lips, face and eyes)	**Gastroenterology**
Gastrointestinal	• Gastro-oesophageal reflux
• Oral pruritis	• Loose or frequent stools, with blood or mucus
• Angioedema (lips, tongue and palate)	• Abdominal pain
• Nausea, vomiting, diarrhoea, colicky abdominal pain	• Constipation
Respiratory	• Perianal redness
• Upper respiratory symptoms (nasal itching, sneezing, rhinorrhoea, or congestion)	• Infantile colic
• Lower respiratory symptoms (cough, chest tightness, wheezing or dyspnoea)	• Food refusal or aversion
Other	• Pallor and tiredness
• Signs and symptoms of anaphylaxis or other systemic allergic reactions	• Faltering growth

Diagnosis

➤ An **allergy-focused history** should be taken (Box 5.3).

➤ **Elimination diet** and subsequent food challenge are the gold standard for diagnosing food allergy.

➤ **Food challenge**, although commonly performed, is less reliable that other tests except in young infants (see section on milk allergy, below). Atopy patch testing or oral food challenge should not be used to diagnose IgE-mediated allergy in primary-care or community settings.

➤ **Skin prick test (SPT) or radioallergosorbent blood test (RAST)** evaluate the presence of IgE for specific allergens. In infants < 1 year of age, a positive SPT or positive RAST is significant because IgE is usually not detectable at this age, whereas a negative test result does not exclude allergy. In older children, the reverse is true: a positive SPT or positive RAST does not necessarily indicate that a specific food is the cause of symptoms. Results of these tests should always be interpreted in the context of the clinical history.

BOX 5.3 Food allergy-focused clinical history

Ask about:

● Any personal or family history of atopic disease
● The feeding history (breast or formula) and age of weaning
● Any foods suspected of allergy, and those avoided and why
● Age of first onset, speed of onset and setting of reaction. Who has raised the concern and suspected the food allergy?
● Duration, severity and frequency of symptoms
● Cultural and religious diet factors that affect the child's diet
● Details of previous treatment including any medications
● Any response to the elimination and reintroduction of foods

---

Management

➤ The child and parents should receive information that is relevant to the type of allergy, including the risk and management of severe allergic reaction.

➤ Allergy tests should not be offered without first taking an allergy-focused clinical history. Tests should only be undertaken by competent healthcare professionals and where there are facilities present for resuscitation.

➤ The only definitive treatment for food allergy is eliminating the offending food item (normally for 2–6 weeks). Most gastrointestinal symptoms resolve within a few days; although some symptoms, particularly food-induced enteropathy, may take a few weeks before resolving. An elimination diet may be followed by a possible planned re-challenge. A dietitian should be involved.

➤ Children with a history of severe or frequent allergy should be supplied with injectable adrenaline and antihistamine. (See section on severe allergic reactions and anaphylaxis, below.)

➤ Patients should be given information on support groups (see below).

Prevention
The American Academy of Pediatrics recommends the following:
➤ Breast-feeding ideally for 12 months or longer, but for at least 6 months. If breast-feeding is not possible, hypoallergenic formula (see section on milk allergy, below) is to be given. Mothers should avoid eating peanuts and tree nuts while breast-feeding.
➤ Gradual introduction of solid foods from age 6–12 months. If parents choose to start giving their babies solid foods before the age of 6 months, nuts, eggs, fish and shellfish should not be included. The use of formulas based on cow's milk in early infancy and the introduction of solid foods before the age of 4 months have been associated with the development of cow's milk allergy and atopic diseases.
➤ Solid foods should be added one at a time, with several days before introduction of a second solid food.
➤ It is best to start with iron-fortified rice cereal mixed with breast milk; then cooked, puréed and strained fruits and vegetables. It is advisable to avoid eggs until the age of 2 years, and peanuts and shellfish until the age of 3 years.
➤ Allergy to kiwifruit has increased; and it should be avoided during the first few years of life.

Prognosis
➤ Most children grow out of a cow's milk allergy, and the prognosis is far better in children than in adults.
➤ Young children with the most common causes of allergy (milk, eggs, wheat and soya) are expected to grow out of their allergy by the age of 4–5 years. Allergy to fish, shellfish, peanuts and tree nuts may continue into adulthood. The above foods constitute about 90% of all food allergies.
➤ About 20% of children with peanut allergy are expected to outgrow this allergy. However, the current recommendation is lifelong avoidance of peanuts.

SPECIFIC FOOD ALLERGIES
Milk allergy
Core messages
➤ Food allergy, particularly cow's milk protein allergy (CMPA), is an increasing problem worldwide. Between 5% and 15% of infants and young children develop symptoms suggesting CMPA.[2] The incidence of CMPA is much lower (about 0.5%) in babies that are exclusively breast-fed.
➤ There is no pathognomonic symptom for CMPA, but the main symptoms are urticaria, and wheezing angioedema occurring within 2 hours of ingestion (IgE-mediated reaction). Gastrointestinal symptoms (e.g. abdominal pain, colic, and diarrhoea) are the predominant symptoms of non-IgE-mediated milk allergy.
➤ Currently, the recommendation for infants at high risk of atopic disease is breast-feeding and delaying the introduction of solids.
➤ Due to the many benefits of breast-feeding, clinicians should advise mothers to continue breast-feeding in cases of CMPA but avoid the causal foods in their own diet, such as milk, eggs and peanuts.
➤ If symptoms improve or disappear after an elimination diet, 1 food per week can be reintroduced to the mother's diet. If symptoms reappear, the food responsible should

be eliminated as long as the breast-feeding continues. If the mother wants to wean, her infant should receive one of the formulas below.

➤ Hypoallergenic formulas (Table 5.4) include soy protein formula; extensively hydro-lysed formulas (eHFs) – first choice in cases of CMPA; amino acid formulas (AAFs), which are indicated if the child refuses to drink eHF (eHF has a more bitter taste than AAF). The risk of failure with eHF is up to 10% in children with CMPA.

➤ SPT and/or RAST are especially helpful in CMPA: infants with negative tests at the time of diagnosis become tolerant to the offending protein at a much younger age than those with positive reactions. In addition, a negative SPT and RAST result reduces the risk of a severe acute reaction during challenge.

➤ About 80% of children with CMPA will grow out of their allergy by the age of 4 years.

➤ Management of infants suspected of having CMPA is shown in Fig 5.1.

TABLE 5.4 Hypoallergenic formulas used for CMPA

Formulas	Comments
Soy protein (e.g. ProSobee)	Only 50–80% of children with CMPA can tolerate these formulas. Soya is not recommended in children < 6 months of age
Extensively hydrolysed, eHF (e.g. Nutramigen, Pepti-Junior)	First choice for children with CMPA. It has a bitter taste, so some children refuse it
Amino-acid-based (e.g. Neocate, Nutramigen AA)	Second choice if eHFs fail
Partially hydrolysed	Not recommended

Milk challenge

This procedure should be performed in a hospital with resuscitation facilities.

➤ A drop of the formula is put on the infant's lips.

➤ If no reaction occurs after 15 minutes, the formula is given orally and the dose is increased stepwise: 0.5 mL, 1.0, 3.0, 10, 30, 50, to 100 mL, every 30 minutes. The infant is observed for 2 hours thereafter.

Peanut allergy

Peanuts (*Arachis hypogaea*) can cause severe or even fatal reactions. About 10 people die every year in the UK from peanut allergy. Reactions to peanuts differ from those caused by other foods in the following ways:

They commonly occur in young children (peak age 14–24 months). In the UK, about 1 in 70 children of school age has an allergy to peanuts and 1 in 200 an allergy to tree nuts. Unlike other food allergies, nut allergy is usually permanent. Only 1 in 5 people will grow out of it, usually children with a mild reaction.

➤ Typical immediate allergic reactions include urticaria, oral pruritis, sneezing, cough-ing, choking, wheezing, dyspnoea and hypotension.

➤ Serious reactions in young children often require emergency treatment (one-third of emergency visits to A&E departments with anaphylaxis are caused by peanut allergy).

➤ Peanut intolerance may also occur, with an incidence of about 1 : 300, and usually manifests as bloating or discomfort.

Clinical assessment suggesting suspicion of CMPA

Mild symptoms
- Frequent vomiting and diarrhoea
- Some blood in stools
- Mild atopic dermatitis
- Colic defined as > 3 h per day and > 3 days a week over a period of > 3 weeks

If breast-fed: continue with breast-feeding, start elimination diet in mother (no cow's milk, eggs, peanuts) for 2-4 weeks. Calcium supplement

Improved

- Continue with elimination diet

If formula-fed:
- Consider eHF or AAF
- Consider referral

Severe symptoms
- Failure to thrive due to vomiting and diarrhoea
- Refusal to feed
- Bloody stools, iron deficiency anaemia
- Severe atopic dermatitis
- Severe adverse reaction caused by milk

Referral to paediatric specialist

Not improved

- Resume normal diet in mother
- Consider referral
- Consider eHF or AAF
- Consider alternative diagnosis, e.g. coeliac disease, lactose intolerance, CF

FIGURE 5.1 Management of an infant with CMPA (summarised from Vandenplas et al.[2])

Treatment

Treatment includes:

➤ Avoidance is currently the only available therapy. Foods that contain peanuts include peanut butter, flour, oil (arachis oil is peanut oil), monkey and beer nuts. Peanuts are sometimes found in egg rolls and stir fry (in some Oriental restaurants), nougat and peanut butter ice-creams.

➤ Referral to dietitian.

➤ Ensuring that parents and anyone else who looks after the child are fully educated about the condition.

➤ Wearing medical alert bracelet, e.g. MedicAlert ID tags.

➤ Emergency treatment of allergic reactions (see section on severe allergic reactions and anaphylaxis, below).

➤ The Department of Health (DOH) advises that atopic and breast-feeding mothers and their infants should avoid peanuts. In 2009, the DOH revised their advice as follows:

➣ There is no clear evidence that eating or not eating peanuts during pregnancy, whilst breast-feeding or during early infant life, influences the chances of a child developing peanut allergy

➣ If mothers choose to start giving their baby solid foods before 6 months of age, they should not introduce peanuts, nuts, seeds, eggs, wheat and fish.

➤ Where a child is atopic (e.g. has eczema or an allergy to foods other than peanut) or if there is a history of allergy in the child's family, mothers are encouraged to talk to their GP, health visitor or medical allergy specialist before giving peanuts to the child for the first time because they are at higher risk of developing peanut allergy. They should avoid peanuts until three years of age.

⚑ RED FLAG

- Children with peanut allergy and asthma are at much higher risk of severe or fatal allergic reactions.

Egg allergy

Guidelines on management

➤ Egg allergy has a prevalence of approximately 2% in children and 0.1% in adults.[3]
➤ A clear clinical history and the detection of egg-white-specific IgE (by SPT or RAST) will confirm the diagnosis in most cases.
➤ Egg avoidance is the cornerstone of management.
➤ Egg allergy often resolves, and re-introduction can be achieved at home if reactions have been mild and there is no asthma.
➤ Patients with a history of severe reactions or asthma should have re-introduction carried out under the supervision of an allergy specialist.
➤ All children with egg allergy should receive MMR (measles–mumps–rubella) vaccination.
➤ Influenza and yellow fever vaccines contain egg protein and should only be considered under the supervision of an allergy specialist if there has been severe allergic reaction to eggs.

Consider referral to a paediatric allergy specialist if:

➤ Symptoms do not respond to a single-allergen elimination diet.
➤ The child has confirmed IgE-mediated food allergy and concurrent asthma.
➤ Tests are negative but there is strong suspicion of IgE-mediated food allergy. There is faltering growth with one or more of the gastrointestinal symptoms shown in Table 5.3.
➤ The child has had one or more acute systemic or severe delayed reactions.
➤ There is significant atopic eczema where multiple or cross-reactive food allergies are suspected by the parent or carer.
➤ There are possible multiple food allergies.
➤ There is persistent parental concern about food allergy (especially where symptoms are difficult or perplexing).
➤ Advice is needed on whether an allergic reaction is sufficiently severe to require an EpiPen.

ALLERGIC RHINITIS (AR)

Definition

➤ AR is defined as a history of nasal symptoms lasting at least 1 hour a day on most days and excluding upper respiratory tract infection (URTI) or other structural abnormalities.

➤ Seasonal AR is caused by sensitisation to wind-borne pollens of trees, grasses and weeds. In perennial rhinitis, house dust mites and pets are often the triggers.
➤ Asthma and allergic rhinitis commonly co-exist. Effective treatment of allergic rhinitis can improve asthma control.

Clinical manifestation
➤ Sneezing is frequently paroxysmal and associated with profuse clear rhinorrhoea, nasal obstruction and itching of the nose and pharynx.
➤ The nasal mucosa may be pale, blue or pink. Nasal turbinates are usually oedematous.
➤ Associated eye symptoms include redness, itching and watering eyes.
➤ Nasal polyps may occur in association with asthma and allergic rhinitis. Symptoms related to polyps include nasal blockage and nasal discharge.

Diagnosis
The diagnosis of a typical AR is made by the following:
➤ The history of atopy and the symptoms and signs (as above).
➤ Dark discolouration beneath the lower eyelids (allergic shiners), caused by venous plexus engorgement.
➤ Open-mouth breathing as a result of nasal blockage.
➤ Horizontal nasal crease (allergic salute sign) at the junction of the cartilaginous and bony bridge of the nose as a result of frequent upward rubbing of the nose.
➤ ENT examination is likely to show bilateral clear, mucoid secretions blocking the nasal passage with bluish, pale and swollen mucous membranes and positive nasal deviation and/or polyp.
➤ Response to AR treatment such as antihistamine.
➤ Allergen-specific IgE detected by SPT or RAST. Results of the tests must be interpreted in the context of the clinical history.

Conditions that should be differentiated from AR are shown in Table 5.5.

TABLE 5.5 Differential diagnosis of allergic rhinitis (AR)

Infectious rhinitis (IR)	• Seen mostly in infancy and the early years of life, while AR is more common later on in life
	• History is short in contrast to chronic history in AR
	• Occurs mostly in winter months and there is often a family history of an upper respiratory tract infection
	• Sneezing and eye symptoms may occur in both types of rhinitis, but these are more persistent in AR
Adenoid hypertrophy	• May co-exist with AR
	• Persistent nasal discharge
	• Mouth-breathing, which is worse at night when the child is lying supine
	• Mouth may be kept open during the daytime as well
	• Snoring during sleep; muffled voice; malodorous breath
	• Irritating cough at night

(continued)

Ciliary dyskinisia (immotile cilia syndrome)	• Chronic nasal discharge and congestion, sinusitis. About 1 in 5 patients have nasal polyps
	• Recurrent acute otitis media or chronic serous otitis media
	• Recurrent respiratory infections leading to bronchiectasis. Cough is productive. Often the initial diagnosis is asthma. This is an associated situs inversus in 50% of cases
Foreign body	• Young children may introduce a small object into the nose
	• Unilateral blockage of the nose followed by discharge which is often associated with pain, purulent nasal discharge and bleeding

Management[4]

➤ There is no evidence to support the use of nasal decongestants.

➤ Education on **allergen avoidance** should be provided, including:

➢ Avoid areas of high pollen count. The child's bedroom windows should be kept closed. Initiate measures to reduce house dust mites and moulds, such as washing bedding frequently, using dust-proof covers for pillows and mattress and removing bedroom carpets. Elimination of exposure to pet dander and feathers is essential for a child with perennial allergic rhinitis.

➢ Food avoidance, e.g. milk or eggs, should not be carried out unless the history or tests support these foods as a cause of allergy.

➢ Measures to minimise cat allergen levels may not be associated with clinical improvement as it takes several months for cat allergen to disappear from a home once the cat has been removed.

➢ Books or leaflets for prevention of allergy should be offered.

➤ **Antihistamine** treatment reduces nasal discharge (rhinorrhoea), sneezing and itching, while its effect on nasal blockage is minimal. First-generation sedating antihistamines (Table 5.6) should not be used (except for acute symptoms of allergy and when insomnia is present), as they reduce academic performance. Most of the sedating antihistamines are relatively short-acting but promethazine may be effective for up to 12 hours.

TABLE 5.6 Antihistamines licensed in the UK

Age of patient	Non-sedating	Sedating
> 6 months		Alimemazine (trimeprazine)
> 1 year	Desloratidine	Hydroxyzine hydrochloride
		Chlorphenamine
> 2 years	Cetirizine hydrochloride	Cyproheptadine hydrochloride
	Loratidine	Promethazine
> 6 years	Fexofenadine hydrochloride	
> 12 years	Acrivastine	
	Mizolastine	

➤ **Topical intranasal steroids** are the most effective therapy in children with AR:

➢ Intranasal steroids are superior to antihistamines. They are the first-line treatment for moderate to severe persistent symptoms, nasal polyposis and treatment failures with antihistamine. Table 5.7 shows some topical steroids used for allergic rhinitis.

➤ Starting treatment 2 weeks before the allergen season begins improves efficacy.
➤ Onset of action is 6–8 hours after the first dose; clinical improvement may not be apparent for 2 weeks.
➤ Side-effects are minimal (local irritation, rarely epistaxis) even when taken for many weeks.
➤ The initial dose should be high, 2 sprays in each nostril twice daily. Once the symptoms are controlled, the dose can be reduced to a spray once daily.
➤ Long-term growth studies in children using fluticasone, mometasone and budesonide provide reassuring safety data, unlike beclomethasone. Regular and high doses of beclomethasone may cause a slight reduction in height velocity. For this reason, regular checks of height and weight are indicated when this drug is used.

TABLE 5.7 Some topical steroids used for treatment of allergic rhinitis

Age of patient	Drug name	Availability
> 4 years	Fluticasone proprinate spray	Over the counter
> 5 years	Flunisolide	Prescription only
	Dexamethasone isonicotinate/	Prescription only
	Tramazoline hydrochloride	Prescription only
> 6 years	Mometasone furoate	Prescription only
	Triamcinolone acetonide	Prescription only
	Beclomethasone diproprionate	Over the counter
>12 years	Betamethasone	Prescription only

➤ **Systemic steroids** are rarely indicated, except:
  ➤ for severe nasal obstruction
  ➤ as short-term rescue medication for symptoms uncontrolled by conventional medications.
➤ **Oral steroids** should be used briefly and always in combination with topical nasal steroids. A suggested regimen for children is prednisolone 1 mg/kg for 5–7 days.
➤ **Hyposensitisation.** This method of treatment (performed only in specialised allergy clinics) is mostly used when patients are not responding to the above treatments. It involves frequent injections and the use of increasing quantities of allergenic extracts. Maintenance treatment may last as long as 3–4 years. Satisfactory results of hyposensitisation have been obtained in cases of combined rhinoconjunctivitis if the allergens are clear-cut, like pollens. The most serious side-effect of this method is systemic anaphylaxis. Oral immunotherapy (Grazax or grass pollen allergen extract) has recently been licensed for those aged 5–18 years. One sublingual tablet (75 000 units) is to be taken daily for 4 months before the hay fever season starts and should be continued for 3 years. The first dose should be taken under medical supervision. The drug is expensive and there is insufficient evidence for its routine use.

URTICARIA AND ANGIOEDEMA

Definition

➤ **Urticarias** are a heterogeneous group of disorders which have in common a pathway system involving the release of histamine and the degranulation of mast cells. Clinically, this reaction produces transient erythematous, pruritic and raised wheals, which are characteristic of urticaria.

➤ **Angioedema** indicates extension of the oedema to deeper tissues, and therefore the oedema is more extensive. Histologically, there is a dermal oedema, which in the case of angioedema extends into the subcutaneous tissues and mucous membranes. There is a variable perivascular cellular infiltrate dominated by degranulating mast cells, lymphocytes, neutrophils and eosinophils. In chronic idiopathic urticaria, activated T-helper cells predominate.

Clinical forms of acute urticaria

➤ **Acute idiopathic urticaria.** This may occur with angioedema. Lip and eyelid swelling is common. Although termed 'idiopathic', many cases are caused by acute viral infection. The rash does not usually last longer than 24 hours.

➤ **Acute allergic urticaria.** This is a rapidly occurring urticaria (within 5–30 minutes) mediated by IgE reaction. Common causes include bee and wasp stings, drugs such as penicillin, and foods such as fish.

➤ **Chronic urticaria.** This is defined as either persistent or episodic urticaria lasting longer than 6 weeks. In the vast majority of cases no underlying cause can be identified.

➤ **Cold urticaria.** This is IgE-mediated, and histamine is the most important mediator. Viral infection and drugs such as penicillin are the most common causes of this reaction. Following an application of an ice cube to the arm, there is a typical urticarial skin reaction 10 minutes later.

➤ **Solar urticaria.** This is characterised by diffuse erythema and weal formation in areas of the skin which are not normally exposed, such as the back. Causes of this type of urticaria are numerous and include systemic lupus erythematosus (SLE) and drugs. Some causes are mediated by mast-cell degranulation releasing histamine; in other reactions mast cells are not involved.

➤ **Cholinergic urticaria.** This reaction is triggered by sweating occurring in response to exercise, a hot shower, and even after eating spicy food. Acetylcholine is the important mediator in this type of urticaria. Diagnosis is made by reproducing the urticaria by exercise or raising the body temperature.

➤ **Vasculitic urticaria.** In addition to urticaria, patients have often arthralgia, glomerulonephritis, and gastrointestinal and CNS vasculitis. In contrast to other forms of urticaria, this type of urticaria is often prolonged and lasts more than 24 hours.

➤ **Urticaria pigmentosa.** This disease mostly affects infants and is characterised by an accumulation of mast cells in different sites of the body. Brownish patches occur typically on the chest, and may blister on rubbing. The lesions are often confused with insect bites. However, the lesions in urticaria pigmentosa persist and increase in number for several months.

Hereditary angioedema

Hereditary angioedema is characterised by:

➤ Painless, non-erythematous, non-pruritic swelling which affects predominately the extremities and the face.

➤ The oedema can also affect the intestine, causing episodic severe abdominal pain with vomiting.

➤ Swelling in the pharynx and larynx leads to choking and asphyxiation.

➤ Bronchospasm causing wheezing, coughing and dyspnoea.

The condition is usually triggered by trauma and emotion, and lasts 2–3 days. It is inherited as an autosomal dominant disease.

Treatment

➤ Most cases of urticaria are benign and self-limiting. In about 90% of cases there is no apparent cause.

➤ Avoid any cause if identified (e.g. foods, drugs, cold or solar urticaria).

➤ For mild cases with symptoms such as itching, antihistamine is effective, using preferably the non-sedating options.

➤ For prolonged and more persistent urticaria, a short course of oral steroids (e.g. prednisolone 1–2 mg/kg) is helpful in controlling the symptoms and shortening the course.

➤ For hereditary angioedema, complement C1 esterase inhibitor (C1-INH) concentrate is given. Fresh frozen plasma can abort angioedema by replacing plasma C1-INH.

INSECT STING ALLERGY

Stinging insects causing an allergic reaction include honeybee, wasp, yellow jacket, hornet, mayfly, caddis fly, moths and fire ant. Anaphylactic reaction may be immediate (IgE-mediated) or delayed (T-lymphocytic-mediated). Allergy to bees is most common among beekeepers. Risk factors to predict future reaction following an initial sting are summarised in Box 5.4.

BOX 5.4 Risk factors which predict future allergic reactions to bee sting

● History of atopy
● History of previous reactions
● Positive venom-specific IgE
● Beekeepers or their family members
● Adult age
● History of prior multiple stings
● Short time of reaction onset following the bee sting

Symptoms and signs

➤ **Cutaneous reaction:** the diameter of the reaction is usually < 4–5 cm and lasts < 24 hours. Those individuals who are already sensitised to an insect react with a more severe local reaction and are at risk of anaphylaxis. Local reaction in sensitised individuals includes large erythema and swelling spreading from the site of the sting to involve the subcutaneous tissue. The reaction is due to vasoactive (histamine, acet-ylcholine, kinins) and irritant substances caused by the bite. It is not an IgE-mediated reaction. **Arthus reaction** is a late reaction, 8–12 hours after a sting, and may persist for 2–3 days. It may cause tissue damage, blistering and bruising.

➤ **Inhalant allergy** includes conjunctivitis, respiratory distress resembling asthma, and rhinitis. This is commonly an IgE-mediated reaction.

➤ **Systemic reaction** usually starts within a few minutes of a sting. It may manifest as generalised pruritis, urticaria, angioedema, dyspnoea (due to laryngeal swelling), bronchospasm, hypotension and shock. A whole limb may be involved, with marked swelling and blister formation. If the insect bite was on the lip, tongue or inside the mouth, severe and life-threatening laryngeal oedema may ensue. On average, 4 peo-ple die in the UK every year from anaphylactic reactions to wasp and bee stings.

Diagnosis

Diagnosis is primarily based on:

➤ The **history** of the insect sting and examination of the skin reaction. Severe local reaction has to be distinguished from systemic reaction.

➤ Positive venom skin prick test or the detection of venom-specific IgE antibodies con-firm the diagnosis and may identify the insect responsible for the sting.

➤ The **skin prick test** (SPT) should be performed for the venom of wasp, honey-bee and hornet. The test should be performed according to the manufacturer's recommendations.

➤ **Venom RAST testing** is available, but in general is not indicated with a clear his-tory of sting allergy.

Management

➤ Plants and areas of countryside which attract stinging insects should be avoided by those at high risk of anaphylaxis. Children should wear appropriate clothing and footwear when visiting areas known to have these insects.

➤ Patients with local reaction are treated with cold compresses, oral antihistamine and possible analgesics if there is moderate–severe pain.

➤ Antihistamine should be given for several days.

BOX 5.5 Summary of insect sting reactions

- The severity of the sting reaction depends on the patient's sensitivity, the amount of venom injected and the site of the sting
- In general, children are at lower risk of anaphylaxis than adults
- Families of children with a history of insect allergy should keep antihistamine medicine at home for use in case of an allergic reaction. Adrenaline injection (such as EpiPen injection) should be considered for those with a history of severe reaction
- Although severity of reaction does not correlate well with size of skin reaction or level of IgE, a negative skin reaction and undetected IgE level suggest that allergic reaction is very unlikely
- Immunotherapy can be an effective form of therapy in individuals at risk of insect-sting anaphylaxis

➤ In the case of anaphylaxis: see section below on severe allergic reactions and anaphylaxis.

➤ Children with inhalation allergy should be treated with bronchodilators, steroids and oxygen (*see* later section of Anaphylaxis). Venom immunotherapy is not used for patients with a history of local cutaneous manifestations only, nor for those with venom-negative skin reaction and RAST results, as it is difficult to know which venom should be used.

➤ A summary of sting allergy is provided in Box 5.5.

DRUG ALLERGY (DA)

Definition

➤ Drug allergy is an immunological or non-immunological response to a drug or its metabolites, characterised by production of an adverse reaction with the adminis- tration of a drug and the disappearance of reaction after discontinuation of the drug, with no other cause for the features evident after a careful physical examination and laboratory investigation.

➤ Immunological reactions account for about 10% of drug reactions; the remaining 90% are non-immunological reactions.

➤ Penicillin, muscle relaxants, insulin and other hormones usually act via IgE-mediated mechanisms, whereas opiates, non-steroidal anti-inflammatory drugs (NSAIDs) and radio-contrast media produce angioedema or anaphylaxis by non-IgE-mediated mechanisms.

Diagnosis

History and physical examination

➤ A careful drug history is an essential first step towards an accurate diagnosis and is often sufficient to identify the offending agent.

➤ Drug history should include details of the drug formulation, dose, route and timing of administration. Medical notes, nursing charts, photographs and eye witnesses should be sought and information documented. Over-the-counter (OTC) prepara- tions should be specifically sought.

The following principles need to be considered to help establish the diagnosis:

➤ DA is a diagnosis of exclusion.

➤ Definitive tests to confirm the diagnosis are usually absent, and a re-challenge is generally discouraged.

➤ There is a lack of characteristic pattern after drug re-exposure.

➤ Symptoms may occur immediately following initiation of therapy or may be delayed for 5–7 days; some even as late as 2–6 weeks after exposure.[5]

➤ Diagnosis is suggested by complete or partial disappearance of symptoms after dis- continuation of the offending drug.

➤ Risk factors for developing drug allergic reactions are listed in Box 5.6.

➤ Patients usually do not appear toxic.

➤ Clinical manifestations (Table 5.8) are often cutaneous, such as urticaria or maculo- papular rash. Feverish patients often have a pulse rate that is disproportionately low in relation to the degree of fever (relative bradycardia).

> **BOX 5.6** Risk factors for developing drug allergy
>
> ● Adults > children
> ● Chemical potency of the drug, e.g. antibiotics (particularly beta-lactam), radio-contrast media, NSAIDs
> ● The route of drug administration (topical > IV or oral route)
> ● High dose and frequent exposure to the drug
> ● Concomitant diseases such as infection with HIV and herpesvirus
> ● Family history of drug allergy (genetic factors)
> ● Atopic (self or family history)

TABLE 5.8 Clinical manifestations of a reaction to drug allergy

Clinical manifestation	Possible drugs
Anaphylaxis	Antibiotics, radio-contrast media
Angioedema, urticaria	Penicillin, muscle relaxants, insulin
Toxic epidermal necrolysis	Antimicrobials, sulfonamide
Stevens–Johnson syndrome	Antimicrobials, anticonvulsants (lamotrigine, phenytoin), NSAIDs (especially piroxicam)
Serum sickness	Antibiotics, thiazides, vaccines, phenytoin
SLE-like	Procainamide, isoniazid, chlorpromazine
Photo-dermatitis	Griseofulvin, tetracycline, furosemide
Contact dermatitis	Topical antibiotics, topical antihistamines
Scleroderma-like	Bleomycin

SLE = systemic lupus erythematosus.

Tests

As allergy tests are not available for the majority of drugs, considerable experience is required for the investigation of drug allergy.

➤ High levels of mediators in blood (e.g. tryptase, histamine and leukotrienes) support the diagnosis of anaphylactic reaction.

➤ **RAST test** is only available for a limited number of drugs. The test is useful when positive but difficult to interpret if negative.

➤ **Skin prick test** (SPT) provides evidence for immediate IgE-mediated sensitisation. If the test is negative an intradermal test is carried out, first at a low concentration. If there is no reaction, higher concentrations are used. Of the many tests evaluated for drug allergy, only intradermal skin testing for IgE antibody has been shown to have strong predictive value in patients with a history of penicillin allergy. The intradermal test is more likely to trigger a systemic allergic reaction, and therefore should only be carried out in a hospital setting.

➤ **Patch test** is carried out by placing potential allergens on the patient's back for about 48 hours. It provides evidence for delayed T-cell-mediated reaction and is most useful for contact dermatitis.

➤ **Challenge test.** When SPT or RAST cannot be performed and the diagnosis remains in doubt, a challenge test may be performed by an experienced physician under close supervision and in a hospital setting. In general, however, challenge testing is discouraged, particularly for those drugs which can be replaced by similar drugs, e.g. antibiotics.

Management of acute drug reactions

➤ A safe and alternative drug is given if there is a history of allergy to a particular drug. If there is no alternative drug, the allergy should be confirmed by skin intradermal or prick test before giving the drug.

➤ In an acute drug reaction, the offending drug should be discontinued immediately. If the patients have received multiple medications, these should be all discontinued if they are not essential.

Penicillin allergy

➤ Penicillin is the most common drug causing allergy. Allergy is more common in adults than in children, with a reported incidence in adults as high as 10%.

➤ History of penicillin allergy is a risk factor for allergic reactions, including anaphylaxis. However, most cases of severe allergic reaction or anaphylaxis have no family history of penicillin allergy.

➤ Many patients are erroneously labelled as 'penicillin allergic' after the occurrence of a non-specific rash. It is worth the time and trouble to determine whether the patient's history suggests a true penicillin allergy. The skin rash is often a part of the illness for which the penicillin was administered.

➤ The SPT has a high sensitivity and specificity and may be used to confirm the diagnosis.

➤ Cross-reactivity may occur with other beta-lactam antibiotics such as cephalosporins. About 10% of patients with penicillin allergy will also be allergic to cephalosporins. If a patient has experienced a reaction to penicillin or a cephalosporin that was not IgE-mediated and was not serious, cephalosporin administration is probably safe.

SEVERE ALLERGIC REACTIONS AND ANAPHYLAXIS

➤ Both IgE-mediated and non-IgE-mediated reaction may occur; the former is the most common type of reaction.

➤ Foods, such as peanuts, are the most common cause of anaphylaxis in children. In around a third of cases, the cause of anaphylaxis remains unknown.

➤ The risk of non-fatal incidence of anaphylaxis from insect stings is about 1% in the USA while the risk of non-fatal anaphylaxis from penicillin there ranges from 0.7–10%. In the USA some 100–500 deaths are estimated to occur per year. There are approximately 20 deaths caused by anaphylaxis each year in the UK, and the incidence in the UK is increasing.

➤ Anaphylaxis usually begins within 30 minutes of exposure to some allergens such as IV antibiotics. Food allergy often begins 2 hours after food ingestion. The more rapid the reaction after the allergen exposure, the more serious is the reaction.

➤ The overall prognosis of anaphylaxis is good, with a case fatality ratio of < 1%.

Clinical presentation

➤ Cutaneous warmth or tingling, urticaria, pruritis, periorbital oedema.

➤ Upper airways: symptoms of rhinitis (sneezing, runny nose), conjunctivitis, metallic taste, laryngeal oedema.
➤ CNS: sensation of anxiety or frightening experience, dizziness, syncope.
➤ Gastro-intestinal: nausea, vomiting, abdominal cramps, diarrhoea.
➤ Respiratory symptoms such as shortness of breath, chest tightness, hoarseness, stridor, choking or fullness in the throat. Respiratory arrest is rare, but is a dramatic and potentially lethal consequence of systemic anaphylaxis.
➤ Cardiovascular: tachycardia, arrhythmia.
➤ Life-threatening shock with vascular collapse, hypotension, bronchospasm.

Diagnosis

Factors which increase the risk of anaphylaxis are shown in Box 5.7. There are no specific laboratory tests to establish the diagnosis of anaphylaxis, and so the diagnosis is made clinically and is based on the history, symptoms and signs at presentation. Anaphylaxis is diagnosed when the following criteria are present:
➤ Sudden onset and rapid progression of symptoms
➤ Life-threatening airway and/or breathing and/or circulation symptoms
➤ Skin and/or mucosal changes (e.g. urticaria, angioedema)
➤ Exposure to a known or at least a suspected antigen.

These clinical features of anaphylaxis may need to be **differentiated** from:
➤ Shock, which is often caused by septicaemia with high fever and possible rash
➤ Vasovagal syncope, which may resemble anaphylaxis because of the sudden appearance of pallor, sweating and collapse with possible impairment of consciousness. However, in syncope improvement is rapid; there is usually bradycardia, in contrast to the tachycardia usually present in anaphylaxis. In addition, in syncope there are no associated laryngeal spasms or respiratory symptoms
➤ Angioedema. In general, clinical symptoms in angioedema progress slowly in contrast to the rapid symptomatology in anaphylaxis. Angioedema lacks the diffuse warmth, flushing and vascular collapse seen in patients with anaphylaxis.

BOX 5.7 Factors which increase the risk of anaphylaxis

● Previous anaphylaxis
● Asthma with peanut allergy
● Presence of atopy (personal or family history)
● Drugs (beta-blockers, ACE inhibitors, steroids)
● No adherence to dietary exclusion
● Strenuous exercise after a meal

Emergency treatment

Effective steps include those shown in the algorithm in Fig 5.2:
➤ Patients should be treated using the Airway, Breathing, Circulation, Disability, Exposure (ABCDE) approach.
➤ Oxygenation (high-flow) with monitoring of O_2 saturation.

➤ Supporting of the circulation and tissue perfusion: normal saline 20 mL/kg to be infused within 20–30 minutes.
➤ Early treatment with IM adrenaline, e.g. EpiPen Junior delivering a single dose of 0.15 mg and EpiPen 0.3 mg adrenaline 1 : 1000 respectively (Table 5.9).
➤ Individuals who are at high risk of anaphylactic reaction should carry an adrenaline auto-injector and receive training and support in its use. Two adrenaline pens (such as EpiPen or Anapen Junior) are required if the child attends a nursery or school.
➤ Other medications (if available) include: IV hydrocortisone, IV antihistamine (chlorphenamine).
➤ All those who are suspected of having had an anaphylactic reaction should be referred to an allergy specialist.

TABLE 5.9 Doses for adrenaline, chlorphenamine and hydrocortisone IM injections in anaphylactic shock

Age (years)	Adrenaline	Chlorphenamine	Hydrocortisone
< 6	0.15 mg (0.15 mL)	2.5 mg	50 mg
6–12	0.3 mg (0.3 mL)	5 mg	100 mg
> 12	0.5 mg (0.5 mL)	10 mg	200 mg

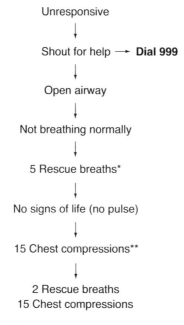

Unresponsive
↓
Shout for help → **Dial 999**
↓
Open airway
↓
Not breathing normally
↓
5 Rescue breaths*
↓
No signs of life (no pulse)
↓
15 Chest compressions**
↓
2 Rescue breaths
15 Chest compressions

*Although ventilation remains a very important component of **CPR**, rescuers who are unable or unwilling to provide this should be encouraged to perform at least compression-only **CPR**. The compression/ventilation ratio at birth remains 3:1

**Use two fingers for an infant < 1 year; use one or two hands for a child > 1 year

FIGURE 5.2 Paediatric Basic Life Support algorithm (Resuscitation Council, 2010)[6]

FURTHER INFORMATION

➤ Allergy UK
  Helpline: 01322 619 898
  www.allergyuk.org
➤ Action Against Allergy
  Helpline: 020 8892 2711
  www.actionagainstallergy.co.uk
➤ Anaphylaxis Campaign
  Helpline 01252 542029
  www.anaphylaxis.org.uk

REFERENCES

1. Sackeyfio A, Senthinathan A, Kandaswamy P, et al. Guidelines: Diagnosis and assessment of food allergy in children and young people: summary of NICE guidance. BMJ 2011; 342. doi: 10.1136.
2. Vandenplas Y, Brueton M, Dupont C, et al. Guidelines for the diagnosis and management of cow's milk protein allergy in infants. Arch Dis Child 2007; 92: 902–908.
3. Clark AT, Skypala T, Leech SC, et al. BSACI guidelines for the management of egg allergy. Clin Exp Allergy 2010; 40: 1116–1129.
4. Scadding GK, Durham SR, Mirakian R, et al. BSACI guidelines for the management of allergic and non-allergic rhinitis. Clin Exp Allergy 2008; 38: 19–42.
5. Mirakian R, Ewan PW, Durham SR, et al. BSACI guidelines for the management of drug allergy. Clin Exp Allergy 2009; 39: 43–61.
6. www.resus.org.uk/pages/pbls.pdf

CHAPTER 6

Haematology and immunology

ANAEMIA

Core messages

➤ Skin colour is mainly determined by its melanin content (itself determined by genetic and racial background). Pallor is caused by a variety of conditions including normal complexion, lack of exposure to sunlight, anaemia, emotional stress or chronic disease (Box 6.1).

BOX 6.1 Classification of anaemia

Microcytic (mean corpuscular volume (MCV) < 70 fL)
- Iron-deficiency anaemia
- Thalassaemia
- Lead poisoning
- Chronic disease (infection, inflammation, tumour)
- Sideroblastic anaemia

Normocytic (MCV 70–90 fL)
- Physiological anaemia
- Haemolytic anaemia (e.g. spherocytosis, G6PD deficiency)
- Haemoglobinopathy (e.g. sickle-cell anaemia)
- Inflammatory bowel disease (e.g. Crohn's disease)
- Hypoplastic/aplastic anaemia
  - ❯ congenital
  - ❯ acquired
- Blood loss
- Haemolytic uraemic syndrome
- Storage disease

Macrocytic (MCV > 90 fL)
- Megaloblastic anaemia (folic acid and Vitamin B_{12} deficiency)
- Malabsorption, anticonvulsant therapy

➤ In neonates, high haemoglobin (Hb) is due to active erythropoiesis in response to low arterial oxygen saturation (AOS) during fetal life. This erythropoiesis ceases abruptly with the rise of AOS at birth. Low erythropoiesis continues for the first 6–10 weeks of a child's life, causing a decline of Hb to 90–110 g/L in full-term and 70–90 g/L in pre-term infants. This decline is termed physiological anaemia that is exaggerated by prematurity.

➤ Iron-deficiency anaemia is common in pre-school children and is defined as an Hb level of less than 110 g/L, a serum iron level of < 14 μmol/L or serum ferritin < 10 mcg/L.

➤ A child with anaemia should be investigated to determine the cause, particularly if the Hb < 80 g/L. Treatment should be initiated without delay (Box 6.2).

This section will only discuss anaemia relevant to primary-care practice.

Recommended investigations

➤ Full blood count (FBC): Hb < 110 g/L indicates anaemia, low MCV (< 70 fL) and mean corpuscular haemoglobin (MCH) (< 26 pg) suggest microcytic, hypochromic anaemia. Normal levels of white blood cells (WBCs) and platelets exclude pathologies such as aplastic anaemia. A blood film may show many spherocytes suggestive of spherocytosis.

➤ Coombs' test for suspected autoimmune haemolysis.

➤ Serum ferritin: low in iron-deficiency anaemia (IDA), normal or high in haemolytic anaemia.

➤ Liver function tests (LFTs): hyperbilirubinaemia suggests acute or chronic haemolysis.

➤ Reticulocyte count (normal reticulocyte beyond 1 week of age is about 1%): high in haemolytic anaemia, and responsive to iron treatment in IDA.

➤ Vitamin B_{12} and folate (MCV > 90 fL) to exclude the most common causes of megaloblastic anaemia.

➤ Spherocytosis can be confirmed by osmotic fragility test.

➤ Hb electrophoresis: HbS in sickle-cell anaemia (SCA); high level of HbF to confirm thalassaemia.

➤ Enzyme estimation in G6PD deficiency.

DIAGNOSTIC TIPS

- All anaemia (even mild) should be investigated as it may indicate a serious underlying disorder.
- In districts or localities with a high rate of socio-economic deprivation, iron-deficiency anaemia is very common. An Hb check should be considered in any child with prolonged feeding or dietary problems.
- Congenital hypoplastic anaemia (Diamond–Blackfan syndrome) manifests at age 2–6 months. It is usually inherited, as dominant or recessive. About 75% of cases respond to corticosteroid therapy.
- By far the most common cause of anaemia is nutritional iron deficiency, which can be easily diagnosed by low Hb, MCV, MCH, and ferritin levels.
- Children with Crohn's disease may present with anaemia alone or with abdominal pain and weight loss as the main clinical presentation.
- Blood loss should be considered as a possible cause of IDA caused by a polyp, peptic ulcer, Meckel's diverticulum, cow's milk protein intolerance and, in some areas, hookworm infestation.
- Uncommon but important complications of haemolytic anaemia include calcium-containing gallstone and susceptibility to aplastic or hypoplastic crisis. This usually occurs in response to parvovirus B19 infection and is accompanied by rapid reduction in Hb.
- It can be difficult to distinguish thalassaemia from IDA, and IDA may co-exist

with thalassaemia. Both have low MCV and MCH. Ferritin is normal or high in thalassaemia.
- $HbA_2 > 3.4\%$ is diagnostic of thalassaemia trait.

BOX 6.2 Guidelines on treatment of anaemia

- Anaemia of prematurity is common, usually normocytic and normochromic and does not respond to iron therapy. Diet should contain iron and folic acid
- Iron supplement should be given to all pre-term infants to prevent IDA until the first year of life. If infants are feeding and growing well, an Hb of 7 g/dL is usually well tolerated
- IDA may have an impact on a child's development. School-age children with IDA may have impaired concentration and activity which affect learning
- Wishes of the parents to add tonics, vitamins or trace metals to iron therapy should be resisted. These have no scientific value
- Treatment with oral iron should be given to all children with Hb < 110 g/L for 4–6 weeks. Suitable preparations include:
  - ❯ Ferrous sulphate drops (25 mg in 1 mL): 0.3–0.6 mL 2–3 times daily
  - ❯ Ferrous sulphate tablets (200 mg): 1 tablet 2–3 times daily
- Iron preparations are an important cause of accidental overdose. Ensure that drugs are kept out of the reach of children. Parents should also be told about common side-effects of iron therapy, including gastrointestinal irritation, constipation. Side-effects decrease if the preparation is taken after meals
- Steps to prevent IDA include:
  - ❯ Continued use of iron-fortified infant formula in the first year of life and not using 'doorstep' cow's milk
  - ❯ Solid food to be introduced by 6 months of age
  - ❯ Tea should not be offered to children
  - ❯ Dietary information includes reduction of milk consumption in older children to improve iron absorption. An iron-rich diet (green vegetables, red meat) should be encouraged
- In macrocytic anaemia, folic acid is given orally in a dose of 1–5 mg/day for 4 months. Folic acid is abundant in many foods, including green vegetables and fruits. Vitamin B_{12} may be given IM (2.5 mg/mL):
  - ❯ Initially: 0.25–1 mg 3 times daily for 2 weeks
  - ❯ Then 0.25 mg once weekly until blood count becomes normal
  - ❯ Then 1 mg every 2–3 months as prophylaxis
  - ❯ Oral vitamin B_{12} 5–10 mg 1 or 2 times/week is less effective and some children do not respond to the oral route
- Children with chronic haemolytic anaemia (e.g. spherocytosis) should receive folic acid 1 mg/day. Full immunisation and oral penicillin should be administered to all children with sickle-cell anaemia
- Referral to a secondary service should be considered in cases of
  - ❯ Unexplained anaemia or a type of haemolytic anaemia
  - ❯ IDA with an Hb < 70 g/L
  - ❯ IDA unresponsive to iron treatment
  - ❯ Secondary anaemia due, e.g., to blood loss

HEREDITARY HAEMOLYTIC ANAEMIA

Glucose 6-phosphate dehydrogenase (G6PD) deficiency

➤ G6PD deficiency is highly prevalent in most parts of Africa, Asia and Southern Europe. It is more common in males than in females. Individuals with G6PD deficiency are susceptible to developing acute haemolytic anaemia when they:
  ➤ Eat fava beans (broad beans), particularly fresh fava (this is termed favism)
  ➤ Take certain drugs (Box 6.3). These should not be taken before testing for G6PD status.

BOX 6.3 Drugs capable of causing haemolysis in patients with G6PD deficiency

Drugs with definite risk of haemolysis in most patients
- Dapsone
- Nitrofurantoin
- Primaquine
- Quinolones (including ciprofloxacin)
- Methylene blue
- Sulfonamides (including co-trimoxazole)

Drugs with possible risk of haemolysis in some patients
- Aspirin
- Chloroquine
- Quinine

SICKLE-CELL DISEASE (SCD)

Core messages

➤ The haemoglobinopathies are a heterogeneous group of more than 1000 genetic disorders divided into two main disease groups:
  ➤ Haemoglobin-variants (e.g. SCD) arising from an alteration in the globin protein structure.
  ➤ Thalassaemias arising from inadequate production of structurally normal globin protein.
➤ SCD is now the most common serious genetic condition in England, affecting more than 1 in 2000 live births.[1] About 350 babies with SCD are born each year in England, and a further 9500 babies are carriers of the disease.
➤ Universal newborn screening (at 5–8 days of life) for SCD and thalassaemia has been established in England since 2006 as part of the newborn dried blood spot screening programme (www.newbornbloodspot.screening.nhs.uk).
➤ GPs should check for the results of the screening test at the 6-week check. The child may be referred for DNA analysis if the diagnosis is unclear.
➤ The basic pathophysiological defect is substitution of valine for glutamic acid at position 6 of the beta-chain, leading to the production of a defective form of haemoglobin known as HbS. HbS is less soluble than the normal HbA, causing red blood cells (RBCs) to sickle at low oxygen levels. The RBCs are too fragile to withstand the mechanical trauma of circulation, leading to haemolysis. The life-span of RBCs in sickle-cell anaemia is 10–20 days (normal RBC life-span is 120 days).
➤ In areas of high prevalence there may be SCD and thalassaemia community centres that provide information, support and advice to families along with genetic counselling and specialist nursing (for a list of centres, *see* www.sct.screening.nhs.uk).
➤ Life expectancy has improved considerably over the last decades, and mortality is now about 1–2% in some areas.

Presentation

See Table 6.1.

➤ Haemolytic anaemia is the first sign of the disease, occurring between 2 and 4 months of age and coinciding with the replacement of the majority of HbF by HbS.

➤ Dactylitis is a common presenting symptom in infants between 9 and 18 months old.

➤ Painful vaso-occlusive episodes, occurring after the age of 2 years, are the most common presentation and are caused by sickle-shaped RBCs blocking the circulation. Avascular necrosis of the femoral and humeral head may occur.

➤ There is susceptibility to overwhelming bacterial infections, e.g. pneumococcal septicaemia (causing sudden death), and *Salmonella* osteomyelitis, which presents insidiously with multiple and symmetrical bone involvement. This enhanced susceptibility results from deficient opsonisation and complement activities and defective splenic phagocytic function (functional asplenia), beginning as early as 3 months of age. Without prompt administration of antibiotics these infections are associated with high mortality.

➤ Strokes affect 5–10% of the paediatric population; the highest incidence is between 2 and 5 years of age. In addition, up to 20% of patients show MRI changes of silent stroke by the age of 20 years. Infarction of the internal carotid/cerebral artery is the commonest site.

➤ Acute splenic sequestration (ASS), often following an acute febrile infection, results from the large amount of blood that is pooled in the spleen.

➤ Acute chest syndrome (ACS) is caused by a combination of pulmonary parenchyma, fat emboli and infection. It is the most common reason for hospitalisation. Infection is predominately due to *Streptococcus pneumoniae*, *Mycoplasma pneumoniae* or *Chlamydia pneumoniae*. Mortality can be as high as 25%.

➤ Recurrent urinary tract infections (UTIs) and vaso-occlusive episodes causing medullary ischaemia, with a loss of renal concentrating ability and acidification that may lead to chronic polyuria manifesting as enuresis and renal failure.

➤ Human parvovirus B19 (HPV B19). In immunocompetent individuals, this virus is the cause of erythema infectiosum, acute symmetric polyarthritis or hydrops fetalis. In patients with chronic haemolytic anaemia, the virus causes aplastic crises that manifests clinically as a further drop in Hb levels.

➤ Priapism, a prolonged and painful penile erection, is often precipitated by fever and/or dehydration. A prolonged attack lasting > 3 hours should be treated as a medical emergency. Repeated episodes cause ischaemia and possible impotence. The condition becomes more common in adolescence.

➤ Liver diseases include jaundice, gallstones occurring in about 50% in children older than 10 years, and liver cirrhosis.

➤ Renal diseases which manifest as proteinuria, haematuria, nocturnal enuresis.

➤ Other, rare, features include leg ulcers, deep venous thrombosis.

➤ Bacterial infections in children with SCA occur in 38% of febrile children. If the cause of the fever is unclear (vaso-occlusive or infection), it is imperative to commence prompt antibiotic therapy. Patients should be informed of the high risk of serious infections and be urged to visit medical facilities promptly for any illnesses associated with fever greater than 38.5°C.

TABLE 6.1 Summary of presentations of SCA

Presentation	Clinical findings
Anaemia	Pallor and lethargy, usual Hb 60–90 g/L. Peripheral target cells, sickle cells, poikilocytes
Dactylitis	Painful, symmetrical swelling of the hands and feet
Infection	Unwell with fever, particularly > 38.5°C, painful bones, meningeal signs
Acute splenic sequestration	Enlargement of spleen, circulatory collapse
Acute chest syndrome	Fever, signs of pneumonia: tachypnoea, grunting
Stroke	Hemiplegia, impaired consciousness
Parvovirus B19 infection	Severe pallor, fever
Priapism	Painful penile erection
Heart/lung	Dyspnoea, cardiac failure, haemic murmur
Hepatic	Cholelithiasis, cholecystitis, pancreatitis
Renal	Nocturnal enuresis, haematuria, proteinuria, urinary tract infection, chronic renal failure

Laboratory findings

➤ SCA is characterised by normocytic, hypochromic anaemia (usual Hb 60–90 g/L, RBC 2–3 million per L), leukocytosis, thrombocytosis, hyperbilirubinaemia, and hyperplastic bone marrow.
➤ The marrow may become aplastic during a sickling crisis or severe infection.
➤ Hb electrophoresis shows mainly HbS with a variable amount of HbF. Blood tests can fail to detect HbS under the following circumstances:
  ➢ Blood transfusion within 3–4 months before testing
  ➢ In children < 3 months of age
  ➢ In cases of polycythaemia.

Management

Management includes:
➤ Education of parents, which includes the need to bring the child to hospital at the onset of acute illness such as fever, sudden pallor.
➤ Ensuring adequate immunisation (Table 6.2).
➤ Ensuring that affected babies have been referred to the local paediatric unit. For multidisciplinary management, *see* Table 6.3.
➤ Physical examination should include checking for anaemia, jaundice, enlarged spleen and cardiac murmur.
➤ Assessment of growth using centile chart.
➤ Children with SCA should be offered annual transcranial Doppler scans from the age of 2 years.
➤ Ensuring lifelong penicillin prophylaxis of phenoxymethylpenicillin (penicillin V)
  ➢ 62.5 mg orally BD in children < 1 year old
  ➢ 125 mg orally BD in children 1–5 years old
  ➢ 250 mg orally BD in children > 5 years old.
➤ Medication: analgesics (paracetamol and ibuprofen) are used to control mild pain in a child who is otherwise well and afebrile or with mild fever. Children with

fever and a temperature > 38.5°C who appear to be in severe pain or seriously ill should be promptly transferred to hospital for IV antibiotics (such as ceftriaxone). Hydroxyurea (hydroxycarbamide) 10–20 mg/kg once daily, taken orally, reduces the frequency of painful crises by 50%. Deferasirox is an effective oral iron chelator to treat transfusional iron overload.

➤ Transfusion is urgently required for acute problems such as stroke, ACS, ASS and parvovirus infection. Regular blood transfusion for mild anaemia is generally discouraged to avoid iron overload.

TABLE 6.2 Recommended immunisation in SCA

Age	Immunisation
2 months	DTaP/Hib/IPV, PCV 13
3 months	DTaP/Hib/IPV, Men C
4 months	DTaP/Hib/IPV, PCV 13, Men C
12 months	Hib/Men C, hepatitis B*
13 months	MMR, PCV 13, hepatitis B*
18 months	Hepatitis B*
12–13 years (girls)	HPV (3 injections)
13–18 years	Tetanus booster
2, 7, 12 and 17 years	Pneumovax* (pneumococcal vaccine)
Annual influenza immunisation from 6 months of age*	

DTaP = diphtheria, tetanus, acellular pertussis; Hib = *Haemophilus influenzae* type B; HPV = human papillomavirus vaccine; IPV = inactivated polio vaccine; Men C = meningitis C; MMR = measles, mumps, rubella; PCV 13 = a conjugate vaccine which contains 13 serotypes of pneumococci.

* These are in addition to the normal schedule of vaccinations.

TABLE 6.3 Multidisciplinary management of SCD (*see* NHS guidelines)[1]

Primary care trust	Commissioning of acute and community medical services, including CAMHS
GPs	Register details from newborn screening programme
	Prescribe penicillin as appropriate
	Provide primary care for common childhood illnesses
	Be aware of signs and symptoms that need emergency hospital assessment
	Prescribe analgesics in conjunction with paediatricians
Practice nurse	Administer conjugate pneumococcal vaccine at 2, 4 and 13 months (as per routine immunisation) + annual flu vaccination
Health visitor	Routine health promotion advice and screening
	Targeted visit
	Link with specialist nurse counsellor
School nurse	Routine health promotion advice and screening
	Liaison with school staff re extra needs of children and awareness of symptoms and signs
	Link with specialist nurse counsellor

(*continued*)

Community paediatrician	Liaison with local authority (social services and education)
	Assessment of children with developmental delay
	Coordination with community services in cases of chronic disability, e.g. strokes
	Maintenance of disability register
Specialist nurse/Nurse practitioner	Specialist support to families
	Training and support of community nurses
	Liaison with primary care and hospital services
	Support of care in the home
Child and Adolescent Mental Health Service (CAMHS)	Provision of clinical psychology assessment and management, neurophysiology services
Education	Regular awareness training for school staff
	Early recognition of learning difficulties and chronic health problems
	Assessment by educational psychologist
Social services	Recognition of 'child in need'
	Registration on Children's Disability Register
	Respite care where appropriate

Sickle-cell trait

➤ This is a heterozygous HbS disorder (HbS is between 20 and 45%) which usually follows a benign clinical course. Under conditions of severe hypoxia (e.g. high altitude or general anaesthesia), symptoms of vaso-occlusive crisis may occur such as bone pain or splenic infarction.

 RED FLAG

- Any child with SCA who presents with cognitive impairment or learning difficulties should have an MRI scan to exclude silent stroke. This occurs in about 20% of patients by the age of 20 years.

Homozygous beta-thalassaemia (thalassaemia major)

Core messages

➤ Homozygous beta-thalassaemia is the most severe form of the thalassaemia syndrome. It is a chronic haemolytic anaemia characterised by a genetically defective production of the beta chain of Hb, which leads to hypochromic, microcytic anaemia, with HbF as the predominant haemoglobin present.

➤ Clinical features are the consequence of:
  ➢ Severe anaemia causing pallor, jaundice, splenomegaly and decreased growth. Cardiac failure may rapidly occur unless therapy ensues.
  ➢ Expanded bone marrow, causing thickening of the cranial bones and maxillary hyperplasia.

➤ The clinical course is dominated by regular transfusions (usually from between 6 months and 2 years) and subsequent absorptive iron overload, causing cardiomyopathy, liver diseases (e.g. cirrhosis, portal hypertension) and endocrinopathies (e.g. diabetes, hypothyroidism, hypoparathyroidism, hypogonadism, and growth hormone deficiency).

➤ Transfusions on a regular basis to maintain Hb above 100 g/L is the main therapy. Haemosiderosis requires elimination with iron-chelating drugs.

➤ Bone-marrow transplantation is curative.

Laboratory findings include hypochromic microcytic anaemia, with a large number of nucleated erythroblasts, target cells and basophilia. Levels of HbF, serum iron, ferritin and unconjugated bilirubin are elevated.

Thalassaemia trait (minor thalassaemia)

➤ Children are usually asymptomatic and do not require blood transfusions. Occasionally there may be tiredness and fatigue. Mild haemolysis may cause iron overload, particularly in the liver.

➤ Hb levels are usually 2–3 g/dL lower than normal, with an MCV of < 70 fL and an MCH of < 30 pg. Iron levels are either normal or elevated (unless there is associated iron-deficiency anaemia).

➤ Diagnosis is established by an elevated HbA of 3.4–7%.

> ### RED FLAG
>
> ● Children with thalassaemia trait are often overlooked and misdiagnosed as having iron-deficiency anaemia, and may be inappropriately treated with iron. Therefore, thalassaemia has always to be considered in any microcytic, hypochromic anaemia before iron is commenced.

PURPURA AND BLEEDING DISORDERS

Core messages

➤ Blood clotting mechanisms are complex, but primarily are based on vascular response (vasoconstriction and retraction of blood vessels), decreased blood flow to the affected area, platelet clot formation, and activation of coagulation factors to form fibrin to stabilise the clot.

➤ Purpura indicates extravasation of blood into the skin or mucosal membranes. Lesions are not raised. Purpura is due to vasculopathy, thrombocytopathy or coagulopathy, or a combination of these mechanisms.

➤ Depending on their size, purpuric lesions are either petechiae (pinpoint haemorrhages <1 cm, usually) or ecchymoses (> 1 cm in diameter).

➤ In contrast to exanthem and telangiectasia, purpura does not blanch on pressure (Fig 6.1 – *see* Plate section). It may be a benign condition or an indication of a serious underlying disorder (Box 6.4).

➤ In neonates, petechiae are commonly observed on the presenting part during delivery, particularly if the delivery was traumatic. In late infancy and toddlerhood, bruises frequently occur over bony prominences such as the shins, knees and forehead.

BOX 6.4 Classification of purpura

Non-thrombocytopenic purpura
- Henoch–Schönlein purpura
- Physical abuse, trauma, vomiting
- Infection (e.g. meningococcal septicaemia (MCS))
- Vascular purpuras (e.g. von Willebrand's disease)
- Drugs

Thrombocytopenic purpura
- Idiopathic thrombocytopenic purpura (ITP)
- Bone marrow infiltration/failure (e.g. leukaemia)
- Wiskott–Aldrich syndrome
- Haemolytic uraemic syndrome
- Kasabach–Merritt syndrome (thrombocytopenia with haemangioma)

Coagulation disorders (bleeding disorders)
- Hereditary coagulation defects (haemophilia A and B)
- Liver disease
- Ehlers–Danlos syndrome (an inherited connective tissue disease)
- Malabsorption

Recommended investigations

➤ Urine to screen for renal involvement in Henoch–Schönlein purpura (HSP).

➤ FBC: to confirm isolated thrombocytopenia; on blood film, blasts suggest leukaemia.

➤ LFT and urea and electrolytes (U&E) for underlying renal and liver disease.

➤ Coagulation screen: bleeding and clotting time; partial thromboplastin time (PTT) (screen for factor VIII; haemophilia); prothrombin time (PT) (for factors VII, V, X); clotting factors (e.g. VIII and IX); vWf (von Willebrand factor).

PRACTICE POINTS

- Baseline tests for most purpuras should include FBC, peripheral blood smear, PT and PTT. Additional tests should be performed according to baseline screening test results.
- Infants up to the age of 3–4 months have physiological prolongation of PTT. Normal values for screening tests are shown in Table 6.4.
- Distribution of the purpura can offer important clues to the diagnosis. In meningococcal septicaemia (MCS), lesions are often on the neck and chest; in HSP, the lesions are predominately on the shins, feet and buttocks; in idiopathic thrombocytopenic purpura (ITP), there is bruising and bleeding from the gums and mucous membranes.
- Of all diseases with purpura, those caused by sepsis and meningococcal disease are the most serious and require urgent referral.
- Whenever there are unexplained bruises, non-accidental injury (NAI) should always be suspected. Lesions are suspicious when they are found in areas of the body not normally subjected to injury (trunk, buttocks, and cheeks). Additional clues for NAI should be sought: inflicted cigarette burns, retinal haemorrhages and intra-oral injury, and skeletal examination should be performed. Referral for radiological skeletal survey may be indicated.

- Any purpura with pallor is likely to be serious: urgent referral is required to exclude leukaemia.
- ITP typically affects children 1–4 years old with sudden generalised petechiae and bleeding from the gums and mucous membranes, in response to a preceding viral infection 1–4 weeks previously.
- Haemophilia A and B are the most common clotting-factor deficiencies that can be diagnosed by prolonged PTT. PT, platelets and bleeding time are normal.
- Von Willebrand's disease is the most common hereditary bleeding disorder, with a prevalence of around 1% of the population. It is characterised clinically by excessive bruising, recurrent epistaxis and menorrhagia. Laboratory findings include prolonged bleeding time and PTT (often), normal PT and thrombocytes count and abnormal assay of von Willebrand factor.

TABLE 6.4 Normal values for screening tests in an infant with bleeding*

Test	Pre-term infant	Term infant	Child > 2 months old
Platelets × 10^9/L	150 000–400 000	150 000–400 000	150 000–400 000
Prothrombin time (seconds)	14–22	13–20	12–14
Partial thromboplastin time (seconds)	35–55	30–45	25–35
Fibrinogen 1.5–3.0 g/L	150–300	150–300	150–300

* Note that these normal values may vary from one laboratory to another.

DISORDERS OF IMMUNITY

The child with recurrent infections

➤ Children commonly present to primary care with recurring infections. The vast majority of these infections (about 95%) are caused by viral infections and are not caused by immunodeficiency.

Group 1: healthy children

➤ At least 50% of these children are healthy young children who have an average of 6–8 respiratory infections per year and who have no known significant underlying cause (such as immunodeficiency) for their infections. This rate of infection is increased to 2- or 3-fold when there is:

  ➣ increased exposure to viral infections at daycare or other group settings
  ➣ exposure to passive smoking.

Group 2: atopic children

➤ About 25–30% of children with frequent infections have atopy, with a tendency towards increased susceptibility for infection. Allergic rhinitis may be mistaken as chronic or recurrent URTIs. Coughing and wheezing are frequent and often mistaken as bronchitis or pneumonia rather than reactive airway disease or asthma. These children are also immunocompetent.

➤ The majority of infections are viral in origin (the mean duration of viral respiratory symptoms is 8 days), with mild symptoms.
➤ Bacterial infections are rare.
➤ The infection responds rapidly to appropriate treatment.
➤ There is rapid recovery from infection and the child is well between infections.
➤ Normal growth and development.
➤ Normal physical examination and laboratory findings.

Group 3: children with an underlying cause
About 10% of children with frequent infections have an underlying chronic disease or anatomical defect other than atopy or immunodeficiency, including:
➤ Acid reflux with frequent vomiting and aspiration into the lungs
➤ Children with neurodisability with aspiration and frequent pneumonia
➤ Congenital heart disease with left-to-right shunt, which increases susceptibility for increased infections
➤ Cystic fibrosis with frequent infections of the respiratory system.

Group 4: children with immunodeficiency
About 5–10% of the remaining children with frequent infection have an underlying immunodeficiency.

Immunodeficiency disorders
➤ Immunodeficiency disorders include a variety of diseases that cause increased susceptibility to infection, malignancies and autoimmunity. About 5–10% of children with recurrent infections have immunodeficiency. Box 6.5 gives a short classification of these disorders.

BOX 6.5 Classification of immune deficiencies with examples of disorders

● B-cell immune deficiency (50–75% of cases)
  ❯ Congenital (mostly inherited), secondary agammaglobulinaemia and hypogammaglobulinaemia
  ❯ Selective IgA deficiency
● Combined B- and T-cell immune deficiency (about 25%)
  ❯ Ataxia telangiectasia
  ❯ Wiskott–Aldrich syndrome
● T-cell immune deficiency (about 5%)
  ❯ Thymic hypoplasia (DiGeorge syndrome)
  ❯ Defective cytokine production
● Phagocytic cell immune deficiency (primary deficiency: about 1%)
  ❯ Neutrophil defects
  ❯ Chronic granulomatous disease
  ❯ Spleen dysfunction/asplenia
● Complement immune deficiency (about 1–2%)
  ❯ Hereditary angioedema

➤ Overall incidence of immunodeficiency is about 1 : 10 000 children.
➤ B-cell immunodeficiency disorders are the most common. Children commonly present after the age of 6 months with increased bacterial infections (e.g. otitis media, pneumonia) and poor growth. Viral or fungal infections are not usually increased (Box 6.6).
➤ Selective IgA deficiency affects as many as 1 in 333 people, and is often asymptomatic. In some children it can cause increased respiratory, digestive and genitourinary infections.
➤ Initial evaluation of a child with frequent infections includes a detailed history, thorough examination and appropriate screening tests (Table 6.5).

BOX 6.6 Clinical presentation of a child with immunodeficiency

- Healthy child with a family history of immunodeficiency
- Serious infections which respond poorly to conventional treatment
- Two or more bacterial infections such as pneumonia, sepsis or meningitis
- More than 3 episodes of otitis media, cellulitis or lymphadenitis in 1 year
- Recurrent tissue or organ abscess
- Infection with an opportunistic organism
- Recurrent muco-cutaneous candidiasis
- Recurrent hospitalisation requiring IV antibiotics for treatment
- Poor growth, failure to thrive
- Persistent lymphopenia

TABLE 6.5 Screening tests for a child with recurrent infections

Immunological tests	To exclude
1. **FBC, peripheral film, CRP**	
Normal neutrophil count	Neutropenia, leukocyte adhesion defect, phagocytic cell defect, T-cell defects
Normal lymphocyte count	T-cell defects
Normal platelets count	Wiskott–Aldrich syndrome
Normal CRP or ESR	Bacterial or fungal infections
Absent Howell-Jolly bodies	Asplenia
2. **Screening tests for B-cells**	
Normal immunoglobulin	B-cell defects
Normal antibody titres to tetanus or *H. influenzae*	
3. **Screening tests for T-cells**	
Normal lymphocyte count	T-cell defects
Positive *Candida albicans* skin test	
Normal thymic shadow (chest X-ray)	

📂 **RED FLAGS**

In any child suspected of having immunodeficiency, particular attention should be given to:
- Immunisation history, which should include any adverse effects from vaccination, particularly live virus vaccination as well as vaccine failure such as the occurrence of chickenpox in a varicella-vaccinated child
- Medications: current and past history should also be noted, particularly immunosuppressive drugs such as corticosteroids.

NEUTROPENIA

Core messages

➤ **Leucopenia** (WBC count less than 4000) occurs frequently in response to a viral infection. Normal values of leucocytes and their main components are shown in Table 6.6.

TABLE 6.6 Normal values for WBCs, neutrophils and lymphocytes $\times$ 10^9/L

Blood element	Normal range	Mean
WBCs		
Neonate	5.0–19.5	11.4
1 year old	6.0–17.5	11.4
4 years old	1.5–15.5	9.1
10 years old	4.5–13.5	8.1
Neutrophils		
Neonate	1.8–5.4	3.6
1 year old	1.5–8.5	3.5
4 years old	1.5–8.5	3.8
10 years old	1.8–80	4.4
Lymphocytes		
Neonate	2.9–9.0	5.6
1 year old	4.0–10.5	7.0
4 years old	2.0–8.0	4.5
10 years old	1.5–6.5	3.1

➤ **Neutropenia**, defined as a polymorphonuclear (PMN) leukocyte concentration of less than 1000×10^9/L, results from either impaired cell production of bone marrow or increased peripheral utilisation. The main causes of neutropenia are listed in Table 6.7. Neutropenia of $< 500 \times 10^9$/L is severe. Box 6.7 lists high- and low-risk factors for developing serious infections.
➤ **Transient neutropenia** (lasting < 2 weeks) is commonly associated with viral infection and usually occurs during the first 1–2 days and lasts 3–8 days.
➤ **Specific symptoms** of neutropenia are lacking. Children may present with:
  ➤ High fever in association with cellulitis, painful ulceration of the mouth and peri-rectal area, sinusitis, otitis media, soft-tissue infection requiring drainage or incision, and recurrent pneumonia

➤ More-severe infections including hepatic abscess and septicaemia.

➤ **Cyclic neutropenia** is a sporadic or familial disorder, characteristically recurring every 3 weeks, each episode lasting 3–6 days. The condition is caused by mutations in the gene encoding neutrophil elastase (ELA2). It is characterised by:

➤ Risk of infections ranging from mild to serious during the neutropenic phase. When there are no symptoms, neutrophils are usually normal

➤ Many patients experiencing significant improvement as they grow older

➤ Good response to prophylactic antibiotics and granulocyte colony-stimulating factor (G-CSF); these are effective treatments.

TABLE 6.7 Main causes of neutropenia

Causes	Diseases
Congenital	Benign ethnic neutropenia (Afro-Caribbean)
	Fanconi syndrome, associated with pancreatic insufficiency (Shwachman–Diamond syndrome)
Acquired	
Viral infections	Human herpes-6, rubella, HIV
Bacterial	Typhoid and paratyphoid, brucellosis
Drugs	Anti-thyroid, anticonvulsants, phenothiazines
Autoimmune diseases	SLE, autoimmune neutropenia
Splenomegaly	Thalassaemia
Anaemia	Advanced megaloblastic anaemia
Cyclic neutropenia	(see text)
Storage diseases	Glycogen storage disease
Bone marrow failure	Malignancy, cytotoxic therapy (see next section)

BOX 6.7 Risk factors for infections in patients with neutropenia

High risk for developing serious infections
- Neutropenia <500 mm^3
- Neutropenia >10 days
- History of splenectomy
- Secondary to cytotoxic therapy
- History of bone marrow transplantation
- Association with malignancy
- Associated fever >39°C

Low risk for developing serious infections
- Isolated neutropenia
- Intact other immune systems
- Viral-induced
- Associated with solid tumours
- Chronic benign neutropenia

LYMPHOPENIA

➤ The proportion of lymphocytes increases rapidly during infancy, reaching an average of 60% by 2 years of age.

➤ Lymphopenia is usually associated with a reduction in the number of CD4 or helper T-lymphocytes (60–65% of lymphocytes are CD4).

➤ Inherited causes of lymphopenia include cases with combined immunodeficiency; while acquired lymphopenia includes HIV infection, treatment with cytotoxic drugs or corticosteroids, and systemic lupus erythematosus (SLE).

➤ Isolated lymphopenia is usually asymptomatic.

RED FLAGS

- Neutropenia in association with an unwell/febrile child requires urgent referral.
- If the patient is well and afebrile and there is no associated anaemia and/ or thrombocytopenia, FBC may be repeated in 24–48 hours; and if neutropenia persists, the child may require an urgent outpatient appointment.

FURTHER READING

1. NHS Sickle cell and Thalassaemia Screening Programme. sickle-cell disease in childhood: standards and guidelines, October 2010. www.sct.screening.nhs.uk/cms.phpfolder=2493

CHAPTER 7

Malignancy

INTRODUCTION

➤ Approximately 1500 children will develop cancer per year by the age of 15 years in the UK, or 1 in 550–600 children. Acute leukaemia accounts for a third CNS and for a fourth of all childhood cancers.

➤ Cancer guidelines aim to:
  ➢ Help GPs identify patients who are likely to have cancer and who therefore require urgent assessment by a specialist
  ➢ Help GPs identify patients who are unlikely to have cancer and who may be managed in primary care or require non-urgent referral
  ➢ Facilitate appropriate referral between primary and secondary care for patients whom GPs suspect may have cancer.

➤ The original 'Urgent Suspected Cancer' referral guidelines launched by the DOH in 2001 were a radical departure from the then usual referral practice within the NHS. GPs were required to fax an 'Urgent Suspected Cancer' referral to a designated cancer unit within 24 hours of seeing the patient and of making the decision to refer.

➤ A review in 2006 of all cancer cases showed a dramatic increase in the number of referrals, though the number of patients actually diagnosed with cancer stayed at about 30%.

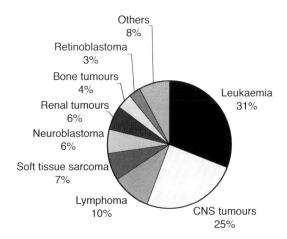

FIGURE 7.1 Percentages of childhood cancers. Relative distribution of main cancer groups among children aged 0–14 years in Great Britain 2001–2005, based on data provided by the National Registry

➤ The criteria, based on NICE guidelines, allow GPs scope to investigate patients urgently before referral and to address their anxiety.
➤ GPs are asked to ensure that their patient is able to attend an appointment within the 2 weeks from the referral being made.

TYPES OF CHILDHOOD CANCER

Figure 7.1 illustrates the distribution of childhood cancers in Great Britain.

RISK FACTORS FOR CANCER

In most cases no risk factor can be identified. It is likely that development of cancer involves both genetic and environmental factors. Known risk factors are shown in Tables 7.1 and 7.2.

TABLE 7.1 Some genetic and environmental risk factors for developing cancer

Factor	Cancer type
Genetic susceptibility	Retinoblastoma
Ionising radiation	Leukaemia
Benzene, nickel, asbestos	Leukaemia, mesothelioma
Immunosuppressant drugs	Lymphoma
Intramuscular iron injection	Sarcoma at injection site
Hepatitis B, C	Hepatic carcinoma
Epstein–Barr virus	Burkitt's and Hodgkin's lymphomas
HIV	Kaposi sarcoma, non-Hodgkin's lymphoma

TABLE 7.2 Malignancies associated with some familial/genetic diseases

Tumour	No of cases per annum	Likely age affected (in years)	Associated conditions
Acute leukaemia	370 (total)	2–4	Down's syndrome
(lymphatic or myeloid)	310		
	60		
Brain tumour	280	Any age	Neurofibromatosis type 1
Lymphoma	50	10–14	Ataxia telangiectasia, immunodeficiency
Soft-tissue sarcoma	80	< 4	Gardner's syndrome, neurofibromatosis type 1
Nephroblastoma	70	< 5	Beckwith–Wiedermann syndrome, hemihypertrophy, aniridia
Bone sarcoma	60	10–14	Li–Fraumeni syndrome
Retinoblastoma	30	< 1	Familial/heritable
Neuroblastoma	80	< 4	Beckwith–Wiedermann syndrome
Hepatoblastoma	10	< 1	Familial adenomatous polyposis coli

ASSESSMENT OF SUSPECTED CANCER

➤ Early detection of cancer is crucial to improve patients' chances of survival.
➤ A thorough history and physical examination are the key to diagnosis.
➤ In patients with typical cancer symptoms, tests should not be carried out by the GP as this could delay referral.
➤ In patients with less-typical symptoms, tests might be needed and should be carried out urgently.
➤ An urgent referral should be made if tests are not readily available.
➤ A GP should be able to demonstrate:
  ➤ Knowledge of cancer referral guidelines and protocols, both local and national (www.nice.org.uk/CG027)
  ➤ Knowledge of the symptoms and signs of early presentation of cancer
  ➤ Knowledge of the appropriate investigations
  ➤ Knowledge of the ethical dimensions of treatment and investigation choices
  ➤ Ability to establish a constructive relationship with the patients and their families
  ➤ Ability to provide support while waiting for the appointment.

Alarming signs of childhood cancer requiring urgent referral

➤ Continued, unexplained weight loss, or loss of appetite
➤ Functional loss, e.g. decreased activity and playfulness, sleep disturbance
➤ Worsening headaches, often with early-morning vomiting
➤ Impaired consciousness
➤ Cranial nerve abnormalities
➤ Gait abnormalities, leg weakness
➤ Increased swelling or persistent pain in bones, joints, back or legs
➤ Lump or mass, especially in the abdomen, neck, chest, pelvis, axilla
➤ Development of unexplained bruises, bleeding or rash
➤ Recurrent or persistent unexplained infections
➤ A whitish colour behind the pupil, acute squint or eye vision changes
➤ Constant tiredness or paleness
➤ Recurrent or persistent fevers of unknown origin
➤ Unexplained new-onset seizure
➤ Blood tests or X-rays suggesting malignancy.

Signs that worry parents which are usually not cancer

➤ Lymphadenopathy, especially in the neck. This is so common that it is almost normal. Worrying signs include associated lingering fever, weight loss and decreased appetite. A firm or hard mass, matted or fixed to the skin or underlying structures, should suggest malignancy. Biopsy, full blood count (FBC) and chest X-ray are essential investigations.
➤ Headaches, usually due to either migraine or tension, are a very common problem, occurring in about 50% of children aged 7 years and 80% of children aged 15 years. Although most causes of headaches in children are benign, it is essential to consider an underlying systemic disease. Worsening headaches presenting in the morning, which are exacerbated by stooping or straining, suggest increased intracranial pressure (ICP). Neuro-imaging is not indicated on a routine basis in children with recurrent headaches where physical examination is normal. It should, however, be

considered with abnormal neurological examination, progressive headaches or co-existing seizure.

➤ Although petechial rash can be a very serious sign of infection, it is more often due to physical trauma such as hard bouts of coughing or vomiting. In these instances the petechiae are usually over the neck and face. Assessing associated signs such as general condition (toxic or well) and the presence of fever are clues to exclude serious illness.

MANAGEMENT OF CANCER

Core messages

➤ Parents are the best observers of their child's symptoms. Persistent parental concern should be sufficient reason for referral, even if the primary healthcare professional considers the symptoms are most likely to have a benign cause.

➤ The outcome for children with cancer has dramatically improved over the past few decades, in part because of effective chemotherapy – more than 7 in 10 children with cancer can now be cured. Chemotherapy is used more often in children than in adults because childhood malignancy is more responsive to chemotherapy than adult malignancy, and because they can better tolerate its adverse effects. Radiotherapy, on the other hand, is not often used in children because they are more vulnerable than adults to its late adverse effects.

➤ During the course of cancer treatment, almost all children experience some pain. Pain relief is an essential component of cancer care (see below).

Support for child and family

(See also the section on grief and bereavement, below.)

Adequate emotional and financial support is invariably needed for the family of a child with cancer. Relationships within the family may become disturbed and siblings may be neglected. Parents and children will need help in expressing their feelings of anxiety, guilt, anger and depression. Tutoring should be encouraged and children should not fall behind in their schooling. In the UK, CLIC Sargent and a number of local charities provide invaluable support by funding specialist nurses and social workers as well as offering financial assistance. They provide practical support during treatment in hospital and at home (see list of charities provided below).

➤ Once the diagnosis is established, the management plan must be carefully explained to parents. Children should be given as much information as they can understand. Effects of treatment, e.g. loss of hair during chemotherapy, should be fully explored. It is usually necessary to repeat an explanation several times before the family fully understands.

➤ There are several organisations and charities which offer information and support, and respite, palliative and terminal care for children and young people with cancers. They also offer hospice services which include short breaks and daytime activities enabling families to have a break, help symptom control and pain relief in addition to support. Examples are: www.rainbows.co.uk, www.childrenwithcancer.org.uk/childhood-cancer (See also the list of organisations and charities provided below.)

MANAGEMENT OF SYMPTOMS

Pain management

Successful pain management requires a systematic approach using the ABCs of pain (Table 7.3). Children aged 3–7 years will be able to describe the severity of pain. Children aged 8 years and older can use visual analogue pain scales accurately, where 0 is no pain and 10 is the worst pain possible.

➤ Pain should be managed in a stepwise manner as recommended by the World Health Organization (WHO) – paracetamol, non-steroidal anti-inflammatory drugs (NSAIDs) and opioids.

➤ Oral medication is often appropriate unless there is severe nausea, vomiting, dysphagia, weakness or impaired consciousness.

➤ Paracetamol, NSAIDs or an opioid such as codeine or dihydrocodeine, alone or in combination, may be helpful in the control of mild to moderate pain.

➤ Opioids remain the mainstay of severe cancer pain management.

➤ When used as the sole analgesics, high doses are often required, which may be associated with troublesome side-effects particularly sedation, constipation and even respiratory suppression.

➤ Unfounded fear of addiction can lead physicians to administer opioids only as a last resort. As a result, children may not receive the potent analgesics required to relieve severe cancer pain.

TABLE 7.3 The ABCs of pain in children

Assess	Pain is best assessed by directly asking children about its character, location, frequency, duration and intensity
	Infants and toddlers show their pain only by how they look and act
	Facial expression measures are useful in neonates
Body	Physical examination should include thorough checking of the body for potential pain sites
Context	The impact of family, environmental factors and healthcare on the child's pain
Document	Recording the location and intensity of pain on a regular basis
Evaluation	Regular assessment of the effectiveness of pain interventions and modification of the treatment plan accordingly

Medications for pain

➤ It is common for children to require a combination opioid and an adjuvant.

➤ Codeine and dihydrocodeine are weak opioids and are potentially constipating.

➤ Morphine, diamorphine and fentanyl are the mainstay of opioid treatment in children. Fentanyl causes less constipation and sedation than morphine. Table 7.4 shows opioid doses, and Table 7.5 shows guidelines for pain treatment according to the tumour site.

TABLE 7.4 Opioid dosage guidelines

Opioid	Route	Dose	Frequency
Codeine	Oral	0.5–1 mg/kg/dose (maximum 240 mg)	4- to 6-hourly
Morphine			
Short-acting	Oral	0.15–0.3 mg/kg/dose	4-hourly
	Solution, e.g. Oramorph	10 mg/5 mL	4-hourly
	Suppository	10 mg and 20 mg	As required
	Injection	0.2 mg/kg/dose	SC or IM, IV (over ≥ 5 minutes) and infusion
Long-acting	Tablet, e.g. MST Continus	5 mg (white) 10 mg (brown) 15 mg (green) 30 mg (purple) 60 mg (orange) 100 mg (grey) 200 mg (green)	12-hourly
	Suspension	20 mg, 30 mg, 60 mg, 100 mg and 200 mg (all per sachet)	12-hourly
Diamorphine	Intranasal spray	Powder to be dissolved in water to provide 0.2 mL of solution	As required
Fentanyl	Lozenge patch (12, 25, 50, 100 mcg)	15 mcg/kg (maximum 400 mcg), releasing 12, 25, 50 and 100 mcg/h for 72 hours	As a single dose

TABLE 7.5 Specific pain sites and proposed drug treatment

Site	Treatment
Bone pain	Ibuprofen, diclofenac, opioids, radiotherapy
Muscle spasm	Diazepam, baclofen, botulinum toxin (for chronic or frequent spasm)
Neuropathic pain	Antidepressants, anticonvulsants, ketamine, dexamethasone
Abdominal pain	Hyoscine butylbromide (colicky abdominal pain is often resistant to opioids)

Mouth care

➤ All children should undergo a dental assessment at the time of cancer diagnosis and before chemotherapy commences. This should be ideally done by a paediatric dentist or a dental hygienist.
➤ All children diagnosed with cancer should be registered with a general dental practitioner or community dental services. Immunosuppressive status can lead to dental abscess and possible sepsis.
➤ The general advice should be to brush the teeth at least twice a day, with a fluoride toothpaste. For babies with teeth, the parents should be instructed on how to clean the mouth with an oral sponge.
➤ A dental assessment should be undertaken every 3–4 months.

Nausea and vomiting

➤ Two of the most common side-effects of chemotherapy are nausea and vomiting.

➤ The chemotherapy trigger zone (CTZ), which is located in the medulla, stimulates the vomiting centre in the medulla oblongata.

➤ Chemotherapeutic agents are presumed to release emetic transmitters (e.g. serotonin, dopamine, etc) which bind to receptors in the CTZ.

➤ Most anti-emetics function as competitors of these transmitters by binding to the

TABLE 7.6 Some drugs used to treat nausea and vomiting due to chemotherapy

Drug	Route	Dose	Frequency	Comments
Cyclizine	Oral or IV	0.5–1 mg/kg/dose	TDS	This is particularly effective in centrally mediated nausea and vomiting
	Rectal	12.5, 25 and 50 mg	TDS	
	Injection	50 mg by IV or SC infusion	Up to TDS	
Ondansetron (Zofran)	IV or SC infusion	0.15 mg/kg/dose; 1–12 years: 5 mg/m²; 12–18 years: 8 mg	Before chemo-therapy	Most effective if there is damage to gut mucosa (post-chemotherapy and radiotherapy)
	Oral	1–12 years: 4 mg 12–18 years: 8 mg	BD–TDS	
Prochlorperazine (Stemetil)	Oral (tablet or syrup)	2–5 years: 1.25–2.5 mg 5–12 years: 2.5–5 mg 12–18 years: 5–10 mg	TDS	Severe dystonic side-effects may occur
	Buccal	2–5 years: 1.25–2.5 mg 12–18 years: 3–6 mg	BD	
	IM	5–12 years: 5–6.25 mg 12–18 years: 12.5 mg	TDS	
Metoclopramide (Maxolon)	Oral (syrup 5 mg/5 mL; tablet 10 mg)	1 month–1 year: 1 mg/kg/dose	BD	Extrapyramidal side-effects may occur
		1–3 years: 1 mg	BD-TDS	
		3–5 years: 2 mg	BD or TDS	
		5–9 years: 2.5 mg	TDS	
		9–15 years: 5 mg	TDS	
		15–18 years: 10 mg	TDS	
Domperidone	Tab or suspension	Up to 35 kg bodyweight: 0.25–0.5 mg/kg/dose	TDS or QDS	Domperidone is less effective than metoclopramide but has less risk of extrapyramidal side-effects
		Bodyweight 35 kg and over: 10–20 mg		
Dexamethasone	Oral	0.1–0.15 mg/kg/dose	BD for 5 days	Enhances the anti-emetic effect of metoclopramide and ondansetron, as well as acting as an appetite-stimulator
	Suspension (2 mg/5 mL); IM	0.1–0.4 mg/kg/dose	OD–BD	

BD = twice daily; OD = once daily; TDS = three times daily.

receptors, therefore preventing binding of the transmitters themselves. For this reason, using anti-emetics prior to administration of emetogenic chemotherapy is important.

➤ Management of nausea and vomiting includes:
  ➢ Monitoring the number of vomiting episodes and assessing the degree of dehydration
  ➢ Encouraging oral intake of liquids
  ➢ Drugs, used as provided in Table 7.6.

Constipation

➤ Causes of constipation in children undergoing cancer treatment are immobility, relative dehydration and opioid therapy.
➤ Stool softeners (such as lactulose or magnesium hydroxide) in combination with a stimulant (docusate, senna or sodium picosulfate) are often required.
➤ Oral naloxone can help in opioid-induced constipation.
➤ Macrogols (e.g. Movicol) are being increasingly used.

Other symptoms and sleep disturbance

(*See* Table 7.7.)
It is worth trying non-pharmacological measures, including:
➤ Keeping to regular bedtime routines.
➤ Bedtime routines may include quiet activities such as cuddling and reading a story.
➤ Keeping lights dim in the evening as bedtime approaches.

If these measures fail, the medications shown in Table 7.7 may be used.

TABLE 7.7 Summary of symptom treatment

Symptom	Medication	Per dose
Pain or dyspnoea	Morphine	*See* Table 7.3
Agitation	Lorazepam (or midazolam)	0.05–0.1 mg/kg (injection or tablet)
Anxiety	Midazolam	0.5 mg/kg
Pruritis	Chlorphenamine	1–4 mg (depending on age) 4- to 6-hourly
Nausea and vomiting	Prochlorperazine	1.25–10 mg
	Ondansetron	4 mg (8- to 12-hourly)
Diarrhoea	Loperamide	0.1–0.2 mg/kg, 3–4 times daily
Sleep disturbance	Melatonin	2.5–5 mg at bedtime
Excessive secretions	Hyoscine hydrobromide	10 mcg/kg (maximum 300 mcg 4 times daily)

Metabolic and haematological manifestations of cancer therapy

Table 7.8 shows some metabolic and haematological abnormalities which may occur during chemotherapy. When an abnormality is found, consultation with the cancer team is indicated. However, if finding a combination of these abnormalities, an urgent consultation is needed.

TABLE 7.8 Some metabolic and haematological manifestations which may occur after chemotherapy

	Features	Causing
Metabolic	Hyperuricaemia	Uric acid nephropathy, gout
	Hyperkalaemia	Cardiac arrhythmia
	Hyponatraemia	Lethargy, seizure
	Hypercalcaemia	Nausea, polyuria
Haematological	Anaemia	Pallor, weakness
	Thrombocytopenia	Petechiae
	Neutropenia	Infection, sepsis
	Disseminated intravascular coagulation (DIC)	Haemorrhage

CANCER TYPES

Leukaemia
Children usually present with a relatively short history, of weeks rather than months. The presence of one or more of the following symptoms or signs requires investigation with an urgent FBC and blood film:
➤ Pallor
➤ Fatigue
➤ Unexplained irritability
➤ Unexplained persistent fever
➤ Persistent, unexplained upper respiratory tract infection, particularly if associated with mouth ulcers
➤ Persistent or unexplained bone pain
➤ Unexplained bruises.

The presence of the following requires **immediate referral**:
➤ Unexplained petechiae or bleeding
➤ Severe anaemia
➤ Hepatosplenomegaly.

Brain tumours
Patients with brain tumour typically present with one or more of the following:
➤ Signs of increased ICP
  ➣ Morning headache
  ➣ Vomiting
  ➣ Diplopia
  ➣ Nystagmus
  ➣ Mood changes, poor school performance
  ➣ Papilloedema
  ➣ VI cranial nerve palsy (lateral rectus palsy)
  ➣ Bulging fontanelle (infant)
  ➣ Increased head circumference (infant).
➤ Focal neurological signs
  ➣ Focal seizure

➤ Cerebellar ataxia
➤ Hemiparesis.
➤ Endocrinopathies, e.g. diabetes insipidus.

🏳 **RED FLAGS**

In brain tumour:
- The headache typically occurs in the morning and is relieved with standing and vomiting.
- The headache is typically dull, generalised, steady or progressive, and worsened by coughing, sneezing or defecation.
- The associated vomiting may be a prominent symptom. In some cases children have even been subjected to a series of gastrointestinal investigations as a result.
- Any diplopia warrants prompt evaluation; it may signal the onset of a serious intracranial disease.
- Although diplopia is a common symptom in posterior fossa tumour, children rarely complain of it as they are able to suppress the image of the affected eye. Instead, head tilting may occur in an attempt to align the two images.

Lymphoma
Hodgkin's lymphoma:
➤ May present with non-tender cervical and/or supra-clavicular lymphadenopathy. The history is long (months). Only a minority have systemic manifestations such as itch, night sweats and fever.

Non-Hodgkin's lymphoma
➤ Typically shows a more rapid progression, and may present with lymphadenopathy, breathlessness, superior vena cava obstruction or abdominal distension.

🏳 **RED FLAGS**

For lymphoma:
- Non-tender, firm or hard, rubbery lymph nodes, matted or fixed to the underlying tissue.
- Finding of a lymph node > 2 cm (particularly if > 3 cm) in maximum diameter.
- Associated with other signs of systemic manifestations such as fever or weight loss.
- Involvement of axillary lymph nodes with absence of signs of infection.
- Lymph nodes in mediastinum or hilar area in chest X-ray.
- Enlargement of the left supraclavicular node suggests malignancy such as lymphoma or rhabdomyosarcoma arising in the abdomen.
- Enlargement of the right supraclavicular node suggests intrathoracic lesions.

Neuroblastoma

➤ Neuroblastoma is the most common extracranial solid tumour of childhood, accounting for 7% of all cases. Over two-thirds of cases occur during the first 5 years of life (median age 2 years).
➤ Children differ in presentation of the disease:
  ➤ An abdominal mass arising from the adrenal medulla may extend beyond the midline of the abdomen. An abdominal plain X-ray or ultrasound scan may detect stippled calcification in the adrenal gland. Intravenous urography (rarely used nowadays) may show inferior displacement of the kidney without distortion of the pyelocalyceal system.
  ➤ Metastasis into the skull (producing signs of increased intracranial pressure and lytic lesions), tubular bones (producing pain and tenderness), the liver (causing rapidly growing abdominal mass), the orbit (causing proptosis), or the skin (subcutaneous nodules) may occur during the neonatal period.
  ➤ Horner's syndrome (meiosis, ptosis, enophthalmia and anhydrosis) may be seen.

Nephroblastoma

This is the second most common malignant retroperitoneal tumour in children, occurring at a rate of 7.5 cases per million children in the USA. The tumour commonly presents as an abdominal mass in a young child (median age 3 years), often detected by a parent (in over 80% of cases). Other presentations include fever (reported incidence 23–50% of cases), haematuria and hypertension (caused by renin secretion). Cough and dyspnoea may occur due to pulmonary metastasis.

Soft-tissue sarcoma

A mass at almost any site.

Bone Tumours

➤ Limbs are the most common sites.
➤ Persistent bone pain, localised or diffuse, particularly pain which requires analgesics and limits activity.
➤ Plain X-ray is usually helpful.

Retinoblastoma

(*See* Fig 7.2.)

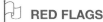 RED FLAGS

- Beware of family history of retinoblastoma (in about 15% of cases) and occurrence of visual problems in children.
- Beware of a new squint or change in the sharpness of the eyesight.
- Beware of a white pupil that does not reflect light.
- Pain suggests secondary glaucoma.
- Retinoblastoma is almost always fatal without treatment; its cure rate is 90% or higher when it is promptly recognised and referred.

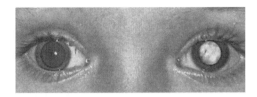

FIGURE 7.2 Abnormal red reflex in the left eye, caused possibly by congenital cataract or retinoblastoma (Image courtesy of the Childhood Eye Cancer Trust)

GRIEF AND BEREAVEMENT

Grief and bereavement reflect a state of deep and intense sadness and mourning after the loss of a loved one. The grief process depends on the relationship with the person who died. Unlike adults, bereaved children do not experience continual and intense emotional grief reactions, although this is age-dependent:
➤ Children before the age of 6 years see death as a kind of sleep. The child cannot fully separate death from life. Although the children often know that death occurs physically, they think it is temporary, reversible and not final.
➤ Children aged 6–9 years may react differently. They often react with learning difficulties, develop anti-social or aggressive behaviour and tend to withdraw from others.
➤ After the age of 9 years, children will have increased anxiety about their own death. Physical reactions are more intense than in younger children, and include sleeping disturbance and a change in appetite.

Breaking the news is best achieved by:
➤ A parent or someone known to or trusted by the child telling him or her of the death soon after it has occurred, using touch to comfort and console. Children can handle sad news much better than they are given credit for by adults.
➤ Using simple factual words such as 'dead' or 'has died' rather than 'gone to heaven' or 'slipped away', which are confusing.
➤ Preparing children gently to make choices about if and how they want to say 'goodbye', e.g. placing a favourite toy or flowers in or on the coffin or writing a letter of farewell.
➤ Informing the child's school of the death and asking for the support of teachers as necessary.

Children need support, most of which comes from friends and family. Doctors, nurses and charity organisations are also an important source of support. This is best given by people who have been trained in bereavement work with expertise in work with bereaved children. Such people are found in charity organisations which include:
➤ The Child Bereavement Charity (CBC) which provides specialised support, information and training to all those affected when a child dies or when a child is bereaved. In addition, the charity provides books, DVD, videos and a confidential listening service to anyone affected by the death of a child or who is caring for a bereaved child.
Tel: 01494 568900
www.childbereavement.org.uk

➤ The Childhood Bereavement Network which is a national, multi-professional organisation providing help for bereaved children and young people.
Tel: 020 7843 6309
www.childhoodbereavementnetwork.org.uk

➤ Winston's Wish which provides services to bereaved children and young people and their families in the UK.
Helpline: 08452 03 04 05
Tel: 01242 515157
www.winstonswish.org.uk

➤ The Compassionate Friends (TCF) which is an organisation offering bereaved families understanding, support and encouragement after the death of a child. They also offer support, advice and information to other relatives, friends and professionals who are helping the family.
Helpline: 08451 23 23 04
Tel: 0845 120 3785 (National Office)
www.tcf.org.uk/localsupport.html

➤ The Department for Work and Pensions offers information on 'bereavement and the law' in the form of a helpful leaflet entitled 'What to do after a death in England and Wales'
www.dwp.gov.uk/docs/dwp004.pdf

ORGANISATIONS AND CHARITIES WHICH SUPPORT CANCER PATIENTS

➤ CLIC Sargent Head Office
Horatio House
77–86 Fulham Palace Road
London W6 8JA
Tel: 0300 330 0803
www.clicsargent.org.uk

➤ CLIC Sargent Scotland Office
5th Floor, Mercantile Chambers
53 Bothwell Street
Glasgow G2 6TS
Tel: 0141 572 5700
www.clicsargent.org.uk

➤ CLIC Sargent Northern Ireland Office
3rd floor
31 Bruce Street
Belfast BT2 7JD
Tel: 028 9072 5780
www.clicsargent.org.uk

➤ Macmillan Cancer Support
89 Albert Embankment
London SE1 7UQ
Tel: 0808 808 00 00
www.macmillan.org.uk/Home.aspx

➤ Children with Cancer UK
51 Great Ormond Street
London WC1N 3JQ
Tel: 020 7404 0808
Fax: 020 7404 3666
www.childrenwithcancer.org.uk

➤ Rainbow Trust Children's Charity
6 Cleeve Court
Cleeve Road
Leatherhead
Surrey KT22 7UD
Tel 01372 363438
www.rainbowtrust.org.uk

CHAPTER 8

Gastrointestinal diseases

MOUTH ULCER

Core messages

➤ Mouth ulceration is common and usually painful; it is caused by a variety of conditions (Box 8.1).

➤ Most mouth ulcers in young children are caused by viral infection, including acute herpetic gingivostomatitis (AHG), while aphthous ulcers are more common in older children and adults (affecting about 20% of the population), with a tendency to recur in contrast to AHG.

➤ Management of mouth ulcers (Box 8.2) includes pain relief, maintenance of fluid and nutrition intake, and early resolution.

BOX 8.1 Causes of mouth ulcers

Viral infections
- Acute herpetic gingivostomatitis (AHG)*
- Hand–foot–mouth disease*
- Other viral infections, e.g. varicella, cytomegalovirus (CMV)*
- Herpangina caused by coxsackie virus
- HIV infection
- Stevens–Johnson syndrome

Bacterial/fungal causes
- Histoplasmosis
- Fungal infection
- Necrotising ulcerative gingivostomatitis

Autoimmune/connective causes
- Systemic lupus erythematosus (SLE)
- Inflammatory bowel disease (Crohn's disease)
- Behçet's disease
- Reiter's syndrome (uveitis, conjunctivitis, arthritis)
- Periodic fever syndrome (e.g. PFAPA)

Miscellaneous causes
- Drugs, e.g. chemotherapy, NSAIDs
- Trauma (including child abuse, chemical burns)*
- Aphthous ulcers*
- Neutropenia (cyclic), aplastic anaemia
- Lichen planus
- Mouth cancer

* These are the most common causes of mouth ulcers.

BOX 8.2 Management of mouth ulcers

- Most mouth ulcers do not require specific treatment
- Food should be soft or liquidised; hard and salty foods such as crisps should be avoided
- Corticosteroids may be used to reduce the inflammatory changes. Beclomethasone as a liquid (rinsing the mouth for 2 minutes 2–4 times daily). Hydrocortisone muco-adhesive buccal tabs: 1 lozenge 4 times daily (2.5 mg)
- Antimicrobial mouthwash is commonly prescribed as an antiseptic and inhibitor of plaque formation on the teeth
  > Chlorhexidine gluconate mouthwash: rinse mouth with 10 mL for 1 minute twice daily
  > Saline mouthwash, for its cleansing effect. This can be prepared by dissolving half a teaspoonful of salt in a glassful of warm water
- If mouth ulcers are very painful, paracetamol or ibuprofen can be used. Benzydamine (Difflam) may be used either as a mouthwash or a spray to provide local analgesia. Calgel (containing 0.33% lidocaine as anaesthetic and cetylpyridinium 0.1% as antiseptic) is commonly used
- For severe herpetic gingivostomatitis, oral aciclovir is prescribed:
  > 100 mg 5 times daily for 5 days (age 1 month–2 years)
  > 200 mg 5 times daily for 5 days (age > 2 years)
- Severe aphthous ulceration may respond to rinsing the mouth with the contents of a 100 mg doxycyline capsule (mixed with a small amount of water) 4 times daily in a child > 12 years of age
- Good hygiene of the oral cavity reduces recurrences of ulcers

Recommended investigations

(Investigation is rarely needed but should be considered in the case of unexplained ulcers, their unusual appearance, severity or persistence after 7–10 days.)
- Full blood count (FBC):
  - neutropenia, including cyclic neutropenia
  - anaemia likely in Crohn's disease
  - leukopenia, anaemia and thrombocytopenia in systemic lupus erythematosus (SLE)
- C-reactive protein (CRP): elevated in bacterial infectious disease and in Crohn's disease
- Serological tests for HIV infection
- Dark-field microscopy for spirochetes (*Borrelia vincentii*)
- Tests for autoimmune diseases, e.g. anti-nuclear antibodies
- Scraping for fungal infection; if positive, tests for immunity are required.

PRACTICE POINTS

- Herpangina can be differentiated from AHG as follows: herpangina has more-posterior lesions (tonsils, tonsillar pillars, uvula, pharyngeal wall and soft palate), while in AHG the lesions affect the cheeks, gingiva and tongue.
- Benign aphthae tend to be small in size (< 1 cm) and self-limiting, while large

aphthae are difficult to heal and may often be associated with more-serious disorder, e.g. HIV infection. HIV also causes oral candidiasis and periodontitis.

- Necrotising ulcerative gingivostomatitis is rare in healthy children but may occur in association with poor dental hygiene. It may mimic AHG, but dark-field microscopy will detect spirochetes. Penicillin therapy is indicated.
- Mouth ulcers are common in Crohn's disease, but rare in ulcerative colitis. The mouth lesions may precede intestinal manifestations.
- Oral lichen planus in children is rare and occurs in about 50% of people with lichen planus on the skin. Lesions consist of painless, whitish streaks on the mucous membranes (Wickham's striae) which become painful once they produce ulcers.

RED FLAGS

- A child with herpetic mouth ulcers is highly infectious and may infect another child with atopic dermatitis resulting in eczema herpeticum.
- Multiple mouth ulcers may be the first sign of neutropenia or aplastic anaemia. FBC is urgently required.
- Oral manifestations of child abuse include broken teeth, lip injury, or tears to the lingual frenulum. This possibility should always be suspected if the injury is not compatible with the history.
- Oral gels (e.g. Bonjela), which are used to treat oral ulcers, may contain salicylate salts. They should not be given to children below 12 years of age as they may cause Reye's syndrome.
- Clinicians should be suspicious of a mouth ulcer persisting for over 4 weeks. Cancer of the mouth can sometimes start with a mouth ulcer which does not heal.

ACUTE ABDOMINAL PAIN

Core messages

➤ Acute abdominal pain is a common complaint caused by a variety of conditions (Box 8.3). The main objective in dealing with an affected child is to differentiate between benign, self-limited conditions such as constipation or gastroenteritis, and more life-threatening surgical conditions such as intussusception or appendicitis.

➤ The term 'acute abdomen' refers to an acute intra-abdominal condition which is likely to require a surgical intervention. The use of sedation or analgesia does not increase the risk of misdiagnosis.

➤ Pain originating from the liver, pancreas and upper intestine is typically felt in the epigastric area; pain originating from the small intestine or appendiceal inflammation is felt typically in the peri-umbilical area (innervation from the T10 level of the spinal cord segment); and pain from the distal colon and urinary tract is felt in the supra-pubic area.

➤ Extra-abdominal conditions, such as pneumonia or pharyngitis, are important causes of abdominal pain.

BOX 8.3 Causes of acute abdominal pain

Diseases which can be managed in primary care
- Gastroenteritis
- Infantile colic
- Gastro-oesophageal reflux

- Constipation
- Urinary tract infection (uncomplicated)
- Gilbert's syndrome

Diseases which may require referral
- Mesenteric adenitis
- Referred pain (e.g. pneumonia, hip synovitis)
- Crohn's disease

- Urinary tract infection (atypical)
- Hepatitis
- Sickle-cell crisis

Diseases which require urgent referral
- Appendicitis
- Gallstones
- Renal stones
- Incarcerated hernia

- Intussusception
- Pancreatitis
- Intestinal obstruction
- Diabetic ketoacidosis (DKA)

Recommended investigations

➤ Urinalysis with urine culture to confirm urinary tract infection (UTI). Dipsticks: the presence of positive nitrite and leucocytes suggests UTI, while their absence makes the diagnosis unlikely; ketones with glycosuria raise the possibility of diabetic ketoacidosis (DKA).

➤ Stool culture: bacterial gastroenteritis; viral antigen detection for rotavirus.

➤ FBC: leucocytosis suggests inflammatory causes; marked leukocytosis (leukaemoid reaction) is seen occasionally in pneumonia.

➤ CRP or erythrocyte sedimentation rate (ESR) for bacterial infections such as UTI.

➤ Liver function tests (LFTs) to diagnose hepatitis.

➤ Blood glucose, urea and electrolytes (U&E) and blood gases to rule out DKA with a history of polydipsia and polyuria (part of management in hospital).

➤ Abdomen X-ray may show signs of impacted stool in constipation or signs of intestinal obstruction.

➤ Abdominal ultrasound for suspected cases of renal or gallstones.

PRACTICE POINTS

- Abdominal examination should be performed gently. Careful hands-off inspection is the first step, followed by taking a non-intimidating position sitting down or kneeling to be at the same level as the child. A young child is best examined in a parent's arms or lap. Distracting the child while palpating the abdomen is very helpful. It is worth asking the child to point with his/her finger to the area 'where it hurts most'.
- The closer the pain to the umbilicus, the less likely it is to be caused by organic disease.
- The primary objective of managing a child with acute abdominal pain is to

exclude a surgical condition, especially appendicitis. Typically, the pain of appendicitis:
  ○ starts around the umbilicus
  ○ radiates to the lower right abdomen
  ○ causes tenderness and rebound effect in the lower right abdomen
  ○ worsens when coughing or jumping
  ○ is followed, not preceded, by vomiting
  ○ is constant and presents as an acute abdomen in case of perforation of the appendix. Children typically have longer history of pain, greater systemic effect, high fever, more-generalised tenderness and minimal or absent bowel sounds.
● The differential diagnosis between functional and organic causes of abdominal pain is shown in Table 8.1.
● Extra-abdominal conditions can present as abdominal pain e.g. spine or hip lesions.
● The typical abdomen in gastroenteritis is non-distended, soft or mildly tender but with little or no guarding, and is cramping in nature rather than constant, usually occurring prior to developing diarrhoea.
● Mesenteric adenitis is often associated with a viral upper respiratory tract infection. Stool culture may be positive for bacteria, particularly *Yersinia*.

RED FLAGS

● Gastroenteritis may mask appendicitis.
● Abdominal pain in DKA may mimic appendicitis.
● Extra-abdominal examination is important, as tonsillitis and lower-lobe pneumonia can produce abdominal pain and mimic abdominal emergencies.
● Any acute abdominal pain that makes the child miserable and ill requires careful assessment.
● A young child with mild abdominal pain and vomiting who has clinical signs of dehydration but no ketones in the urine may have an inborn error of metabolism. Urgent referral is required.

TABLE 8.1 Differential diagnosis between functional and organic causes of acute abdominal pain (AP)

Clinical features	Functional AP	Organic AP
Family history of AP	More likely positive	Likely negative (except inflammatory bowel disease (IBD))
Psychological factors/anxiety	More likely	Less likely
Site of pain	Usually central; often epigastric	Usually at flanks, upper or right lower quadrant area, supra-pubic
Abnormal symptoms such as fever, vomiting or loss of weight	Usually absent	Often present

Clinical features	Functional AP	Organic AP
Severe pain, persistent, significant, worsening pain, awaking child at night	No	Likely
Abnormal signs	Usually absent	Present
Abnormal tests	Absent	Present

RECURRENT ABDOMINAL PAIN

Core messages

➤ Recurrent abdominal pain (RAP) is a very common symptom, estimated to affect around 10% of school-age children. RAP is responsible for about 40% of referrals to paediatric gastroenterology clinics. The symptom is significant because it is responsible for a high rate of morbidity, missed school days, high use of health resources and parental anxiety. Typical age of occurrence is 5–14 years.

➤ RAP is defined as pain severe enough to interfere with activity, intermittent, and at least 3 recurrent episodes occurring over a 3-month period (Apley's criteria). Apley in 1958 estimated that only 8% of patients with RAP had organic pathology after extensive investigation. Nowadays, a higher estimate is accepted, mainly because irritable bowel syndrome (IBS) has been recognised as an important cause of RAP and because of a high rate of detecting pathology by the newer imaging technologies.

➤ Causes of RAP are shown in Box 8.4. The most common causes are functional abdominal pain, food intolerance/allergy, IBS, and abdominal migraine.

➤ Recurrent crying episodes in an infant who draws the legs up and appears to be in pain are defined as colic and not RAP.

BOX 8.4 Causes of RAP

Functional causes
- Infantile colic (evening colic)
- Functional (psychogenic, e.g. school phobia)
- Food intolerance/allergy (e.g. to milk)
- Abdominal migraine
- IBS
- Gilbert's syndrome

Organic causes
- Parasites (e.g. *Giardia*)
- Gastro-oesophageal reflux
- IBD (Crohn's disease, ulcerative colitis)
- Coeliac disease
- Recurrent UTI
- Sickle-cell anaemia (SCA)
- Meckel's diverticulum
- Pancreatitis
- Stones in the urinary system and gall bladder
- Peptic ulcer
- Lead poisoning
- Familial Mediterranean fever (FMF)
- Porphyria

Recommended investigations

➤ Urinalysis: haematuria may suggest renal stones; leucocytes and nitrite suggest UTI.

➤ Stool for parasites and culture.

➤ FBC with CRP: useful in excluding inflammation and infection; anaemia in sickle-cell anaemia.

➤ LFTs to diagnose hepatitis, Gilbert's disease.
➤ Coeliac screening tests in blood (e.g. anti-tTG antibodies and anti-endomysial anti-bodies of immunoglobulin A).
➤ Faecal antigen testing in stool for *Helicobacter pylori*.
➤ Abdominal ultrasound scan for renal or gallstones.
➤ Endoscopy, if organic gastrointestinal cause suspected.
➤ Technetium-99 isotope scan for Meckel's diverticulum.

PRACTICE POINTS

● The distinction between organic disease, functional and emotional disorders can be difficult; overlap between them may co-exist.
● Meckel's diverticulum, remnant of the omphalomesenteric duct, is present in about 2% of the population. This is usually asymptomatic but may present with painless rectal bleeding, intestinal obstruction, intussusception or RAP.
● Abdominal migraine is diagnosed by at least 5 attacks fulfilling the following criteria:
  ○ Episodic midline abdominal pain, peri-umbilical or poorly localised
  ○ Dull pain of moderate or severe intensity, lasting 1–72 hours
  ○ Normality between episodes
  ○ Association with 2 of the following 4 symptoms: anorexia, nausea, vomiting and pallor
  ○ Not attributed to another disorder.
● Familial Mediterranean fever (FMF) is an autosomal recessive disease; patients present with abdominal pain due to peritonitis. About 6–10 hours later fever occurs, followed by recovery within 24–72 hours. Symptoms rapidly respond to 0.6 mg of colchicine.
● Pain in constipation is often over-diagnosed. The diagnosis should not be made until other diagnoses have been excluded.
● Parasites such as *Giardia* are a common and important cause of RAP in developing countries.
● The commonest cause of RAP is functional abdominal pain. Typical features are:
  ○ Healthy appearance of the child
  ○ Central abdominal pain, with no guarding, rebound or rigidity, and without abnormal physical sign such as fever
  ○ Investigation reveals no organic cause
  ○ Child is well between episodes.

🏳 RED FLAGS

● A child known to have recurrent functional abdominal pain may later present with an acute abdomen and should not be dismissed without adequate reassessment.
● RAP may be an unusual presentation of child sexual abuse. If suspected, the child should be admitted to hospital and the admitting team made aware of your concerns.

BOX 8.5 Management of recurrent abdominal pain (RAP)

- Most children with RAP have mild symptoms which are successfully managed in primary care
- A thorough assessment with full history, examination and investigation should be performed at the outset. Repeated investigations should be avoided unless for new symptoms
- Eliciting parental concerns, explanation and reassurance
- RAP will require follow-up and usually cannot be dealt with in a single consultation. Referral, as shown in Box 8.3, may be required but repeated referral except for new symptoms should be avoided
- Psychogenic causes of RAP should be diagnosed on positive grounds, not simply by excluding organic disease. Once diagnosis is established, it is inappropriate to tell the parents 'the cause is psychological', but it is of great comfort to support the parents by offering reassurance that their child is healthy and the symptom will not affect his/her wellbeing
- Food intolerance/allergy is the second most common cause of RAP (after psychogenic causes). Eliminating the suspected food item (particularly milk or wheat) for about 2 weeks is the best diagnostic and therapeutic tool. Blood or skin testing is of limited value. Addition of dietary fibre has not been shown of value. Referral to a paediatric dietitian should be considered
- Severe cases (e.g. causing frequent absence from school) may require referral for cognitive–behavioural therapy
- Medications have limited value. Analgesics such as paracetamol are frequently prescribed. Peppermint oil may be beneficial for some cases of IBS. Pizotifen appears of some benefit for abdominal migraine but can cause sedation and weight gain

ABDOMINAL DISTENSION

Core messages

➤ Abdominal distension is defined as an increase in girth of the abdomen caused by air, fluid, stool, mass or organomegaly. It is a common clinical finding, particularly in neonates, that must be evaluated carefully.

➤ History is of paramount importance: duration of the distension (acute or chronic), any weight loss, diarrhoea or vomiting; is the vomiting bile-stained?

➤ The priority is to exclude life-threatening surgical causes of abdominal distension such as intestinal obstruction Box 8.6.

Recommended investigations

(Need for investigation is determined by the history and clinical findings.)

➤ FBC, CRP. Blood culture to rule out sepsis.

➤ Plasma protein and albumin, U&E for cases with malabsorption and malnutrition or ascites. Tests for coeliac disease.

➤ A stool microscopy for *Giardia*, pus cells, fat droplets.

➤ Plain abdominal X-ray for intestinal obstruction, calcification in nephroblastoma and detection of faecal masses in severe constipation.

➤ Ultrasound scan to confirm intra-abdominal tumour, renal or ovarian lesions.

➤ Barium enema may suggest Hirschsprung's disease; rectal biopsy confirms it.
➤ CT or MRI to evaluate abdominal masses.
➤ Sweat test for cystic fibrosis.

BOX 8.6 Main causes of abdominal distension

Physiological
- In toddlers (usually mild)

Intestinal causes
- Malabsorption (coeliac disease, cystic fibrosis, *Giardia*)
- Intestinal obstruction
- Constipation
- Hirschsprung's disease

Non-intestinal causes
- Abdominal mass (e.g. neuroblastoma)
- Glycogen storage disease
- Ascites (e.g. nephrotic syndrome)
- Ovarian cyst
- Kwashiorkor (in the tropics)
- Imperforate hymen

PRACTICE POINTS

- Mild abdominal distension in a toddler who is thriving and well is very common and normal.
- A lower intestinal obstruction (e.g. Hirschsprung's disease) usually presents with abdominal distension and late vomiting, while upper intestinal obstruction presents with early vomiting and no or little distension.
- A long history of abdominal distension associated with poor weight gain and loose motions is very suggestive of malabsorption; disaccharidase deficiency and coeliac disease are the most common causes. If the disease becomes chronic, deceleration in height ensues.
- Repeated vomiting may cause bilious vomiting in the absence of intestinal obstruction. However, bilious vomiting usually indicates obstruction below the second part of the duodenum.
- Rare but important causes of abdominal distension in infants and toddlers include neuroblastoma and nephroblastoma.
- Causes of abdominal distension in the tropics differ from those in developed countries; parasites (e.g. *Giardia*, worms) should be considered in children arriving from tropical countries.
- Hydronephrosis and multicystic dysplastic kidney commonly cause abdominal masses, but rarely abdominal distension.

RED FLAGS

- Abdominal distension is usually a sign of serious disease requiring urgent referral, with the exception of physiological abdominal distension in toddlers.

- Malabsorption and coeliac disease often present with failure to thrive or poor weight gain.

RECURRENT VOMITING

Core messages

➤ Vomiting is a forceful action accomplished by a downward contraction of the diaphragm along with tightening of the abdominal muscles against an open sphincter, expelling gastric contents. Unlike vomiting, regurgitation indicates discharge of gastric contents without effort or nausea.

➤ Retching signals the beginning of vomiting. These steps are coordinated by the medullary vomiting centre, which receives afferent signals from the gastrointestinal tract, the blood stream, the equilibrium system of the inner ear and the CNS.

➤ Because vomiting is a very common symptom in children, it should be evaluated in the clinical context with other associated symptoms. Clinicians should assess the severity of the vomiting, looking for signs of dehydration and an underlying cause. In this section, only vomiting as a major symptom is discussed.

BOX 8.7 Gastrointestinal and other causes of vomiting

Gastrointestinal causes
- Swallowed blood or fluid during delivery
- Pyloric stenosis (PS)
- Gastroenteritis
- Appendicitis
- Peptic ulcer
- Intestinal obstruction
- Gastro-oesophageal reflux
- Medications (e.g. antipyretics, antibiotics)
- Inflammatory bowel disease
- Rotavirus and norovirus infection

Cranial causes
- Meningitis
- Increased intracranial pressure (e.g. tumour)
- Subdural haematoma
- Migraine

Systemic causes
- Systemic infection (e.g. pneumonia, urinary tract infection)
- Inborn errors of metabolism (e.g. galactosaemia)
- Periodic syndrome (cyclic vomiting)
- Renal or biliary colic
- Rumination

Recommended investigations

Investigations may include:

➤ Urine for reducing substance to diagnose galactosaemia; blood gases, aminoacids and other metabolic screen tests may be required for inborn error of metabolism.

➤ Blood for FBC, CRP and U&E for more-persistent vomiting. Leucocytosis and high CRP suggest bacterial infection (e.g. sepsis, pneumonia).

➤ Stool for microscopy and culture for significant gastroenteritis.

➤ Abdominal and chest X-ray is useful in intestinal obstruction.

➤ Abdominal ultrasound scan may confirm pyloric stenosis.

PRACTICE POINTS

- About 50% of neonates and infants regurgitate or vomit several times a day after feeding. If they are well otherwise, thriving and the vomit looks like curdled milk, a diagnosis of gastro-oesophageal (GO) reflux can be made.
- Most infants with GO reflux recover by age 6–12 months; rare complications include oesophagitis, aspiration pneumonia and abnormal neck and head posturing (Sandifer syndrome).
- Children with GO reflux vomit during or immediately after feeding, in contrast to pyloric stenosis when the vomiting is delayed for at least 15–30 minutes and is usually projectile, starting in the first 2–3 weeks of life in a baby who appears hungry with visible gastric peristalsis.
- A palpable pyloric 'tumour' (present in about 50% of cases) is pathognomonic for pyloric stenosis. It can be palpated as an 'olive' in the right upper quadrant. Ultrasound is a very useful tool in experienced hands. A pylorus thickness > 4 mm detected by ultrasound scan suggests the diagnosis.
- Pain usually precedes vomiting in appendicitis and intestinal obstruction.
- Cyclic vomiting is characterised by frequent episodic vomiting with symptom-free intervals. A family history of migraine supports the diagnosis. Inborn errors of metabolism should be considered.
- Anti-emetics and antidiarrhoeal drugs should be avoided. Diagnosing the underlying cause of the vomiting is far more important than spending time exploring the British National Formulary (BNF) for anti-emetics. An exception is chemotherapy and occasionally migraine-induced vomiting.
- Management includes fluid replacement (see the section on diarrhoea, below).

RED FLAGS

- Inborn errors of metabolism should be considered in the differential diagnosis of any ill neonate who presents with poor feeding, lethargy, vomiting and convulsion in early life. The condition is often lethal unless prompt treatment is initiated. Early referral is essential.
- Complications from severe vomiting include dehydration, hypochloraemic hypokalaemic alkalosis or bleeding from tears in the distal oesophagus.
- Although bilious vomiting occasionally occurs after severe vomiting, the symptom is serious and usually suggests intestinal obstruction requiring immediate referral.

VOMITING BLOOD (HAEMATEMESIS)

Core messages

➤ Haematemesis is much less common in children than in adults because of the rarity of GI cancers in children. It usually indicates a bleed from a site proximal to the ligament of Treitz of the duodenum (proximal GI tract).

➤ When haematemesis is caused by brisk bleeding, it usually indicates an arterial source, while coffee-grounds emesis results from bleeding that has slowed or stopped, allowing conversion of the red colour of haemoglobin (Hb) to brown haematin by gastric acid.

➤ The causes of haematemesis (Box 8.8) vary accordingly to the age of the child and whether there are other associated symptoms.

➤ Haematemesis (usually associated with nausea, the act of vomiting, pain and possible tenderness of the abdomen) must be differentiated from haemoptysis (associated with cough, frothy colour, crackles on lung auscultation, and evidence of pulmonary disease) and swallowed epistaxis (blood present in the nose, dripping into the posterior nasopharynx).

BOX 8.8 Causes of haematemesis

Swallowed blood
- Swallowed blood from cracked nipple during breast-feeding
- Swallowed maternal blood during birth
- Swallowed blood from e.g. epistaxis

Oesophageal/gastric
- Mallory–Weiss syndrome
- Oesophagitis (GO reflux)
- Oesophageal varices (usually large haematemesis)
- Gastric erosion or ulcer
- Gastric tumour
- Meckel's diverticulum
- Drugs

Systemic
- Haemophilia
- Thrombocytopenia

Recommended investigations
➤ FBC for anaemia suggesting chronic blood loss; thrombocytopenia suggests a haematological cause of the haematemesis.

➤ Coagulation studies (prothrombin time (PT), partial thromboplastin time (PTT), clotting factors, LFTs) for bleeding or coagulation disease.

➤ The Apt test will determine whether the haematemesis is maternal (blood denatures with alkali) or fetal (blood does not denature with alkali) in origin.

➤ Abdomen plain X-ray is useful for necrotising enterocolitis, foreign body.

➤ Abdominal ultrasound scan is the first line of imaging for suspected intussusception; if confirmed, an enema is used for reduction.

➤ Endoscopy for upper GI bleed.

PRACTICE POINTS

- Mallory–Weiss tear (linear laceration at the gastro-oesophageal junction) was described in 1929 in association with alcohol bingeing in adults. GO reflux remains one of the most common causes of this tear in children. Mallory–Weiss tear may occur after a single episode of vomiting. Children with portal hypertension or hepatic insufficiency are at high risk of developing this tear.
- In the majority of cases of haematemesis, the history will suggest the likely diagnosis and the tests required.

- The most common cause of haematemesis in a well full-term baby is the swallowing of maternal blood during delivery or from the breast. Inspection of the mother's breast or expressing of milk will suggest the diagnosis.
- Haematemesis caused by medications, particularly non-steroidal anti-inflammatory drugs (NSAIDs), is underreported; it is always worth taking a detailed history of the recent intake of drugs.
- Management in primary care includes assessing whether or not shock is present (e.g. capillary refill time (CRT), clammy skin, agitation or lethargy, tachycardia with weak pulse, blue fingernails). Resuscitation with IV fluid and urgent admission are needed.

RED FLAGS

- Haematemesis is always a frightening experience for parents. There should be a low threshold for admitting the child.
- Aspirin should not be given to children (except in certain indications, e.g. Kawasaki disease) because of the risk of GI bleeding and Reye's syndrome. Parents may not be aware that many over-the-counter cough remedies and analgesics contain aspirin.

RECTAL PROLAPSE

Core messages

➤ Rectal prolapse (RP) refers to a protrusion of the rectal mucosa through the anus; when the protrusion includes the rectal wall, it is termed procidentia.

➤ RP is usually noted after defecation during the first few years of life. RP is uncommon after the age of 4 years.

➤ RP is more common in tropical and developing countries due to the high prevalence of diarrhoea, malnutrition and parasitic infestation.

➤ One of the most important causes of RP in industrialised countries is cystic fibrosis (it occurs in about 20% of CF patients), and RP is the first manifestation of the disease in one-third of these patients.

BOX 8.9 Conditions associated with RP

Intestinal
- Chronic constipation
- Chronic diarrhoea (e.g. coeliac disease, ulcerative colitis)
- Connective tissue disorders (e.g. Ehlers–Danlos disease)

- Intestinal parasites
- Repair of imperforate anus
- Hirschsprung's disease
- Idiopathic

Systemic
- Malnutrition
- Chronic cough

- Cystic fibrosis
- Meningomyelocele

➤ The primary-care doctor should view RP as a symptom caused by a variety of conditions rather than a specific disease (Box 8.9).

➤ Chronic rectal prolapse can progress to ulceration, bleeding and inflammation (proctitis).

PRACTICE POINTS

- Incidence of rectal prolapse decreases as children grow older, and conservative management is usually successful. Approximately 90% respond to conservative management. Spontaneous resolution is less likely after the age of 4 years.
- Parents should be taught how to reduce rectal prolapse, as it is likely to recur (Box 8.10). Gloves and lubricant should be provided.

BOX 8.10 Management of rectal prolapse (RP)

- A sweat test is indicated in all children with RP who present without a known underlying cause
- Prolonged sitting on a potty and straining in older children should be avoided
- Management is directed towards the underlying cause. Those with constipation should be aggressively treated with laxative and diet, including high-fibre diet
- The prolapse should be reduced promptly after its occurrence. One way to reduce the RP is to hold the prolapsed bowel with lubricated gloved fingers and push it back in with gentle, steady pressure. If the bowel is slightly oedematous, pressure for several minutes may be necessary
- Prompt surgical referral is required for an irreducible prolapse or request routine referral for failed conservative management

---

RED FLAGS

- Rectal prolapse is usually painless or associated with mild discomfort. Pain suggests complications such as ulceration, ischaemia or proctitis.
- RP needs to be differentiated from rarer causes of prolapse resembling RP: prolapsed intussusception, haemorrhoids and prolapsed polyp. The last appears as a dark, plum-coloured mass in contrast to the lighter pink mucosa appearance of an RP.

LOWER GASTROINTESTINAL BLEEDING (RECTAL BLEEDING)

Core messages

➤ Small-intestine bleeding is rare in contrast to bleeding from the upper or lower GI tract.

➤ Beyond the neonatal period, anal fissures are the most common cause of rectal bleeding. These present with painful defecation and small blood streaks on the surface of the stool. Other causes are shown in Box 8.11.

➤ Haematochezia, passage of bright-red blood, usually indicates a bleed from a site below the ligament of Treitz of the duodenum, i.e. the blood has not been in contact with gastric juice.

➤ Bright blood mixed with loose stools suggests a bleeding site above the anus (colitis, e.g. infectious or ulcerative colitis).

➤ Melaena, the passage of black tarry stools, usually indicates an acute upper GI bleed.

BOX 8.11 Main causes of rectal bleeding

Swallowed blood
● Swallowed maternal blood or from epistaxis*

Gastric/oesophageal causes
● Peptic ulcer
● Any cause of haematemesis
● Mallory–Weiss syndrome
● Oesophagitis (GO reflux)

Intestinal causes
● Anal fissure*
● Intussusception*
● Polyps (juvenile colonic polyps, familial adenomatous polyposis coli), haemangioma
● Henoch–Schönlein purpura*
● Colitis, e.g. ulcerative colitis, allergic colitis, bacterial gastroenteritis*
● Sexual abuse causing, e.g. proctitis
● Milk-protein intolerance*
● Meckel's diverticulum
● Drugs*
● Peutz–Jeghers syndrome
● Rectal foreign body
● Haemorrhoids

Systemic causes
● Vitamin K deficiency, e.g. haemorrhagic disease of the newborn
● Thrombocytopenia
● Hereditary haemorrhagic telangiectasia
● Haemolytic uraemic syndrome (HUS)

* These are the commonest causes.

Recommended investigations

➤ FBC: anaemia suggests chronic blood loss or acute massive bleeding or haemolytic uraemic syndrome (HUS). Anaemia with high CRP suggests inflammatory bowel disease; thrombocytopenia suggests disseminated intravascular coagulopathy or idiopathic thrombocytopenic purpura.

➤ LFTs for liver cirrhosis.

➤ High urea and creatinine suggests HUS.

➤ Clotting studies for coagulopathies such as haemophilia.

➤ Apt test to differentiate maternal from fetal blood.

➤ Stool testing for occult blood to confirm or exclude bleeding; culture will rule out infective colitis.

➤ Abdominal plain X-ray is useful in suspected cases of intussusception.

➤ Sigmoidoscopy/colonoscopy is indicated in suspected polyps.

PRACTICE POINTS

- Rectal bleeding in a healthy neonate is most often maternal in origin, with blood swallowed during either delivery or breast-feeding. The baby is well without signs of shock.
- Neonatal peptic ulcer may be caused by hyperalimentation or drugs such as indomethacin, used for patent ductus arteriosus (PDA) closure. Neonatal stress ulcer has been linked with antenatal dexamethasone given for lung maturity in pre-term infants.
- Anorectal disorders such as fissures, distal polyps and haemorrhoids are the most common causes of GI bleeding producing bright-red blood.
- An upper GI bleed can cause bright-red rectal bleeding if the bleeding is massive and the intestinal transient time is short.
- Juvenile colonic polyp is the cause of rectal bleeding in 3–4% of cases and is the commonest GI tumour in childhood. It usually presents between 2 and 8 years of age.
- GI bleeding is less common with Crohn's disease than with ulcerative colitis. The former presents with the triad of anaemia, loss of weight and abdominal pain.
- The most important distinguishing factors in determining the cause of rectal bleeding are: age of the child, the presence or absence of anal pain during blood passage, and the presence or absence of diarrhoea.
- Iron, charcoal, licorice, blueberries and bismuth preparations can cause a black appearance of the stool which may be mistaken as melaena.

RED FLAGS

- Sexual abuse in children may present as GI bleeding, e.g. peri-anal tears, irregular tags, dilated anal tone or proctitis.
- Although juvenile colonic polyps are usually benign, dominantly inherited familial polyposis (familial adenomatous polyposis coli, Gardner syndrome and Peutz–Jeghers syndrome) are pre-malignant polyps requiring referral for possible resection. Children with a positive family history need monitoring and genetic counselling.
- Children with Henoch–Schönlein purpura may present with severe pain, leading to laparotomy. This may occur if the abdominal pain precedes the skin rash and joint manifestations. Therefore, the buttocks, arms and legs should be searched thoroughly for skin petechiae.

PERSISTENT DIARRHOEA

Core messages

➤ Diarrhoea is very common in children and in most cases is infectious in origin. It is defined as an increase in the daily fluid losses of stool, and is usually associated with frequent stools. Acute diarrhoea lasts < 7 days; persistent diarrhoea 1–4 weeks and chronic diarrhoea > 4 weeks. Causes are listed in Box 8.12.

➤ Most diarrhoeal diseases in children living in developed countries are viral, mild and self-limiting, and do not require hospitalisation or laboratory evaluation. In developing countries, diarrhoea is often severe with high mortality.

➤ In young children who are ill enough to require hospitalisation and in those with persistent diarrhoea for > 5 days, laboratory investigation of the stool is indicated to determine the cause of the diarrhoea.

➤ Children presenting with loose, frequent stools may have an infection elsewhere, e.g. UTI or appendicitis.

BOX 8.12 Causes of persistent diarrhoea

Physiological causes
- Breast-fed 'diarrhoea'
- Toddler's 'diarrhoea'

Infectious causes
- *Bacterial*
  - ❭ Enteropathogenic *Escherichia coli*
  - ❭ Enteroaggregative *E. coli*
  - ❭ Non-typhoidal *Salmonella*
- *Virus*
  - ❭ Cytomegalovirus and other viruses
- *Parasites*
  - ❭ *Giardia lamblia*
  - ❭ *Cryptosporidium* spp.
  - ❭ *Ascaris lumbricoides*

Non-infectious causes
- Antibiotics-induced (e.g. pseudomembranous colitis)
- Post-infectious secondary lactose/cow's milk protein intolerance
- Malabsorption (e.g. coeliac disease, cystic fibrosis)
- Inflammatory bowel disease (IBD)
- Overflow in constipation
- Irritable bowel syndrome (IBS)
- Acrodermatitis enteropathica
- Münchausen syndrome by proxy

Recommended investigations
➤ Stool for bacterial culture, and viral antigen (rotavirus).
➤ Stool tested with Clinitest tablet for reducing substances (indicating lactose intolerance if positive).
➤ Blood U&E is indicated if there are signs of dehydration.
➤ HIV test if chronic diarrhoea.

PRACTICE POINTS
- Toddler's diarrhoea is common and may be misdiagnosed as gastroenteritis. These children are healthy and thriving, passing 3–5 soft stools daily which often contain undigested food particles (e.g. carrots, whole peas).
- Mothers are usually good historians. Ask about urine frequency and colour to estimate the degree of dehydration (Table 8.2). The principal complication from diarrhoea is dehydration. If a child is alert and playful, the degree of dehydration is unlikely to be significant.
- Large amounts of watery diarrhoea in association with cramping central abdominal pain and vomiting is typical for gastroenteritis, whereas small frequent stools, lower abdominal pain with blood in stool are very suggestive of colitis. Table 8.3 provides some differential diagnostic clues.

- Persisting diarrhoea is often due to lactose/milk protein intolerance. Temporary withdrawal of milk and dairy products is usually diagnostic and therapeutic. Clinitest confirms the diagnosis of lactose intolerance.

TABLE 8.2 Rapid assessment of severity of dehydration

Mild (3–5%)*	Alert or restless, thirsty, moist or mild dryness of mucous membranes, concentrated urine (orange colour)
Moderate (6–9%)	Restless or lethargic, reduced or absent tears, sunken eyes, skin turgor (reduced skin elasticity), deep respiration, rapid and weak pulse, normal or slightly prolonged capillary refill time (CRT), reduced urine output (oliguria); urine contains ketones
Severe (> 10%)	Circulatory collapse, CRT > 3 seconds

* The percentage refers to loss of bodyweight; there are no symptoms or signs of dehydration if there is < 3% dehydration.

TABLE 8.3 Clues in differentiating some conditions presenting with diarrhoea

Appendicitis	Predominately diffuse abdominal pain, localising later to right iliac fossa (RIF), tenderness and guarding on palpation of abdomen
	Diarrhoea not severe and diminishing
Bacterial gastroenteritis (GE) (usually in summer)	
Shigella, *Escherichia coli* 017:H57, *Yersinia campylobacter*	Systemic manifestations usually present, e.g. high fever, crampy abdominal pain
Amoeba (in endemic areas)	Stool: blood and mucus, no vomiting. Faecal white blood cells (WBCs) present
	High C-reactive protein (CRP), WBCs
Toxigenic *E. coli*, traveller's diarrhoea, cholera, *Clostridium*	Systemic manifestations as above
	Stool: watery, no blood or mucus, absent faecal WBC
Viral GE (usually in winter)	
Rotavirus and norovirus (in winter)	Systemic manifestations usually mild; no or low-grade fever
	Stool: watery diarrhoea with vomiting, no blood
	Normal or mildly elevated CRP, WBCs
Inflammatory bowel disease	
Crohn's disease	Associated intermittent abdominal pain with weight loss, anaemia and high CRP
Ulcerative colitis	Older children (> 10 years of age) are usually affected; relapsing and remitting bloody diarrhoea with mucus
	Stool culture for bacteria negative

Management of diarrhoea

➤ Initial treatment consists of replacement of fluid and electrolyte loss (Table 8.4). This is best accomplished by oral rehydration solution (ORS), e.g. Dioralyte sachets dissolved in 200 ml of fresh drinking water.

➤ Children with signs of moderate or severe dehydration should be admitted to hospital for intravenous fluids.

➤ If lactose intolerance or cow's milk protein intolerance is suspected, extensively hydrolysed formulas (eHFs), such as Nutramigen, are the first choice. Amino acid formulas (AAFs), such as Neocate, are indicated if the child refuses to drink eHF (eHF has a more bitter taste than AAF). The risk of failure with eHF is up to 10% in children with cow's milk protein intolerance.

➤ Antibiotic therapy is usually not required except in:
  ➤ Severe systemic manifestations which suggest a bacterial cause – *Shigella* (trimethoprim-sulfamethoxazole (TMP-SMZ), e.g. Septrin); *Campylobacter* (erythromycin); cholera (doxycycline). *Yersinia* probably requires no antibiotics. *Escherichia coli* species such as enteropathogenic *E. coli* are treated either with TMP-SMZ or a quinolone (e.g. ciprofloxacin).
  ➤ Infants < 3 months of age with *Salmonella* gastroenteritis should be treated with a third-generation cephalosporin or a quinolone, depending on the regional resistance pattern.
  ➤ Patients with *Giardia* and *Entamoeba histolytica* infection are treated with metronidazole. *Cryptosporidium* infection does not require antibiotics.

➤ Vitamin A and zinc supplementation should be considered for those with deficiency.

TABLE 8.4 Fluid replacement in dehydration

Mild dehydration	Oral 50 mL/kg administered over 4 hours, followed by maintenance fluid of:
	100 mL/kg/24 h for children with a bodyweight < 10 kg;
	50–75 mL/kg/24 h for a bodyweight of 10–20 kg;
	20–50 ml/kg/24 h for a bodyweight > 20 kg
	(Fluid replacement can be done at home)
Moderate/severe dehydration	Requires hospitalisation

⚑ RED FLAGS

- Laxative-induced diarrhoea, as seen in Münchausen's syndrome, is rare but should not be missed. The diarrhoea is usually chronic or recurrent. There is an underlying psychiatric disturbance in the carer of the child.
- Intussusception may follow gastroenteritis. A change in the pattern of illness, with more regular, severe paroxysms of abdominal pain, bloody stools and progressive lethargy, will make the diagnosis of gastroenteritis unlikely.
- Assessment of the severity of dehydration is particularly difficult in obese children and in diabetic ketoacidosis (DKA).
- Some children who present with 'diarrhoea' have constipation with overflow. The stools in this case are smaller in volume, adherent and offensive. Symptoms of constipation can be elicited.

CHRONIC CONSTIPATION

Core messages

➤ Constipation is a term used to describe infrequent (< 3 defecations per week) and hard stools which are difficult to pass. It is a common complaint which accounts for some 25% of visits to paediatric gastroenterologists. It is either functional (in 95% of cases) or organic (in 5% of cases). The latter often presents in the first few weeks of life. Usual causes of constipation are listed in 8.13.

➤ Encopresis involves bowel movement in inappropriate places at least once a month for a period of > 3 months in children older than 4 years of age. Peak age is 2–4 years. Faecal soiling involves seepage of stool into the child's underpants.

➤ Physical examination of a child with constipation should routinely include palpation of the abdomen for faecal mass and examination of the anal area for fissure, anorectal malformation (e.g. ectopic anus) and sacral anatomical abnormalities.

➤ In general, breast-fed babies have more frequent stools than bottle-fed babies. However, infrequent defecation may occur in some breast-fed babies who may not have a stool for 5 days and even longer. The stools are usually soft and easy to pass. This is not constipation, and does not require intervention as long as the babies are thriving, feeding well, have no abdominal distension and pass stools without pain or blood. Straining during defecation is normal.

➤ In older children, the most common reason is withholding stool for fear of having a bowel movement following an experience of painful defecation.

BOX 8.13 Usual causes of constipation

Intestinal causes
- Normal variant in breast-fed babies
- Chronic constipation
- Irritable bowel syndrome
- Hirschsprung's disease

Systemic causes
- Prolonged febrile illness with inadequate fluid intake
- Increased output (e.g. polyuria, vomiting)
- Neurodisability (cerebral palsy, myotonica dystrophica)
- Metabolic (e.g. hypercalcaemia, renal tubular acidosis, hypokalaemia)
- Anal fissure
- Hypothyroidism
- Drugs, such as narcotics, antidepressants
- Lead poisoning
- Botulism

RECOMMENDED INVESTIGATIONS

Investigations which may be considered include:

➤ Urinalysis to exclude associated UTI.

➤ Thyroid function tests (TFTs), serum calcium, U&E to exclude hypothyroidism, hypercalcaemia or hypokalaemia.

➤ Serum lead level if clinically indicated.

➤ Plain abdominal X-ray, which may show distended rectum (megacolon).

➤ MRI for spinal cord disorders such as tethered spinal cord, which is a malformation of the spinal cord often associated with spina bifida.

➤ Rectal biopsy if there is clinical suspicion of Hirschsprung's disease.

PRACTICE POINTS

- Over 90% of healthy neonates pass a stool in the first 24–48 hours of life; a delay of > 48 hours is abnormal.
- Although rectal examination should not be a routine procedure in paediatric practice, it is indicated in suspected Hirschsprung's disease: an empty rectum may suggest the diagnosis while a rectum full of hard stool suggests chronic constipation. Before performing rectal examination, explain the procedure and the reason for it to the child and parents, and offer a chaperone.
- Faecal soiling may be mistaken as diarrhoea. Parents should receive information about the mechanism causing the stool overflow. This is to be differentiated from diarrhoea by:
  - ○ Frequent small quantities of stool, which are sticky and hard to remove
  - ○ Symptoms (such as painful defecation, passing hard stools) and signs (such as palpable stool masses in the abdomen, anal fissure) of constipation are present.
- By far the most common cause of constipation is functional. Organic diseases, including Hirschsprung's disease (failure to thrive with distended abdomen), hypothyroidism (other symptoms and signs are usually present), hypercalcaemia (elfin face in hypercalcaemia), renal tubular acidosis (failure to thrive, vomiting), are rare in practice.
- Children with constipation typically withhold stool to avoid painful defecation. Parents wrongly interpret this as pushing. Doctors should give an explanation why this is not the case.
- Stool impaction is common; symptoms include:
  - ○ Child has not passed a stool for days but frequently soils with liquid overflow
  - ○ Child is uncomfortable and distressed, often not eating well
  - ○ Impacted stool masses on palpation of the abdomen.

Management of constipation is shown in Box 8.14.

BOX 8.14 Guidelines on management of constipation

- Exclude organic causes of constipation by history and physical examination
- Parents of chronically constipated children should be told that there is usually no quick solution for constipation, and long-term treatment is often required: while 60–70% of children recover within 1–2 years, some 30% may need longer-term treatment with laxatives
- Faecal soiling (involuntary seepage of a small amount of stool) is usually caused by chronic rectal retention. It is treated by evacuating the rectum and laxatives for several months (see below). Constipation is often under-treated with inadequate doses of laxatives given for too short a time
- Routine radiography and anorectal manometry are not recommended for evaluation of children with constipation
- Encourage a diet rich in fibre, e.g. porridge or high-fibre cereals such as Weetabix or Shredded Wheat, and fruit with every meal. Sweets and desserts should not be offered until the child has eaten a piece of fruit

- Increase fluid intake in the form of water as the main drink. Squash, fizzy drinks and milk (in toddlers and older children) should be limited

Medications

- Osmotic laxatives such as macrogols (also called polyethylene glycols; such as Movicol Paediatric Plain) or lactulose
- Stimulants, e.g. sodium picosulphate, senna and sodium docusate, are usually prescribed in addition to osmotic laxatives
- For stool impaction, Movicol Paediatric Plain is very useful:
  - › 2 sachets on day 1
  - › 4 sachets for 2 days
  - › 6 sachets for 2 days
  - › 8 sachets for 2 days
  - › A child older than 5 years can take up to 12 sachets daily.

Each sachet should be mixed in a quarter of a glass of water; total daily dose to be taken over a 12-hour period

Based on NICE guidelines.[1]

Referral to secondary care is required in:
- ➤ A baby who has not passed a stool after 48 hours
- ➤ Vomiting, abdominal distension, severe stool impaction, suspected child abuse, e.g. peri-anal injury or ulceration, severe abdominal pain
- ➤ An associated abnormal neurological finding
- ➤ Weight loss, failure to thrive, associated urinary symptoms
- ➤ Failure to respond to treatment.

RED FLAGS

- Chronic constipation with overflow is often overlooked and undertreated.
- It is important to differentiate organic causes from the much more common functional causes: the former usually manifest during the first few weeks of life with features which include delay in passing meconium, failure to thrive, and abdominal distension.

JAUNDICE

Core messages

- ➤ Physiological jaundice (apparent clinically in natural sunlight if total bilirubin is > 35 μmol/L) affects almost all neonates during the first few days of life. The hyper-bilirubinaemia is always indirect, i.e. unconjugated.
- ➤ Jaundice appearing after 3 or 4 days of life suggests an infection, e.g. UTI or sepsis.
- ➤ Jaundice in neonates after the first week of life suggests breast-milk jaundice, biliary atresia, infection or metabolic disorders, e.g. galactosaemia or hypothyroidism (Box 8.15).
- ➤ After the neonatal period, viral hepatitis remains the most common cause of jaundice

worldwide. Hepatitis A virus (HAV) used to be a common infectious disease, but its incidence has declined significantly in developed countries.

➤ The prevalence of hepatitis B (HBV) and C (HCV) and other hepatotropic viruses has increased worldwide, causing chronic liver disease and primary hepatocellular carcinoma. An estimated 300 000 new cases of HBV infection occur in the USA each year.

➤ The most important risk factor for acquisition of HBV is vertical transmission from an infected mother to her infant. In mothers who are positive for both HBsAg and HBeAg antigens, approximately 90% of their infants become chronically infected if untreated.

➤ Xanthochromia (carotenaemia) caused by excessive carotene deposits in the skin can mimic jaundice.

BOX 8.15 Common causes of jaundice

Neonatal period
- Physiological
- Haemolytic (e.g. Rh or ABO incompatibility, spherocytosis)
- Breast-milk jaundice
- Congenital hepatitis (e.g. cytomegalovirus, toxoplasmosis)
- Crigler–Najjar syndrome
- Biliary atresia

Infancy and childhood
- Infection
  > Infectious hepatitis (e.g. HAV, HBV), malaria, mononucleosis, leptospirosis, brucellosis, typhoid fever, yellow fever
- Metabolic/endocrine causes
  > Wilson disease, galactosaemia, hypothyroidism
- Drug/herbal-induced
  > E.g. paracetamol overdose
  > Reye syndrome
- Miscellaneous
  > Gilbert's syndrome, autoimmune hepatitis, obstructive jaundice (e.g. by gallstones), cystic fibrosis, Dubin–Johnson syndrome and Rotor syndrome

---

Recommended investigations

(The tests below should be considered if the jaundice is high, persistent or unexplained.)

➤ Urine: Clinitest for reducing substances will suggest galactosaemia, and culture to confirm UTI.

➤ FBC: Hb low in haemolysis; leucocytosis suggests infection; reticulocytosis suggests haemolysis.

➤ LFTs: conjugated hyperbilirubinaemia (normal: < 20% of the total bilirubin of < 17 µmol/L) indicates hepatocellular disease such as hepatitis. Unconjugated hyperbilirubinaemia with otherwise normal LFTs (including transaminases) is very suggestive of Gilbert's syndrome. Positive direct Coombs' test on the infant suggests ABO or Rh– incompatibility.

➤ Serological tests for hepatitis viruses.

➤ Blood group and Rh status of the mother and infant.

➤ Tests for intrauterine infections (TORCH complex (toxoplasmosis, other, rubella, cytomegalovirus, herpes simplex))).

➤ Abdominal ultrasound scan to rule out bile obstruction (e.g. choledochal cyst).

➤ Other tests include isotope scan with technetium, and liver biopsy.

PRACTICE POINTS

- Breast-milk jaundice (incidence 15–40% in breast-fed infants) is simply physiological jaundice, which may persist for weeks. It is not a disease and mothers should be encouraged to continue breast-feeding as long as the child is thriving with normal stool colour and is otherwise asymptomatic. It is a diagnosis of exclusion.

- There is a lack of correlation between bilirubin levels and kernicterus in pre-term infants, i.e. kernicterus can occur at lower levels of bilirubin in these infants because of altered permeability of the blood–brain barrier by hypoxia, hypoglycaemia and other risk factors.

- There is no evidence that a well full-term baby without haemolysis will get any ill-effects from a bilirubin < 400 μmol/L.

- Direct-reacting (conjugated) bilirubin is water-soluble, not fat-soluble, and therefore it does not damage the brain tissue to cause kernicterus. It is, however, associated with serious diseases, such as congenital hepatitis and biliary atresia.

- Infectious hepatitis is the most common cause of jaundice worldwide. Jaundice is present in only 10–20% of those with HAV; in 25% of those with HBV and in <1 in 3 of cases of HCV (anicteric hepatitis). A child with jaundice should therefore not be diagnosed with hepatitis on the basis of hyperbilirubinaemia. An increased transaminase level is essential in diagnosing hepatitis. Differentiation of common causes of jaundice is shown in Table 8.5.

- A neonate born to an HBsAg-positive mother should receive three HBV vaccines: the 1st dose accompanied by 0.5 mL of hepatitis B immune globulin (HBIG) before leaving the nursery, the 2nd dose at age 1 month and the 3rd dose 6 months after the 1st dose. Guidelines for vaccination are provided in Table 8.6 and Box 8.16.

- Extra-hepatic symptoms of a child with HBV infection include arthralgia, urticaria, arteritis, glomerulonephritis and aplastic anaemia.

- Gilbert's syndrome is the most common cause of unconjugated hyperbilirubinaemia in older children, affecting up to 5% of the population. It is an autosomal recessive condition caused by reduced activity of the enzyme glucuronyltransferase. It is a benign condition and should be differentiated from haemolytic disease (by an increased reticulocyte count).

- Neonates with jaundice should have a serum bilirubin estimation (usually done by the midwife).

Indication for referral should include the following:

➤ Infants with a total bilirubin > 285 μmol/L or a conjugated bilirubin > 25 μmol/L.

➤ Any child with jaundice who is unwell or feverish.

➤ Unexplained or prolonged jaundice.

➤ Jaundice due to hepatocellular or haemolytic disease.

RED FLAGS

- A conjugated bilirubin of 34 μmol/L or greater indicates serious disease and is never physiological. It may be caused by neonatal hepatitis secondary to congenital infection (e.g. rubella, cytomegalovirus) or biliary atresia. It is urgent to determine the cause of direct hyperbilirubinaemia in an infant before irreversible damage to the liver occurs. Urgent referral is essential.
- Babies born to parents from parts of the world where HBV is endemic are offered three HBV vaccinations as above, but not HBIG.

TABLE 8.5 Differential diagnosis of common causes of jaundice

Disease	Distinguishing features	Diagnosis
Hepatitis A, B	80% are asymptomatic	Abnormal LFT, high serum transaminases, positive for IgM
	When symptomatic: mild fever, malaise, nausea, abdominal pain, dark urine and acholic stool	
Mononucleosis	100% fever, pharyngitis, lymphadenitis	Positive for EBV-IgM, monospot
Gilbert's syndrome	Usually asymptomatic and discovered by ↑ indirect bilirubin; otherwise normal LFT; normal reticulocyte	Accident; occasionally presents with fatigue and mild abdominal pain
Haemolytic anaemia (e.g. G6PD deficiency)	Usually asymptomatic; haemolysis in response to an infection, food (broad beans/favism) or drugs	Hyperbilirubinaemia is indirect with high reticulocytosis
Drug-induced hepatitis	Symptoms similar to those in infectious hepatitis	Abnormal LFT, negative IgM for viruses, history of drug intake
Autoimmune hepatitis	Symptoms similar to those in infectious hepatitis, pallor because of anaemia	Positive auto-antibodies, anaemia
Yellow skin	Asymptomatic, no jaundice of the sclera	Normal LFT

EBV = Epstein–Barr virus; IgM = immunoglobulin M; LFT= liver function test

TABLE 8.6 Interpretation of screening tests for HBV

Tests	Results	Interpretation
HBsAg	Negative	Susceptible
Anti-HBc	Negative	
Anti-HBs	Negative	
HBsAg	Negative	Immune due to natural infection
Anti-HBc	Positive	
Anti-HBs	Positive	
HBsAg	Negative	Immune due to HBV – Hepatitis B vaccination
Anti-HBc	Negative	
Anti-HBs	Positive	

Tests	Results	Interpretation
HBsAg	Positive	Acutely infected
Anti-HBc	Positive	
IgM-anti-HBc	Positive	
Anti-HBs	Negative	
HBsAg	Positive	Chronically infected
Anti-HBc	Positive	
IgM-anti-HBc	Negative	
Anti-HBs	Negative	

BOX 8.16 Guidelines for HBV vaccination

Babies whose mothers have had acute hepatitis B during pregnancy or are positive for HBsAg should have immediately after delivery:
- Hepatitis B vaccination, and
- Hepatitis B immunoglobulin given at the same time but preferably at a different site

Babies whose mothers are positive for HBsAg and for e-antigen should receive:
- Vaccination only
- Hepatitis B immunoglobulin given in addition if the baby is < 1.5 kg bodyweight

Vaccine should also be given to children at high risk of contracting hepatitis B, including:
- If close family contacts are carriers of HBsAg
- Haemophilia
- Chronic liver disease or renal disease including those receiving haemodialysis
- Patients of daycare or residential accommodation or custodial institutions
- Foster carers and their families
- Adopted from countries with a high prevalence of HBV

REFERENCE

1. Diagnosis and management of childhood constipation: summary of NICE guidance. BMJ 2010; 340. www.bmj.com/content/340/bmj.c2585.full

CHAPTER 9

Respiratory diseases

RESPIRATORY NOISES

Core messages

➤ Respiratory noises are extremely common and often difficult to differentiate from each other. Children may make multiple noises at a given time, which can be intermittent or alternating within minutes. The noise may also depend on the child's sleeping position (polyphonic noises) or whether he/she is awake or asleep.

➤ Clinicians should be familiar with a few common noises including snuffle, wheeze, stridor, rattle, grunt and snore (Table 9.1). An error in recognising specific types of noise will lead to diagnostic and therapeutic errors.

➤ Imitating a wheeze, stridor or whoop to parents can be a help in identifying the right noise.

➤ Snuffles and stridor are caused by obstruction of the extrathoracic airways (nose, pharynx, larynx and the extrathoracic portion of the trachea), while wheezing is caused by intrathoracic obstruction.

TABLE 9.1 Summary of common respiratory noises

Noise	Description
Snuffles	Commonly due to a blocked nose in children < 6 months of age, usually caused by normal mucus collected in the nose and not by infection
	No treatment is usually required. Increased humidity, frequent smaller feeds and saline drops may help
Wheeze	Indicates intrathoracic airway obstruction, heard mainly during expiration.
	Bronchodilators are the mainstay of treatment
Stridor	Consists of harsh inspiratory sound caused by extrathoracic airway obstruction. Acute stridor with involvement of the vocal cords (hoarseness) is usually caused by croup; without vocal cord involvement is usually caused by laryngomalacia. Epiglottitis is a rare but potentially life-threatening disease
Rattle	Coarse irregular sound mainly heard in inspiration, caused by secretions in the trachea or major bronchi subsequent to viral (rarely bacterial) infection and, occasionally, gastro-oesophageal reflux or sputum retention often found in neuromuscular diseases
Snore	Inspiratory and irregular noise caused by partial obstruction of the naso-oro-pharynx
Grunt	Short expiratory sound caused by partial closure of the glottis during expiration. It is an important sign of pneumonia

PRACTICE TIPS

- Acute snuffles are mostly caused by a viral infection; if persistent, this may be due to allergic rhinitis, adenoid hypertrophy or 'normal' snuffly noises of infancy.
- Persistent snuffles are inspiratory and nasal, and are so common in early infancy that they can be regarded as normal. They are often misdiagnosed as a 'cold'. They normally resolve by 6 months of age.
- In older children with persistent nasal snuffles, polyps need to be excluded. Cystic fibrosis is an important underlying cause.
- The term 'snuffles' was first used for children with congenital syphilis. Although this infection is rare, it is on the rise. It mainly presents with the triad of anaemia, snuffle and splenomegaly.
- Expiratory grunts are usually a more serious sign associated with respiratory distress syndrome in neonates and pneumonia in older children.
- The association of hoarseness and stridor suggests an obstruction at the vocal cords of the larynx, such as in croup. Hoarseness in laryngomalacia is not present because the vocal cords are not involved. If a cough is present, it suggests the trachea is involved.
- Laryngomalacia is the most common cause of chronic stridor, usually starting soon after birth and resolving at the age of 12–18 months. It does not require laryngoscopy unless there are atypical features such as failure to thrive, persistent cough, hoarseness of the voice or feeding problems.

STRIDOR

Core messages

➤ Stridor occurs subsequent to an acute upper airway obstruction, commonly caused by viral infection (croup or laryngotracheobronchitis), or without a history or the presence of fever or signs of a viral infection (spasmodic croup). Other causes are listed in Box 9.1.

➤ Symptoms of viral croup and spasmodic croup are usually mild and transient, and recovery within a few days is the likely outcome. Management of less-severe degrees of upper airway obstruction is shown in Box 9.2.

➤ More-severe degrees of obstruction occur with bacterial infection and produce

---

BOX 9.1 Main causes of stridor

Acute transient stridor

- Laryngotracheobronchitis (viral croup)
- Spasmodic croup
- Angioedema
- Epiglottitis
- Bacterial tracheitis (staphylococcal infection)
- Aspiration of foreign body
- Laryngospasm (hypocalcaemic tetany)

Persistent stridor

- Laryngomalacia
- Vocal cord paralysis
- Tumour, e.g. papilloma, haemangioma, nodule

rapidly progressive respiratory distress, worsening cough, irritability, restlessness, nasal flaring, subcostal and intercostal recession, and potential risk of death.

➤ The obstruction is more serious in infants and young children than in older children because of the smaller airway.

🚩 RED FLAGS

- A child with croup who rapidly becomes unwell with high fever has either developed an extension of the infection into the respiratory tract, bacterial tracheitis as a complication of the viral croup, or has bacterial epiglottis. Urgent admission is required.
- In contrast to viral croup, epiglottitis is a potentially lethal condition because of rapidly progressing obstruction leading to severe hypoxia. The voice is muffled or there may be a mild stridor. Typically the child has not been immunised against *Haemophilus influenzae*. Urgent referral is required.
- In cases of viral croup or epiglottitis, throat inspection, including the use of a tongue depressor, may result in sudden cardiorespiratory arrest and therefore should be omitted.
- A young child (typically 6 months to 2 years of age) with sudden choking or coughing which may occur with or without stridor or hoarseness should be suspected of having a foreign body.

BOX 9.2 Management of croup

- Most children with acute viral croup or spasmodic croup can be managed at home
- The child should be disturbed as little as possible. If admission becomes necessary, a parent should be allowed to stay with the child
- The child should be observed carefully for worsening symptoms of respiratory distress
- The use of steam from a shower or vaporiser at home is often effective
- Drug treatment of croup includes:
  - ❯ Budesonide administered by nebuliser, 2 mg as a single dose or in 2 divided doses separated by 30 minutes. This can be repeated in 12 hours
  - ❯ Dexamethasone 0.15 mg/kg or prednisolone soluble 1–2 mg/kg administered by mouth in primary care or before a transfer to hospital
- Nebulised adrenaline is indicated for severe croup. This should not be administered in primary care; urgent referral is essential
- Antibiotic treatment is not indicated for viral or spasmodic croup
- **Urgent admission** to hospital is indicated in cases of:
  - ❯ Suspected epiglottitis
  - ❯ Progressive or severe stridor
  - ❯ Marked tachypnoea, as this may be the first sign of hypoxia
  - ❯ Severe respiratory distress (e.g. obvious suprasternal recession)
  - ❯ Restless or drowsy child
  - ❯ High fever or toxic-appearing child
  - ❯ Feeding or swallowing difficulty
  - ❯ Poor air entry on auscultation
  - ❯ Concerned parents

UNEXPLAINED SHORTNESS OF BREATH AND ASTHMA

Core messages

➤ Dyspnoea is a common symptom of a variety of cardiopulmonary diseases (Box 9.3). Asthma is the most common cause. In older children, psychological factors are often the underlying cause. Congestive cardiac failure is an important but rare cause of dyspnoea at any age of childhood.

➤ Dyspnoea rarely occurs in isolation. Accompanying features include cough, wheezing, tachypnoea and subcostal recession.

➤ Children may describe dyspnoea as 'getting tired easily', or 'can't keep up with other kids'. It may occur spontaneously or during certain activities such as exercise, or during feeding in infants.

➤ Wheezing is not usually a symptom of pneumonia, while grunting with flaring of alae nasi is a very important sign of pneumonia.

➤ The differentiation between cardiac and pulmonary causes of dyspnoea can be difficult. The presence of a murmur, liver enlargement and relative tachycardia favours cardiac causes. Oxygen saturation usually improves rapidly with administration of oxygen in pulmonary disease, but makes little difference in cardiac disease.

BOX 9.3 Main causes of severe dyspnoea

- Pulmonary:
  - ❭ Undiagnosed asthma
  - ❭ Viral-induced wheeze/ bronchiolitis
  - ❭ Pneumonia
  - ❭ Pulmonary oedema
  - ❭ Pulmonary embolism
  - ❭ Inhaled foreign body
  - ❭ Pleural effusion
  - ❭ Congenital malformations, including hypoplasia
  - ❭ Pneumothorax

- Cardiac:
  - ❭ Congestive cardiac failure (CCF)
  - ❭ Myocarditis, pericarditis
  - ❭ Hypertrophic obstructive cardiomyopathy
- Metabolic acidosis such as diabetic ketoacidosis
- Neuromuscular
- Psychogenic

Recommended investigations

➤ Initial assessment should include:
  - ➤ oxygen saturation monitoring (oximetry)
  - ➤ respiratory rate
  - ➤ peak expiratory flow rate
  - ➤ blood gases in severe cases when admitted to hospital.

➤ Spirometry can differentiate between *obstructive* (decrease in flow) and *restrictive* (decreased lung volume) causes of chronic dyspnoea.

➤ Chest X-ray is a helpful investigation. It may show hyperinflation (asthma, bronchiolitis); collapse or consolidation (pneumonia); pneumothorax. However, a chest X-ray in the absence of a clinical indication should not be part of the initial diagnostic work-up, to avoid radiation exposure.

➤ Echocardiography and ECG in patients with suspected heart disease.

PRACTICE TIPS

- Enquire about symptoms associated with exercise such as running, cycling or exposure to cooler weather.
- An important cause of dyspnoea is bronchiolitis and bronchitis. A clear distinction between them in the first 2 years of life is difficult and usually of no therapeutic significance. Antibiotic treatment is administered if there is evidence of bacterial infection, such as an unwell child with fever of >39°C or pulmonary infiltration on a chest X-ray.
- Features that favour bacterial rather than viral pneumonia:
  - Absence of upper respiratory tract infection
  - More-rapid and severe symptoms
  - Absence of wheeze
  - Fever > 38.5°C
  - Tachypnoea – although this sign is present in both types of pneumonia (Table 9.2), the respiratory rate tends to be higher in bacterial than in viral pneumonia.
- The decision to refer to hospital a child with dyspnoea due to asthma can sometimes be difficult. As a guide, oxygen saturation in air of > 95% and peak expiratory flow measurements of > 70% of expected (in a child > 5 years of age) suggest that the child can be managed at home.
- Dyspnoea during exercise is frequently caused by asthma. Measurement of the peak expiratory flow (PEF) in children > 5 years of age before and after exercise supports the diagnosis.
- If psychogenic hyperventilation or dyspnoea is suspected, especially in adolescent girls, enquire about other related symptoms such as swallowing difficulty, suggesting globus. Respiratory rate and oxygen saturation are normal.
- Management of dyspnoea includes identifying any underlying cause and reassurance of the patient. If the diagnosis is unclear, a trial with a bronchodilator may be justified.

TABLE 9.2 Normal and abnormal respiratory rates in children

Age	Respiratory rate (breaths/min)	WHO definition of pneumonia (value for respiratory rate, breaths/min)
< 2 months	40–50	> 60
< 1 year	30–40	> 50
1–2 years	25–35	> 40
2–5 years	25–30	> 40
5–12 years	20–25	> 40 for older children
>12 years	15–20	

ASTHMA

Asthma is diagnosed by recurrent episodes of coughing and wheezing, usually triggered by exercise, viral infection or inhaled allergens. Diagnostic features of asthma are provided in Box 9.4. Although most children who present with recurrent wheezing and cough have asthma, conditions mimicking airway obstruction are listed in Table 9.3.

BOX 9.4 Clinical diagnostic features of asthma

- More than one of the following symptoms: wheeze, cough, dyspnoea, chest tightness, particularly if these are frequent and recurrent; are worse at night; occur in response to pets, cold or damp air, or with emotions
- Personal and family history of atopic disease
- Response to bronchodilators or inhaled or oral steroids (2 mg/kg daily to maximum of 40 mg) for 2 weeks supports the diagnosis. Alleviation of symptoms usually occurs 3–7 days after initiation
- Over the age of 6 years, ask the patient to perform and record serial peak flow measurements at home. Variability > 20% is diagnostic

---

TABLE 9.3 Summary of main conditions mimicking asthma

Disease	Diagnostic clinical clues
Cystic fibrosis	Is the second most common chronic airway disease after asthma (incidence: 1 in 2500)
	Severity and progression of the disease is highly variable: respiratory symptoms may not appear until adolescence; symptoms and signs of malabsorption may not be present.
	Finger clubbing is an important diagnostic clue
	Little or no response (clinical and lung function) to a short course of bronchodilator and steroids
Ciliary dyskinisia	Persistent cough almost since birth, in association with persistent or recurrent otitis media
	Situs inversus (Kartagener's syndrome) is present in about 50% of patients
	May present with purulent sputum production due to bronchiectasis
Foreign body	Commonest in 1- to 3-year-olds, the child being previously asymptomatic
	There is usually sudden onset of respiratory distress with choking, cough and asymmetric air entry or wheezing
	Symptoms may persist or disappear for a period to present later with abscess formation, bronchiectasis or pneumonia
	An obstructing object may occlude a bronchus causing atelectasis, which can be detected by dullness on lung percussion, diminished air entry on lung auscultation and typical opacity with well-defined margins on a chest X-ray
Hyperventilation	Usually in adolescents, commoner in girls
	Normal examination of the cardiopulmonary system, normal respiratory rate and normal lung function tests
Immunodeficiency	Recurrent pneumonia, often pyogenic; other recurrent infections
Gastro-oesophageal reflux	Co-existing gastrointestinal symptoms such as vomiting causing aspiration

Management of asthma in primary care

➤ Initial management of a child presenting with asthma is shown in Figure 9.1.

➤ Once the diagnosis of asthma is established, the clinical course will be mild inter-mittent, mild, moderate or severe persistent asthma (Figure 9.2).

➤ Treatment of acute asthma:

> For **mild asthma** attack: 2–4 puffs of salbutamol 100 mcg repeated every 20–40 minutes. Up to 10 puffs may be needed for more-severe attacks, via a spacer. There should be minimal delay between actuation and inhalation. Older children may prefer to use a dry-powder inhaler (DPI) that eliminates the need to coordinate taking a breath and squeezing the canister.

> For a **more severe attack**, increase the salbutamol dose by 2 puffs every 2 minutes according to response, up to 10 puffs.

> Children with an **acute asthma attack at home and symptoms not controlled** by up to 10 puffs or 2.5 mg of nebulised salbutamol should seek urgent medical attention. Additional doses of bronchodilator should be given as needed whilst awaiting transfer to hospital.

➤ Patients with asthma should be offered a self-management plan that focuses on indi-vidual needs, reinforced by a written personalised action plan. Useful action in this plan includes:

> PEF < 80% best necessitates increase of the inhaled steroid

> PEF < 60% best necessitates commencing oral steroid

> PEF < 40% best necessitates seeking urgent medical help.

➤ Good asthma control is associated with low bronchodilator use (less than once a day). Use of 2 or more canisters per month of a beta$_2$ agonist or >10–12 puffs/day is a marker of poorly controlled asthma. High usage of beta$_2$ agonist necessitates review of asthma management.

➤ **Inhaled corticosteroids** (ICSs) are the most effective medication for controlling asthma symptoms by reducing inflammation in the airways. ICSs at or above 400 mcg beclomethasone (BDP) or budesonide per day may be associated with systemic side-effects, including growth impairment and adrenal suppression. Indications for adding corticosteroids are:

> using an inhaled beta$_2$ agonist 3 times a week or more

> patient symptomatic 3 times or more per week

> patient waking 1 night per week, or

> exacerbations of asthma in the last 2 years, e.g. severe exacerbations requiring admission, use of nebuliser or oral corticosteroids.

➤ A starting dose of ICS should be 50–200 mcg twice daily. The dose can be titrated to the lowest effective dose. ICS is more effective when taken twice daily. Some patients with milder asthma and good control can be managed on once daily ICS.

➤ Early use of **oral corticosteroids** in acute asthma can reduce the need for hospital admission. Their effect becomes apparent within 3–4 hours. A soluble preparation of prednisolone is available for those who are unable to swallow tablets. A suitable dose is prednisolone 20 mg for children aged 2–5 years and prednisolone 30–40 mg for those older than 5 years. Patients prone to frequent severe exacerbation should be given an emergency supply of these tablets.

➤ Monitoring of asthmatic children is shown in Box 9.5. Children with asthma should be reviewed regularly by a nurse or doctor with appropriate training in asthma management.

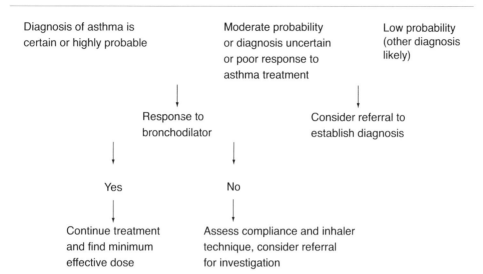

FIGURE 9.1 Summary of initial management of asthma in the primary-care setting

---

BOX 9.5 Annual review of a child with asthma should include:

- Symptoms score
- Exacerbations, oral steroid use, and absence from school/nursery
- Inhaler technique and assessment of inhaler device suitability
  - Children < 3 years of age are likely to require a spacer with attached facemask:
    - Shake the canister for 5 seconds
    - Hold the mask snugly to the face
    - Press down the canister with the index finger
    - If possible, the child inhales slowly and deeply through the mouth
    - If a second inhalation is required, wait 15–30 seconds between puffs. Shake the canister again
  - Spacers should be:
    - Used in children aged 0–5 years
    - Washed in detergent monthly and allowed to dry in air
    - Replaced every 6–12 months if plastic
    - Used for ICS (under 5 years and 5–15 years). The same spacer may also be used for a beta$_2$ agonist
- Concordance (assessed e.g. by reviewing prescription refill frequency)
- Possession of and use of self-management plan
- Exposure to tobacco smoke
- Peak expiratory flow (PEF) record-keeping (using e.g. Mini-Wright peak flow meter), in writing. Normal lung function is present when the PEF is >80% of predicted
- Growth (weight and height centiles)

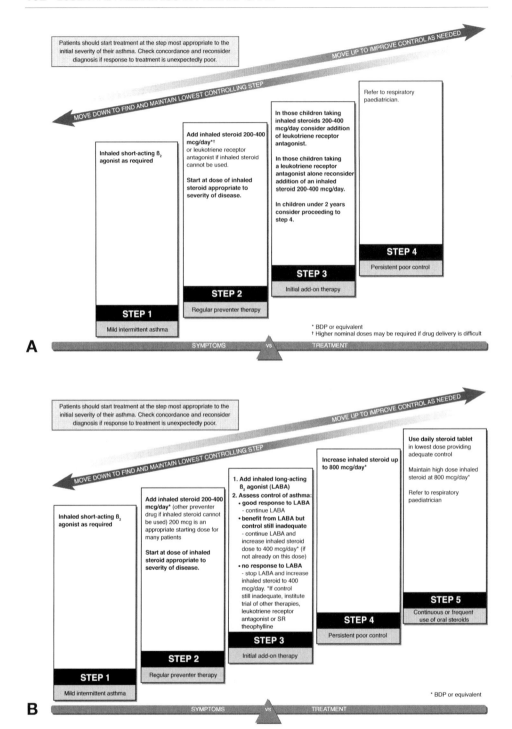

FIGURE 9.2 A: Summary of stepwise management of asthma in children less than 5 years; B: Summary of stepwise management of asthma in children aged 5–12 years. Based on the recommendations of the British Thoracic Society[1] (www.brit-thoracic.org.uk)

BOX 9.6 Common discussion points

Breast milk

A systematic review and meta-analysis involving 8183 children followed for at least 4 years revealed a significant protective effect of breast-feeding against the development of asthma, particularly in children with a family history of atopy.[1] In conclusion: breast-feeding for at least 6 months should be encouraged. Modified milk formulae using hydrolysates have not shown any consistent significant long-term benefits

Foods

There is conflicting data on the association between early introduction of allergenic foods into the infant diet and the subsequent development of allergies; no evidence was identified in relation to asthma

Probiotics

There is absence of evidence of benefit for their use

Immunotherapy

Can be considered in patients with asthma where a clinically significant allergen cannot be avoided. The potential of severe allergic reactions must be fully discussed with patients

Breathing exercises

May be considered for chronic asthma. There are trends for improvement (reduction in bronchodilator use and acute exacerbations) and in quality of life measurements[2]

Aeroallergen avoidance

There is no consistent evidence of benefit from domestic aeroallergen avoidance. Measures to decrease house dust mites have not been shown to have an effect on asthma severity. Families with evidence of house dust mite allergy and who wish to reduce allergen exposure should do the following:
- Have complete-barrier bed-covering systems
- Removal of carpets
- Removal of soft toys from bed
- High-temperature washing of bed linens
- Apply acaricides (pesticides) to soft furnishings
- Have good ventilation with or without dehumidification

Damp and mould

Can cause worsening asthma and should be treated.[3]

Prognosis

The earlier the onset of wheeze, the better the prognosis. The majority of children presenting before the age of 2 years become asymptomatic in mid-childhood. Co-existing atopy is a risk factor for persistence independent of age of presentation.

RED FLAGS

Children who require ≥800 mcg/day BDP/budesonide or ≥400 mcg fluticasone should:
- Have a specific written advice (e.g. steroid alert card) in the event of a severe intercurrent illness or surgery.
- Be under the care of a paediatrician for the duration of treatment.

BOX 9.7 Indication for specialist referral (*see* also Fig 9.1)

- Moderate or severe asthma attack (Table 9.4)
- Failure to respond to asthma treatment, particularly inhaled steroid of >400 mcg/day or frequent use of oral steroids
- Diagnosis unclear or in doubt
- Symptoms present since birth, or symptoms related to perinatal problems
- Persistent wet or productive cough
- Excessive vomiting or possetting
- Failure to thrive
- Nasal polyps
- Unexpected clinical findings (e.g. focal signs, inspiratory stridor, dysphagia)
- Parental anxiety or need for reassurance

(Children transported to hospital by ambulance should be treated with oxygen and beta$_2$ agonists during the journey)

TABLE 9.4 The three degrees of severity of asthma in children > 5 years of age

Symptom	Mild	Moderate	Severe
Pulse rate (beats/min)	<120	120–170	>170
Respiratory rate (breaths/min)	<40	40–70	>70
SaO$_2$	>94%	90–94%	<90%
PEF*	>70% of predicted	50–70% of predicted	<50% of predicted
Drowsiness	No	No	Agitated or drowsy
PCO$_2$	Decreased	Normal	Increased
Speech in:	Sentences	Phrases	Difficult or unable to say phrases or words
Subcostal recession	Mild	Moderate	Severe

*Peak expiratory flow measurement can be carried out by children aged ≥5 years.

PCO$_2$ = blood partial pressure of carbon dioxide; SaO$_2$ = oxygen saturation.

Useful websites
➤ British Thoracic Society: www.brit-thoracic.org.uk
➤ Asthma UK: www.asthma.org.uk
➤ Be in Control materials: www.nhs.uk/conditions/asthma-in-children
➤ Scottish Intercollegiate Guidelines Network: www.sign.ac.uk

PERSISTENT COUGH

Core messages

➤ Cough is one of the most common symptoms in children. Cough is defined as acute (< 2 weeks), subacute (2–4 weeks) or chronic (>4 weeks, persistent and daily). Table 9.5 lists the main causes of persistent cough.

➤ A child's cough is rarely productive, therefore the term 'wet cough' rather than 'productive cough' is more appropriate. Cough is also divided into *dry* (e.g. asthma) and *wet–moist* (e.g. bronchiectasis).

TABLE 9.5 Causes of persistent cough

- Upper respiratory tract infection (viral URTI, croup)
- Pulmonary:

○ Asthma	○ Aspiration
○ Pneumonia	○ Alpha-1 antitrypsin deficiency
○ Bronchitis, bronchiolitis	○ Tuberculosis
○ Ciliary dyskinisia	○ Tracheo-oesophageal fistula
○ Inhaled foreign body	○ Severe chest-wall deformity
○ Cystic fibrosis	○ Pertussis
○ Bronchiectasis	○ Congenital lobar emphysema

- Allergy (dust or pollen inhalation)
- Gastro-oesophageal reflux
- Psychogenic
- Drugs (angiotensin-converting enzyme (ACE) inhibitor)

Recommended investigations

➤ FBC: white blood cells (WBCs) and C-reactive protein (CRP) are raised in bacterial infection and sometimes in asthma. Eosinophilia suggests an allergic condition (abnormal if > 4%).

➤ Sputum for culture from children with productive cough.

➤ Lung function testing: using spirometry or peak flow meter.

➤ Chest X-ray is very helpful in diagnosing pneumonia, foreign body. Also very useful in excluding pathology if the presentation does not suggest a clear diagnosis.

➤ Computed tomography (CT) scan of the lung if bronchiectasis is suspected (done in hospital).

➤ Sweat test if cystic fibrosis is suspected (done in hospital).

➤ Gastric pH study for cases suspected of gastro-oesophageal reflux (done in hospital).

PRACTICE TIPS

- A child who presents with cough on exertion only is likely to have exercise-induced asthma. PEF measurements before and after exercise, and with and without salbutamol inhalation, will support the diagnosis of asthma.
- If the cough is persistent and a diagnosis is unexplained, a trial of bronchodilator is justified; inhaled steroids (ICSs) may also help.

- A psychogenic cough is rare but may occur; typically, it never occurs during sleep.
- All children with chronic cough should undergo lung function tests, chest X-ray and pulse oximetry.
- Foreign body (FB) can mimic symptoms of croup and asthma. In any child with prolonged unexplained cough, inhaled FB should be excluded. If missed, bronchiectasis is likely to ensue.
- An underweight child with chronic cough should undergo a sweat test to exclude cystic fibrosis.
- Children with developmental delay who present with persistent cough often aspirate and may develop aspiration pneumonia.

The two conditions associated with persistent cough include:
- **Pertussis (whooping cough)**
  - ○ Typical paroxysmal cough often ending in a 'whoop' noise.
  - ○ Diagnosis is clinical; if uncertain, *Bordetella pertussis* can be cultured from pernasal swab or using PCR (polymerase chain reaction) testing. The latter is more suitable in patients treated with antibiotics.
  - ○ Antibiotic treatment should be started during the first 1–2 weeks of the cough starting and before coughing paroxysms occur, if pertussis is suspected.
  - ○ Erythromycin, clarithromycin and azithromycin are the first choices. Azithromycin is preferred for post-exposure prophylaxis and treatment.
  - ○ Consider adenovirus and other viruses in a child with a pertussis-like cough who is fully immunised.
- **Tuberculosis (TB)**
  - ○ Persistent, unremitting cough, associated with low-grade fever, fatigue, night sweating and weight loss/failure to thrive.
  - ○ Identification of *Mycobacterium tuberculosis* (positive in 30–40% of cases) from sputum, pleural fluid or cerebrospinal fluid (CSF).
  - ○ Positive tuberculin test, using 5 tuberculin units of purified protein derivative. A positive reaction is 5 mm or more induration present after 48–72 hours.
  - ○ Remember that TB is a notifiable disease and should be referred to a specialist.

Management of persistent cough
(*See also* Fig 9.3.)
➤ Cough is usually self-limiting and the focus should be directed at the cause.

The use of over-the-counter (OTC) cough medications, including cough suppressants, are generally of little benefit and place young children at risk of potential side-effects.
➤ **Indication for referral** if the cough:
  ➢ Is significantly interfering with the child's sleep or daily activity
  ➢ Persists and the cause is obscure
  ➢ Is causing considerable anxiety to the parents.

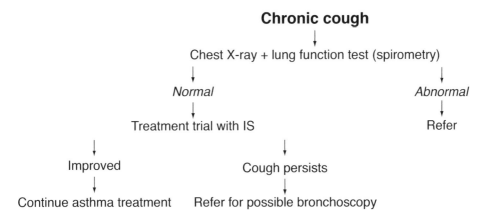

FIGURE 9.3 Summary of cough management

COUGHING UP BLOOD (HAEMOPTYSIS)

Core messages

➤ Haemoptysis is defined as coughing or expectoration of blood or the presence of blood-tinged sputum. In contrast to adults, the causes of haemoptysis in children (Box 9.8) are mostly benign and not life-threatening.

➤ In general, the source of the bleeding is either from the lungs or the bronchial system. The amount of bleeding from the lungs tends to be small compared with bleeding from the bronchi, which produces a larger quantity of blood.

➤ Haemoptysis must be differentiated from epistaxis and haematemesis (Table 9.6).

BOX 9.8 Causes of haemoptysis

Pulmonary

- Vigorous cough
- Pneumonia
- Foreign body (mostly if < 4 years of age)
- Bronchiectasis
- Cystic fibrosis
- TB
- Pulmonary embolism
- Arteriovenous malformation

- Pulmonary tumours (adenoma, hamartoma)
- Goodpasture's syndrome
- Lung abscess, or tuberculosis
- Pulmonary oedema
- Sarcoidosis
- Haemosiderosis
- Mycetoma (fungus ball)

Cardiac

- Left ventricular heart failure

- Mitral valve stenosis

Systemic

- Coagulopathy, e.g. disseminated intravascular coagulation (DIC)

- Hereditary haemorrhagic telangiectasia
- Systemic lupus erythematosus (SLE)

TABLE 9.6 Differentiating haemoptysis from haematemesis

Haemoptysis	Haematemesis
Sputum frothy	Sputum not frothy
Bright-red or pink	Brown or black
No vomiting and nausea	Associated vomiting and nausea
Alkaline pH	Acidic pH
Concurrent lung disease	Concurrent gastrointestinal disease

Recommended investigations

➤ FBC: low haemoglobin (Hb) may confirm anaemia if the bleeding was significant and prolonged; leukocytosis in infection such as pneumonia or auto-immune diseases; low platelets in thrombocytopenia or coagulopathy.

➤ Coagulation study with International Normalised Ratio (INR), prothrombin time (PT) and partial thromboplastin time (PTT) in case of coagulopathy.

➤ Auto-antibody screen may indicate connective tissue diseases.

➤ Sputum cytology for suspected TB or tumour.

➤ Chest X-ray is essential for detecting the majority of causes.

➤ Sweat test for suspected cases of cystic fibrosis (CF).

➤ Bronchoscopy and high-resolution CT scan of the lung may be indicated in unclear cases of suspected haemoptysis or tumour.

PRACTICE TIPS

● After a careful history and physical examination, a chest X-ray should be performed. If the diagnosis is not clear, a referral to a chest specialist should be considered.

● Haemoptysis and high fever is most likely caused by pneumonia.

● Haemoptysis is not uncommon in CF; some 5% of all patients would develop this symptom, which may recur.

● Young children aged < 5 years swallow their sputum and may not present with coughing up of bloody sputum unless the haemoptysis is massive.

● A rare cause of haemoptysis is left ventricular heart failure or mitral stenosis causing pulmonary hypertension.

● Pulmonary embolism may cause haemoptysis. This diagnosis should be considered if there is evidence of deep venous thrombosis (DVT) or the child is at risk of thrombosis, such as sickle-cell anaemia or homocystinuria.

● TB is on the increase in the UK, and should be included in the differential diagnosis of haemoptysis.

Referral

➤ All cases with haemoptysis should be referred except mild self-limiting cases caused by vigorous cough where the child is well and the chest X-ray is normal.

➤ Paediatricians may manage children with haemoptysis as long as the diagnosis is clear, e.g. pneumonia. Unclear cases should be referred to the chest unit to establish the diagnosis and treatment.

REFERENCES

1. British Thoracic Society Guideline on the Management of Asthma, 2008; revised in 2012. www.brit-thoracic.org.uk
2. Cochrane Database Syst Review 2004; (1): CD001277.
3. WHO guidelines for indoor air quality: dampness and mould 2009.

CHAPTER 10

Cardiology

CORE MESSAGES

➤ Congenital heart disease (CHD) in children is caused by a combination of genetic and environmental factors. The incidence of CHD is approximately 1.3%.

➤ It is vital that heart disease is identified as early as possible.

➤ The cardiovascular system (CVS) should be examined soon after birth and at the 6-week check. This must be thorough and include more than simply auscultation for murmurs.

➤ A good clinical assessment can usually decide whether or not a child has CHD. Such an assessment can also spare many children from unnecessary investigations.

➤ The most common cardiovascular problem in GP practice is to assess the clinical significance of a cardiac murmur, which is present in around 40% of pre-school children. The vast majority of such murmurs are innocent.

➤ The main causes of acquired heart disease in children are Kawasaki disease and myocarditis; rheumatic heart disease is very rare in the Western world.

PRESENTATION OF CHD (BOX 10.1)

BOX 10.1 Presentations of CHD

Symptoms
1. Respiratory distress
2. Heart murmur
3. Cyanosis
4. Increased frequency of lower respiratory tract infections
5. Fatigue, exercise intolerance
6. Unusual presentations such as chest pain

---

1. Respiratory distress

Symptoms and signs of respiratory distress such as tachypnoea and subcostal recession may occur in both pulmonary diseases and cardiac failure. Box 10.2 shows features that suggest the presence of heart failure. Symptoms of congestive cardiac failure caused by CHD usually manifest before the age of 2 months.

BOX 10.2 Symptoms and signs of congestive cardiac failure

Symptoms
- Dyspnoea, fatigue, sweating, particularly during feeding or exercise

Signs
- Tachycardia, tachypnoea, subcostal recession
- Heart enlargement (displaced apex beat)
- Heart murmur and gallop rhythm (due to a 3rd heart sound)
- Cyanosis
- Liver enlargement (the liver edge normally should not be more than 2 cm below the costal margin)
- Excessive weight gain, mainly in infants
- Lung oedema causing inspiratory crepitations on auscultation
- Peripheral oedema (late sign)

 RED FLAGS
- When respiratory distress occurs in a newborn or a young infant, always consider CHD as a possible cause.
- Tiredness and sweating during feedings may suggest CHD.

2. Heart Murmur

(see below)

3. Cyanosis

Most newborns with CHD are diagnosed either in utero by ultrasound scan or at the neonatal or 6-week check. Some infants with certain CHD (e.g. coarctation of the aorta or severe pulmonary stenosis) may present with cyanosis at age 1–2 weeks because their CHD is dependent upon patent ductus arteriosus (PDA) for pulmonary blood flow, and the cyanosis appears when the ductus closes. Causes of cyanosis are listed in Box 10.3.

BOX 10.3 Usual causes of cyanosis

Peripheral
- Breath-holding attack
- Cardiac failure (reduction in cardiac output)
- Fever (poor peripheral circulation)
- Raynaud's phenomenon
- Shock (reduction in cardiac output)

Central
- Persistent pulmonary hypertension
- Cardiac failure (if associated with cyanotic CHD)
- Pulmonary (pneumonia, severe asthma, pneumothorax)
- Cyanotic CHD
- Methaemoglobinaemia (congenital as an autosomal recessive inherited condition or due to drug reaction, e.g. nitroglycerin)

PRACTICE POINTS

- Cyanosis caused by arterial desaturation is termed *central cyanosis*, while that associated with normal arterial saturation is termed *peripheral cyanosis*.
- If the differential diagnosis between central and peripheral cyanosis is uncertain, the use of a pulse oximeter is diagnostic: pulse oximetry shows normal readings of 94–100% in peripheral but <85% in central cyanosis.
- Cyanosis is best detected by checking the tongue, nail beds and conjunctiva in natural light. Central cyanosis invariably increases during crying.
- Long-standing arterial desaturation (longer than 6 months) leads to clubbing of the fingernails and toenails.

4. Increased frequency of respiratory infections

CHD with large left-to-right shunt predisposes to lower respiratory tract infections.

5. Fatigue, exercise intolerance

Infants with CHD may tire easily and sweat during feedings. As a result the infant is unable to take full feeds, resulting in poor weight gain. Older children may present with exercise intolerance.

6. Other presentations

Other clinical presentations of CHD include squatting and hypoxic spells, arrhythmia and chest pain. Adult presenting with symptoms of cardiac disease such as angina and peripheral oedema are rare in children but can occur in severe aortic stenosis. Oedema such as peri-orbital and pre-tibial are rare and late manifestations of CHD.

DIAGNOSTIC EVALUATION

History

Careful history includes:
➤ Family history of sudden cardiac death and CHD. If a parent has CHD, the incidence of CHD increases from 1.3% in the general population to 15%. If a sibling has CHD, the risk of a second child having CHD is 2–3%.
➤ Other risk factors are shown in Table 10.1.

Physical examination

➤ **Observation**
  ➤ General appearance, including colour. Is there any obvious syndrome? (Table 10.2.)
  ➤ The chest. Is the left side of the chest abnormally prominent?
  ➤ Finger clubbing (may be normal, or more often caused by cystic fibrosis).
  ➤ Are there signs of dyspnoea, tachypnoea or retraction which may suggest congestive cardiac failure? (Chest retraction is abnormal and usually indicates stiff lungs from pulmonary or cardiac causes.)
➤ **Palpation** of pulses, for thrill, and apex (for evidence of displacement as a sign of heart enlargement). The brachial pulse should be palpated in preference to the radial pulse.

TABLE 10.1 Maternal risk factors predisposing to CHD

Risk factors	Possible CHD
Drug exposure during pregnancy	
Anticonvulsants (phenytoin)	PS, AS, COA
Progesterone, oestrogen	VSD, TGA
Amphetamine	VSD, PDA, ASD, TGA
Alcohol	FAS with VSD, ASD, PDA
Maternal diabetes	Cardiomyopathy
Maternal lupus	Heart block
Congenital infections (e.g. rubella)	PS

AS = aortic stenosis; ASD = atrial septal defect; COA = coarctation of aorta; FAS = fetal alcohol syndrome; PDA = patent ductus arteriosus; PS = pulmonary stenosis; TGA = transposition of great arteries; VSD = ventricular septal defect.

PRACTICE POINT

- Check femoral and dorsalis pedis pulses, which are weak or absent in coarctation of the aorta. They are also weak or difficult to palpate in obese children. It takes practice to feel femoral pulses in neonates and young infants.

TABLE 10.2 Some syndromes associated with CHD

Syndrome	Incidence	CHD
Down's syndrome	40%	ASD
Turner's syndrome	35%	COA
Fragile X-syndrome	50%	ARD, MVP
Cri-du-chat syndrome	25%	VSD, PDA
Marfan's syndrome	80–100%	ARD
Fetal alcohol syndrome	30–50%	ASD, VSD

ARD = aortic root dilation; ASD = atrial septal defect; COA = coarctation of the aorta; MVP = mitral valve prolapse; PDA = patent ductus arteriosus; VSD = ventricular septal defect.

➤ Auscultation (heart murmur)

- ➢ If the child appears likely to cry, auscultate first, even if this is not the ideal way to examine the cardiovascular system
- ➢ Auscultation should focus on the intensity and rhythm of the heart sounds and their variation with respiration. It is abnormal not to have sinus arrhythmia (acceleration of heart rate during inspiration and slowing during expiration)
- ➢ Innocent murmurs are by far the most common findings, occurring in as many as 40% of 3- to 4-year-olds (Box 10.4). Murmurs are uncommon in neonates, and more likely to be serious if non-musical
- ➢ The two important conditions causing continuous murmurs are patent ductus arteriosus and venous hum. The latter is produced by turbulence of blood over

the jugular veins. Venous hum has no pathological significance, and is usually loudest in the neck or right supraclavicular fossa. This murmur is usually heard only in the sitting or upright position, not in the supine position

➤ A heart murmur that is first detected at the 6-week check suggests ventricular septal defect

➤ In the normal child, the split of the 2nd sound widens with inspiration (due to increasing right ventricular stroke volume) and narrows in expiration

➤ Occasionally, pathological murmurs are detected (Box 10.5)

BOX 10.4 Characteristics of innocent murmurs

● Short systolic ejection type of murmur
● No or insignificant radiation to the apex, base or back
● Murmur changes intensity and is usually louder in the supine position
● Murmur quality is vibratory or musical
● Murmur intensifies with increased cardiac output such as exercise and fever; diminishes in standing due to the decrease in stroke volume that occurs in the standing position
● Grade 1 or 2 in intensity (Table 10.3), best heard along the left lower or midsternal border
● Auscultation findings do not suggest heart disease such as pansystolic murmur, diastolic murmur or greater in intensity than grade 2 (Table 10.4)

BOX 10.5 Features of pathological murmur

● Diastolic or late systolic murmur
● Loud murmur > 2/6 in intensity
● Palpable thrill
● Continuous murmur with the exception of venous hum
● A murmur that sounds like a breath sound
● A murmur at the pulmonary area with fixed splitting of the 2nd sound
● Associated with any symptoms or signs of heart disease such as fatigue, shortness of breath, tachypnoea, hepatomegaly

---

TABLE 10.3 Intensity grades of a murmur

Grade 1	Difficult to hear, softer than the heart sounds
Grade 2	Intensity equal to heart sounds
Grade 3	Louder than the heart sounds, no thrill
Grade 4	Loud murmur associated with thrill
Grade 5	Is heard with only the edge of the stethoscope

TABLE 10.4 Types of murmur, including venous hum

Systolic	
Pansystolic	VSD, MR or TR (Fig 10.1)
Early systolic	Small VSD
Late systolic	MVP
Ejection type	AS, PS
Diastolic	AR or PR
Continuous	PDA
Venous hum	Best heard just below the clavicle. It disappears when the child lies down or turns his/her head to the other side. It can be confused with PDA

AR = aortic regurgitation; AS = aortic stenosis; MR = mitral regurgitation; MVP = mitral valve prolapse; PDA = patent ductus arteriosus; PR = pulmonary regurgitation; PS = pulmonary stenosis; TR = tricuspid regurgitation; VSD = ventricular septal defect.

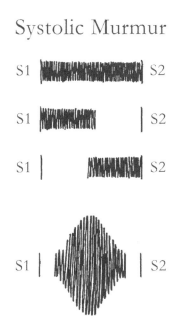

Systolic Murmur

FIGURE 10.1 Subtypes of systolic murmur

➤ **Indications for referral:**
  ➤ Doubt about the significance of a murmur
  ➤ Any murmur which has pathological features
  ➤ A new murmur which was not heard before.

Blood pressure

Blood pressure (BP) measurement can be challenging in children, but is an essential part of the cardiovascular examination. It is important to choose the right size of cuff, which should cover almost all the upper arm, the hand being supinated and then elevated to the level of the heart. Table 10.5 shows normal values for pulse, respiratory rate and BP. Children with coarctation of the aorta often present with hypertension. Blood pressure in the arms and legs should be measured in any child with hypertension to exclude this.

TABLE 10.5 Normal values (average and/or range) for pulse, respiratory rate (RR), and systolic and diastolic BP*

Age	Pulse (beats/min)	RR (breaths/min)	SBP (mmHg)	DBP (mmHg)
Newborn	125	30–40	75	45
	(70–190)		(60–90)	(40–60)
1–12 months	120	25–40	90	60
	(80–160)		(80–100)	(50–70)
5 years	100	15–25	95	60
	(80–120)		(90–115)	(55–75)
12 years	85	15–20	110	65
	(65–110)		(95–125)	(60–80)

* A simple calculation of normal systolic BP (in mmHg) is 90 + the child's age.

Exercise testing

Exercise testing is not commonly used in children, although it can play an important role in evaluating cardiac symptoms. Available testing includes a graded treadmill apparatus and a bicycle ergometer.

Pulse oximetry

Pulse oximetry is a useful method of monitoring oxygen saturation, reflecting the condition of the cardiovascular system. The device is usually applied on a fingertip or earlobe.

Chest X-ray

Chest X-ray may provide information about the cardiac size and shape, and lung vascularity. A cardiac enlargement exists when the maximal cardiac width is more than half the maximal chest width.

ECG

ECG provides important diagnostic information, particularly on cardiac hypertrophy and arrhythmia.

Echocardiography

Echocardiography, or simply an echo, is one of the most commonly used non-invasive diagnostic tests in cardiology. It uses standard 2-dimensional and Doppler ultrasound to create images of the heart and estimate cardiac function, such as calculation of the cardiac output.

CHEST PAIN

➤ Chest pain is a rare presentation of CHD in children, particularly in infants. In older children, chest pain is the second most frequent cause of referral to paediatric cardiologists after cardiac murmur. Box 10.6 lists causes of chest pain

➤ Although chest pain in adults is considered a medical emergency because of the possibility of a myocardial infarction, this is rare in children. The symptom causes, however, a significant parental anxiety and may result in restriction of activities and school absence

➤ The first clinical issue in a child with chest pain is to determine the cause of chest pain and identify patients who can be managed at home (Box 10.7) and those who require referral to a specialist (Box 10.8)

➤ Chronic or recurrent chest pain is likely to be benign and mostly caused by anxiety

➤ Chest pain is a common presentation in teenagers due to anxiety or benign transient intercostal muscle pain

➤ Cardiac causes of chest pain are rare in infancy but may occur in anomalous origin of the coronary arteries or Kawasaki disease

---

BOX 10.6 Causes of chest pain

Non-cardiac causes
- Idiopathic (20–45%)
- Musculoskeletal (15–30%) such as osteochondritis, Tietze's syndrome, direct trauma to the chest
- Anxiety or stress (5–10%)
- Pulmonary (12–20%), e.g. pneumonia, asthma, pneumothorax, pleurisy
- Acid reflux (4–7%)

Cardiac causes (5–10%)
- Severe aortic stenosis
- Mitral valve prolapse
- Pericarditis
- Hypertrophic obstructive cardiomyopathy (HOCM)
- Long Q–T syndrome
- Supraventricular tachycardia (SVT) with very rapid heart rate
- Dissecting aortic aneurysm in Marfan's syndrome

BOX 10.7 Management of chest pain

- Management depends on the underlying cause of the chest pain, requiring a thorough history and physical examination
- Benign and common causes of chest pain, e.g. psychogenic or idiopathic, are more frequently seen at GP surgeries. Reassurance is essential but occasionally it does require further investigation, such as ECG or exercise testing
- The principal management of musculoskeletal chest pain is reassurance, analgesics, rest or a combination of these measures

> **BOX 10.8** Cardiac symptoms and signs that are likely to require referral to the paediatric cardiologist
>
> ● Abnormal ECG
> ● History suggestive of cardiac disease:
>   › Family history of sudden death, genetic disorders of cardiac nature
>   › Sharp, retrosternal pain that often radiates to the left shoulder, is aggravated on supine position or taking a deep breath, and relieved on bending forward (suggestive of pericarditis). Squeezing, tightening, constrictive or pressurising sensation may suggest ischaemic heart disease
>   › Exertional chest pain
>   › Exertional syncope
>   › History of cardiac intervention
> ● Abnormal cardiac findings on physical examination:
>   › Tachycardia, which may worsen on lying down
>   › Muffled heart sounds, gallop rhythm, arrhythmia, click or murmur
>   › Associated palpitations
>   › Tall stature suggestive of Marfanoid appearance

PRACTICE POINTS

● Idiopathic chest pain is the most common cause (20–45%). The condition is defined by the absence of cause after thorough history, physical examination and laboratory testing. It is a diagnosis of excluding an organic disease.

● Chronic (lasting >6 months) or recurrent episodes of chest pain without abnormal findings is likely to be psychogenic. This cause accounts for 5–10% of cases.

● Typical features of non-cardiac chest pain include sharp quality, of short duration and unrelated to exercise.

● Musculoskeletal chest pain often follows physical exercise or trauma, and presents as sharp, burning or stabbing. Pain may worsen with a certain body position, movement or deep breathing. Costochondritis and Tietze's syndrome are caused by inflammation of the cartilage connecting the ribs with the sternum; the latter has localised inflammatory swelling of the affected cartilage of the costochondral, or sternoclavicular joints, mostly involving the 2nd and 3rd ribs.

● Symptoms of chest discomfort, dyspnoea and/or heaviness may suggest exercise-induced asthma. The use of a bronchodilator before exercise is likely to prevent these symptoms and confirms the diagnosis.

● Acid reflux can cause retrosternal or left-sided chest pain, or epigastric pain. The pain often produces a burning sensation.

● Psychogenic causes of chest pain account for 5–10% of cases, and usually present as a dull or sharp pain of short duration and unrelated to exercise. Teenagers are mostly affected. Enquire about psychosocial problems such as loss, a break-up with a friend, bullying, or whether a parent or close relative has had angina or a heart attack.

● Patients with a Marfanoid appearance and chest pain require close attention

because they are at risk of dilation of the ascending aorta and of dissecting aneurysm.
- Chest pain of cardiac origin manifests as a deep heavy pressure, choking or squeezing sensation, and it is usually triggered by exercise. It is not sharp and is not affected by respiration.

SYNCOPE

Syncope requires special attention, as this can be cardiac in origin (around 6% of syncope cases). It is important to distinguish between vasovagal faint and cardiac syncope which may be caused by serious cardiac disease. There are many causes of syncope (Box 10.9). Differentiating features between cardiac and vasovagal syncope are given in Table 10.6.

BOX 10.9 Usual causes of syncope

- Vasovagal faint/autonomic failure
- Unexplained
- Cardiac syncope (e.g. HOCM)
- Seizures (e.g. atonic seizures)
- Head injury
- CNS infection or haemorrhage
- Breath-holding spells (cyanotic and pallid forms)
- Toxins/poisoning/medication
- Hysteria
- Narcolepsy

TABLE 10.6 Differential diagnosis between cardiac and vasovagal syncope

	Vasovagal syncope	Cardiac syncope
Relevant history	Previous episodes	Family history of sudden cardiac death, history of CHD
Sex	Often in girls	Boys or girls
Age	Adolescents, uncommon before age 10–12 years	Any age, more often in teenagers
Prodromal symptoms	Sweating, nausea, vomiting	Palpitations, chest pain or sudden drop attack with no warning
Typical triggers	Long standing on hot days without adequate food or drinks, unpleasant smells or fear	During exercise, e.g. running or swimming

Referral

➤ All cases apart from infrequent vasovagal faint
➤ Frequent vasovagal faints (refer to paediatrician)
➤ Unexplained and cardiac syncope (refer to paediatric cardiologist)
➤ Frequent episodes of syncope irrespective of the aetiology

RED FLAG

- Syncope without warning (drop attack) is very suggestive of cardiac origin. This requires referral for investigation, as recurrence can be fatal.

HYPERTROPHIC OBSTRUCTIVE CARDIOMYOPATHY (HOCM)

HOCM may occur in infants of diabetic mothers, as secondary to obstructive CHD, e.g. severe aortic stenosis, or to storage diseases, e.g. glycogen storage disease or mucopolysaccharidosis, or idiopathic. The condition is usually inherited as an autosomal dominant condition. Patients may be asymptomatic, mildly symptomatic or develop sudden cardiac arrest. It is known as a leading cause of sudden death in young athletes. Box 10.10 lists the main risk factors for sudden death. The cardiac hypertrophy is often massive and particularly involves the interventricular septum.

Clinical findings

➤ Symptoms: none or dyspnoea, chest pain (angina), palpitation, fatigue and syncope
➤ Signs of cardiomegaly (displaced apex, prominent ventricular heave)
➤ There may be no murmur, or a systolic ejection type of murmur of medium intensity (similar to the murmur of aortic stenosis). Murmur increases with standing or during the strain phase of a Valsalva manoeuvre
➤ Carotid pulsation is brisk and jerky

BOX 10.10 Risk factors for sudden death in patients with HOCM

- Family history of HOCM or sudden cardiac death
- Recurrent episodes of syncope
- Previous episodes of aborted cardiac arrest
- A young age at first diagnosis (< 30 years)
- History of SVT or VT
- Ventricular septal thickness > 3 cm

SVT = supraventricular tachycardia; VT = ventricular tachycardia.

RED FLAG

- Once HOCM has been diagnosed in a child, immediate testing of all family members is required.

Diagnosis is made by chest X-ray, ECG (showing the ventricular hypertrophy), echocardiography, cardiac MRI (confirming the septal hypertrophy) and gene testing.

INFECTIVE ENDOCARDITIS

Endocarditis often occurs as a complication of CHD or rheumatic heart disease, but may have no apparent cause. It is either acute or subacute endocarditis. Table 10.7 provides a summary of endocarditis.

TABLE 10.7 Summary of aspects of endocarditis

Risk factors	VSD, aortic valvular diseases, Fallot's tetralogy, PDA and shunts
Bacterial causes in endocarditis	*Streptococcus viridans*, mostly causing subacute endocarditis in patients with underlying CHD
	Staphylococci, mostly causing acute endocarditis in patients with no underlying CHD
	Enterococci, usually occurring in patients undergoing lower bowel or genitourinary procedures
	Pseudomonas in IV drug users
Clinical features	History of CHD with a dental, intestinal or genitourinary procedure
	Symptoms include fever, night sweats, arthralgia, myalgia, weight loss
	Signs include tachycardia, new or changing murmur, embolic signs such as splinter nail bed, splenomegaly, heart failure
Diagnosis	Echocardiography and blood culture
Oral prophylaxis	Amoxicillin: 50 mg/kg 1 h before a procedure
	Clindamycin (20 mg/kg), cephalexin (50 mg/kg) or azithromycin (15 mg/kg) for children with penicillin allergy
	Patients undergoing intestinal or genitourinary procedures are often referred for antibiotic injection such as vancomycin, gentamicin or ampicillin

PDA = patent ductus arteriosus; VSD = ventricular septal defect.

ANTIBIOTIC PROPHYLAXIS FOR DENTAL PROCEDURES

Recommendations for antibiotic prophylaxis for children with CHD undergoing dental and other intestinal or genitourinary procedures have recently changed.[1,2] Antibiotic prophylaxis should be offered to those patients with high-risk cardiac factors:
➤ previous infective endocarditis
➤ cardiac valve replacement surgery
➤ surgically constructed systemic or pulmonary shunt or conduit.

Good oral hygiene is the most important factor in reducing the risk of endocarditis in susceptible individuals.

ARRHYTHMIAS

Sinus arrhythmia

The normal pulse varies physiologically in relation to respiration: it accelerates during inspiration and slows during expiration. It is abnormal for a child not to have sinus arrhythmia.

Long Q–T syndrome

Long Q–T syndrome is either autosomal-dominant-inherited (Romano–Ward syndrome), autosomal-recessive-inherited (Jervell–Lange–Nelson syndrome) or acquired (myocarditis or electrolyte disturbance). Symptoms include:
➤ fainting, especially after exercise or emotional excitement
➤ seizures
➤ ventricular arrhythmia
➤ sudden cardiac arrest.

A heart-rate-corrected Q–T interval of >470 milliseconds supports the diagnosis, whereas a Q–T interval of >440 milliseconds is suspicious. Treatment includes beta-blockers or cardiac defibrillation.

PRACTICE POINTS

- All patients with long Q–T should be referred to a paediatric cardiologist.
- Patients should not participate in competitive sports and activities that place high physical demands on the body.
- All family members should be tested for this syndrome.
- Some drugs can prolong the Q–T interval and should not be used for patients with this syndrome. A full list of these drugs is available from www.qtdrugs.org

Supraventricular tachycardia (SVT)

Paroxysmal SVT is a regular rhythm at a rate of 180–300 beats/min. SVT is usually caused by impulses from the atrioventricular (AV) node re-entering the atria. Infants often present with signs of cardiac failure.

Complete heart block

Complete heart block is associated with a heart rate of about 50 beats/min. The congenital type of heart block is usually caused by an autoimmune disease such as systemic lupus erythematosus (SLE) in the mother, who may or may not have symptoms of SLE.

Brugada syndrome

Brugada syndrome is a genetic disease characterised by cardiac conduction abnormalities (ventricular arrhythmia, first-degree AV block and other ECG findings) and sudden death more commonly in men without a clinically known underlying cause.

FURTHER READING

1. Report of the Working Party of the British Society for Antimicrobial Chemotherapy: guidelines for the prevention of endocarditis. J Antimicrob Chemother 2006, 57: 1035–42.
2. Department of Health. NICE guidance on antibiotic prophylaxis against infective endocarditis, 2008. Gateway reference number 9638.

CHAPTER 11

Urogenital

URINARY TRACT INFECTION (UTI)

UTI is common and around 1 in 10 girls and 1 in 30 boys will have had a UTI by the age of 16 years. Boys have a greater incidence of UTI in the neonatal period and early infancy. Girls overtake boys in the incidence of UTI at the age of 3–6 months.

In a general practice of 10 000 patients with 6 GPs and 100 births per year, each GP will expect to have the following consultation rates for UTI:[1]

➤ 2 consultations a year with a child younger than 5 years
➤ 1 consultation a year with a boy aged 0–14 years
➤ 4 consultations a year with a girl aged 0–14 years.

Definitions

Definitions of terms used in this section are:

UTI

➤ UTI is caused by a single organism of >100 000 colony-forming units per mL.
➤ UTI can be divided into:
  ➤ *Upper UTI*, defined as an infection with a fever of 38°C or higher, which is the most common presentation of UTI in infancy, or
  ➤ *Lower UTI*, defined as a collection of well-recognised symptoms including dysuria, frequency, and supra-pubic pain in toilet-trained children.

Atypical UTI

➤ Seriously ill
➤ Raised creatinine levels
➤ Abdominal or bladder mass
➤ Septicaemia
➤ Poor urine flow
➤ No response to treatment with suitable antibiotics within 48 hours

Recurrent UTI

➤ 2 or more episodes of acute upper UTI
➤ 1 episode of acute upper UTI plus 1 or more episodes of lower UTI
➤ 3 or more episodes of lower UTI

Urine collection

Children presenting with unexplained fever with temperatures of ≥38°C should have the urine tested using the following methods:

➤ A clean-catch urine sample is the recommended method if possible.
➤ Non-invasive methods such as urine collection pads should be used if a clean-catch sample is not obtainable.
➤ Cotton-wool balls, gauze and sanitary towels should not be used to collect urine in children.
➤ Test the urine with dipsticks and/or microscopy and culture. The most significant indicator with dipsticks is the nitrite test, which indicates significant bacteria levels. Normal urine contains nitrates but not nitrites; about 90% of bacteria causing UTIs can convert nitrates to nitrites.
➤ Culture of urine within 4 hours of voiding is likely to give a true indication of the presence or absence of bacteriuria. The results are interpreted as follows:

Microscopy results

	Pyuria +ve	Pyuria –ve
Bacteriuria +ve	Child should be regarded as having UTI	Child should be regarded as having probable UTI; treat with an antibiotic while waiting for culture result
Bacteriuria –ve	Antibiotic treatment should be started if clinically diagnosed with UTI	Child should be regarded as unlikely to have UTI; no antibiotic is required

Dipstick results (particularly useful after the age of 3 years)

Nitrites +ve, leucocytes +ve	Start antibiotic treatment. If high or intermediate risk of serious illness or past history of UTI, send urine sample for culture
Nitrites +ve, leucocytes –ve	Start antibiotic if fresh urine was tested. Send urine sample for culture
Nitrites –ve, leucocytes +ve	Send urine sample for microscopy and culture. Only start antibiotic treatment if there is good clinical evidence of UTI
Nitrites –ve, leucocytes –ve	UTI can be regarded as unlikely; no antibiotics are required

Symptoms and signs

These are given in Table 11.1.

Acute management of children with symptoms suggestive of UTI

➤ **Infants <3 months of age with a possible UTI (high risk of serious illness):**
  ➢ Should be referred immediately to hospital for parenteral antibiotic therapy
  ➢ Urine sample for urgent microscopy and culture or dipstick testing.
➤ **Children >3 months to <3 years (intermediate risk of serious illness):**
  ➢ Consider referral to hospital
  ➢ Urgent urine for microscopy and culture; treatment should be started if microscopy or dipstick testing is positive (as above). A urine sample is to be sent for microscopy and culture

TABLE 11.1 Symptoms and signs in children with UTI

Age group	Symptoms and signs	
	Most common	Uncommon
Children <3 months		
Upper UTI	Fever, lethargy, vomiting, poor feeding, irritability	Failure to thrive, jaundice, haematuria, offensive urine
Children >3 months		
Upper UTI	Fever, abdominal pain, loin pain and/or tenderness	Lethargy, haematuria, vomiting, offensive urine, failure to thrive
Lower UTI	Dysuria, frequent urination, dysfunctional voiding. No systemic features	Fever, malaise, vomiting, haematuria, offensive urine, cloudy urine

> - Treatment with oral antibiotics for 7–10 days, for example trimethoprim or nitrofurantoin (as first-line treatment in primary care). Cephalosporin or co-amoxiclav often used in secondary care
> - If oral antibiotics cannot be used, child should be referred to hospital for IV antibiotics for 2–4 days followed by oral antibiotics for a total duration of 10 days.
> **Children >3 years with cystitis/lower UTI (low risk of serious illness):**
>> - Urine sample for microscopy and culture, or dipstick testing
>> - Treat with oral antibiotics for 3–5 days
>> - The choice of antibiotics should be directed by local antibiotic resistance. Trimethoprim, nitrofurantoin, cephalosporin or amoxicillin are suitable
>> - If the child remains unwell after 24–48 hours, he or she should be reassessed. A urine sample should be submitted for culture and alternative diagnoses should be excluded.

Investigation after an episode of acute UTI

Investigation is as outlined in Table 11.2.[2]

Long-term management and prevention

The main aim of follow-up of children after initial UTI is to prevent recurrent UTI and renal damage. Management includes:

> - Elimination and treatment of dysfunctional voiding and constipation. Children should void more frequently (normal range 4–7 voids/day) and empty the bladder completely
> - Encouraging children to drink more
> - Antibiotic prophylaxis should not be routinely recommended following first-time UTI, but such prophylaxis should be considered for recurrent UTI
> - Children who do not require imaging investigations do not require follow-up
> - Children who remain asymptomatic following an episode of UTI should not routinely have their urine tested for infection
> - Children who have recurrent UTI or abnormal imaging results should be assessed and followed up by a paediatric specialist.

TABLE 11.2 Recommended imaging schedule for infants and children

Test	Responds well to treatment within 48 hours	Atypical UTI	Recurrent UTI
Infants aged <6 months			
Ultrasound during acute UTI	No	Yes	Yes
Ultrasound within 6 weeks	Yes	No	No
DMSA 4–6 months following acute UTI	No	Yes	Yes
MSUG	No	Yes	Yes
Children aged >6 months to <3 years			
Ultrasound during acute UTI	No	Yes	No
Ultrasound within 6 weeks	No	No	Yes
DMSA 4–6 months following acute UTI	No	Yes	Yes
MCUG	No	No	No
Children aged >3 years			
Ultrasound during acute UTI	No	Yes	No
Ultrasound within 6 weeks	No	No	Yes
DMSA 4–6 months following acute UTI	No	No	Yes
MCUG	No	No	No

DMSA = dimercaptosuccinic acid, MCUG = micturating cystourethrogram

URINARY TRACT STONES

Presentation:
➤ Urinary tract infection
➤ Renal colic
➤ Microscopic haematuria (usually an incidental finding on dipsticks)

Management
➤ All patients with renal colic should be seen at the surgery and examined. If the child is acutely ill or in severe pain, urgent referral to hospital is indicated.
➤ Analgesics: either diclofenac orally 1–2 mg/kg or suppository (12.5 mg, 25 mg, 50 mg and 100 mg), or Oramorph (see British National Formulary for Children for dosage) (usually initiated in secondary care).
➤ Urinalysis: usually shows haematuria without significant proteinuria or casts.
➤ Renal ultrasound scan: within 24 hours whenever possible.
➤ Plain abdominal X-ray is not indicated because of the radiation involved and the fact that some stones (cystine and uric acid) are not visible on X-ray film.
➤ Other tests (likely to be performed in hospital) include full blood count (FBC), plasma electrolytes, urea, creatinine, bicarbonate, calcium and phosphate.
➤ Consider **immediate referral** if there is
  ➢ persistent pain
  ➢ associated fever
  ➢ signs of obstruction.
➤ The stone should always be sent for chemical analysis.

There are four options for managing **renal stones**:

➤ Extracorporeal shock wave lithotripsy (ESWL). ESWL shatters most renal stones, but more than 1 treatment may be needed. Minor postoperative complications from this procedure include:
  ➢ bruises at the site of shock wave entry
  ➢ haematuria
  ➢ colic
➤ Percutaneous nephrolithotomy (PCNL)
➤ Ureterscopy
➤ Open surgery.

Postoperative measures include plenty of fluid to dilute the urine and reduction of dietary calcium.

NOCTURNAL ENURESIS

Core messages

➤ Nocturnal enuresis affects over half a million children in the UK.
➤ Only 1 in 6 children with nocturnal enuresis attends surgery to seek advice from a healthcare professional. This is based on the widely held perception that it is a self-limiting problem and children will grow out of it.
➤ Nocturnal enuresis affects 10–15% of children aged 5 years, 5% of those aged 10 years and 1% of those in post-puberty. The spontaneous resolution rate per year is about 15%.
➤ Nocturnal enuresis can have a negative psychological (particularly self-esteem) and social impact on the child. The parents may become intolerant of their child's enuresis, which may lead to increased risk of non-accidental injury to the child. Treatment of enuresis aims to eliminate these adverse factors.

Definitions

These are given in Box 11.1.

BOX 11.1 Definition of terms used in this section

● **Primary nocturnal enuresis** (PNE) is defined as the involuntary voiding of urine during sleep at least 3 times a week in a child 5 years or older who has not achieved consistent night dryness
● **Secondary nocturnal enuresis** is a nocturnal enuresis in a child who has previously been dry for at least 6 months
● **Maximum bladder capacity** (MBC) is calculated by the formula: (age of the child in years $\times$ 30) + 30. A child of 7 years is expected to have an MBC of 240 mL
● **Nocturnal polyuria** is defined as the amount of urine passed during 1 night which measures more than the MBC
● **Overactive bladder** (formerly: detrusor instability) is an uninhibited bladder contraction which manifests as urinary frequency (> 7 times/day), urgency and urge incontinence and which results in a decreased MBC. Children, especially girls, with an overactive bladder are at risk of UTI

Aetiology

➤ Primary enuresis most often represents genetically a developmental delay of bladder control, which resolves in time.

➤ Secondary enuresis requires the exclusion of underlying pathology, e.g. a UTI, diabetes mellitus or anxiety.

Four aetiological factors are commonly involved:

➤ **Genetic:** the risk of nocturnal enuresis in children aged 5 years is 10–15% if neither parent was affected, 40% if one parent was affected and 75% if both had the condition. Research has identified a genetic link to chromosomes 13q, 12q, 8q and 22q.

➤ **Lack of arousal from sleep:** many parents perceive 'deep sleep' to be the cause of their child's bedwetting. As wetting may occur at any stage of sleep cycles, 'deep sleep' cannot be sustained as the cause of bedwetting. Enuretic children have difficulty waking in response to the sensation of a full bladder compared with non-enuretic children.

➤ **Overactive bladder/reduced bladder capacity:** an overactive bladder (caused for example by UTI, dysfunctional voiding, or idiopathic) presents during the daytime as incontinence with symptoms of urgency and frequency. An overactive bladder with or without reduced MBC is present in many enuretic children. Bedwetting occurs when the volume of urine produced exceeds the MBC.

➤ **Nocturnal polyuria and arginine vasopressin deficiency:** normally, there is a decrease in overnight urine production as a result of an increase in plasma levels of the antidiuretic hormone arginine vasopressin (AVP). Some enuretic children are lacking in AVP production at night. The resulting overproduction of urine appears to be a direct result of a nocturnal AVP deficiency.

Investigation

Urinalysis is always recommended, particularly if the bedwetting is of recent origin, there are daytime symptoms, or symptoms are suggestive of possible infection or diabetes mellitus.

Initial management

➤ Offer support, assessment and treatment to all children with bedwetting. Young children (e.g. aged <7 years) should not be excluded from the management of bedwetting on the basis of age alone.

➤ Reassure children and parents that the bedwetting is not the child's fault and that there is overwhelming evidence that the child will become dry.

➤ Punitive measures should not be used.

➤ Address excessive or insufficient fluid intake or abnormal toileting patterns before other treatments:

  ➢ Encourage a healthy daytime fluid intake of 6–7 cupfuls a day (age 5 years, 1000–1400 mL per day; age 9–13 years, 1200–2300 mL per day, age 14–18 years, 1400–2500+ mL per day).

  ➢ Encourage regular voiding, 6–7 times a day including at break times at school.

  ➢ Avoid caffeine-based and blackcurrant drinks from mid-afternoon.

➤ Encourage the child to empty the bladder before bed, and ensure there is access to the toilet at night. A potty by the bed may help.

➤ Discourage the use of nappies or pull-up pants.
➤ Treatment should take into account the patient's needs and preferences.
➤ Consider enuresis alarm or drug treatment depending on the age, the frequency of bedwetting and the motivation of the child and family.
➤ Explain to children and parents that rewards may be offered for agreed behaviour (such as using star charts):
  ➣ drinking recommended levels of fluid during the day
  ➣ urinating before sleep
  ➣ helping to change sheets or taking medication.
➤ Ask about the presence of daytime symptoms, including:
  ➣ daytime frequency (> 7 times/day?)
  ➣ urgency
  ➣ wetting the underwear.

Management of daytime symptoms (with or without nocturnal enuresis)
➤ Initial management (as above).
➤ Always check the urine with dipsticks (and possibly culture), because of the high incidence of UTI.
➤ Treat daytime symptoms before addressing enuresis.
➤ Children are encouraged to urinate every 2 hours and should not delay attending the toilet to urinate if there is an urge to do so.
➤ Consider treatment with oxybutynin; discuss effects and side-effects with parents.

Management of nocturnal enuresis without severe daytime symptoms
➤ Initial management (as above).
➤ If the child wakes at night, encourage him or her to use the toilet before returning to sleep. Planned lifting of the child at regular times may have practical short-term success (and can be used for young people who have not responded to other treatment), but there is no evidence that it promotes long-term dryness.
➤ If there are some dry nights, a positive-reward system may be tried (reward drinking the right quantities during the day, toilet before bed, helping change sheets, but do not take rewards away for wet nights).
➤ The main treatments are enuresis alarm and desmopressin (*see* the summary in Fig 11.1). If there is no response to either desmopressin or enuresis alarm, combination treatment with both can be used.

Enuresis alarm
An enuresis alarm may be considered as first-line treatment if the management above has failed. Alarms can be bought from Education and Resources for Improving Childhood Continence (ERIC; www.eric.org.uk). They may be available for loan through a local enuresis advisor or ERIC.
➤ The alarm is inappropriate if:
  ➣ the child is too young (e.g. younger than 7 years)
  ➣ the bedwetting is infrequent (e.g. < 1–2 wet beds/week)
  ➣ there is a lack of motivation
  ➣ the child is a deep sleeper.

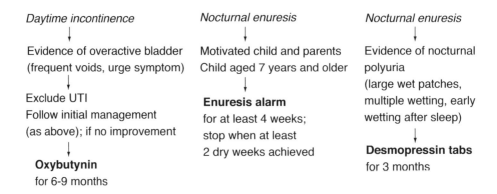

Daytime incontinence
↓
Evidence of overactive bladder
(frequent voids, urge symptom)
↓
Exclude UTI
Follow initial management
(as above); if no improvement
↓
Oxybutynin
for 6-9 months

Nocturnal enuresis
↓
Motivated child and parents
Child aged 7 years and older
↓
Enuresis alarm
for at least 4 weeks;
stop when at least
2 dry weeks achieved

Nocturnal enuresis
↓
Evidence of nocturnal
polyuria
(large wet patches,
multiple wetting, early
wetting after sleep)
↓
Desmopressin tabs
for 3 months

FIGURE 11.1 Summary of daytime and night-time wetting

➤ Assess response after 4 weeks; stop only if there are no early signs of response (significant improvement).
➤ Continue until a minimum of 14 consecutive dry nights have been achieved. Assess and consider alternative treatment after 3 months unless the child is still improving.
➤ Predictors of success:
  ➢ No daytime wetting
  ➢ Normal functional bladder capacity
  ➢ The child feels able to wake during the night
  ➢ The family is prepared to be disturbed at night
  ➢ The child and parents are prepared for longer-term treatment before achieving dryness.

Desmopressin

Offer desmopressin (200 micrograms at bedtime, increased to 400 micrograms if the lower dose is ineffective. Sublingual dose is 120 micrograms at bedtime, increased to 240 micrograms if the lower dose is ineffective) to children with bedwetting if:
  ➢ rapid onset and/or short-term improvement in bedwetting is the priority of treatment
  ➢ an alarm is inappropriate or undesirable
  ➢ there is evidence of nocturnal polyuria (large urine volume)
  ➢ there is no daytime wetting.

Assess response to desmopressin after 4 weeks; stop only if there are no signs of significant improvement.

Parents should be advised that excessive fluid intake while on desmopressin could lead to the rare complication of hyponatraemia.

Referral criteria

➤ Persistent daytime symptoms. Consider referring any child (aged >2 years) who is struggling to remain dry during the day in spite of awareness of the need to pass urine, and who knows how to use the toilet.
➤ History of recurrent UTIs.
➤ Any suspected physical or neurological problems.

➤ Developmental attention or learning difficulties, behavioural or family problems.
➤ Lack of response to treatment.

Further information

ERIC (www.eric.org.uk, Helpline 0845 370 8008, 24 hours a day) produces a number of useful resources for patients and healthcare professionals:
➤ Bedwetting: A Guide for Parents
➤ A Guide to Enuresis
➤ Nocturnal Enuresis Resource Pack
➤ A systematic review of the effectiveness of interventions for managing childhood nocturnal enuresis.

GENITALIA
Groin swelling
Core messages

➤ Swelling of the groin in infants and young children is usually noticed while bathing a child. Lymphadenopathy and inguinal hernia (IH) are the two most common causes (Box 11.2).
➤ An important finding in this area is spermatic cord hydrocele, which is a fluid collection along the spermatic cord, resulting from patent processus vaginalis. It has two types: an encysted hydrocele which does not communicate with the peritoneum, and a communicating hydrocele where the fluid collection communicates with the peritoneum.

BOX 11.2 Main causes of groin swelling

● Inguinal hernia (IH)
● Infectious lymphadenopathy
● Hydrocele of spermatic cord
● Undescended testis (true undescended)

● Femoral hernia
● Testicular feminisation
● Cancerous lymphadenopathy

Recommended investigations

(Diagnosis of groin swelling is clinical, and investigations are usually not required.)
➤ FBC and C-reactive protein (CRP) are occasionally required in case of lymphadenitis (bacterial? leukaemia?).
➤ Ultrasound is useful in differentiating solid mass (lymph node from hydrocele or hernia).
➤ Further tests (such as biopsy) may be required if the lymphadenopathy suggests malignancy.

PRACTICE POINTS

- Children with cystic fibrosis, undescended testes, connective tissue diseases and prematurity (up to 30% of very low birthweight infants) have a high incidence of IH.
- The risk of incarceration from an inguinal hernia (IH) is high during the first 6 months of life. Therefore, urgent referral to a paediatric surgeon should be made for any neonate found to have IH before leaving the hospital.
- Transillumination simply demonstrates the presence of fluid, and of itself is rarely diagnostic since IH may also transilluminate.
- It is important to differentiate between true undescended and retractile (yo-yo) testis. The scrotum in the latter is well developed, while hypoplastic in true undescended testis, and the testis can be manipulated down into the normal scrotal position.
- As undescended testes and IHs commonly co-exist (both due to patent processus vaginalis), an orchidopexy is usually carried out at the same time as hernia repair.
- A child has around 600 lymph nodes but only the minority of them can be palpated, mainly in the neck and sub-mandibular, axillary and inguinal regions. Generalised lymphadenopathy indicates the involvement of at least 2 of these sites.
- Following a repair of IH, a contralateral hernia develops in about 30–40% of cases. The risk rises to 50% if the repair of unilateral hernia is performed within the first year of life.
- An IH which cannot be reduced by manipulation (this occurs in about 5–10% of cases) may occur subsequent to strangulation. This is recognised by:
  - Marked tenderness of a firm mass in a child who inconsolably cries
  - Oedematous skin over the mass, which is often discoloured
  - Signs and symptoms of intestinal obstruction, such as vomiting and abdominal distention.

RED FLAGS

- In adults, it is a common practice to insert the index finger into the inguinal canal to feel for an impulse while the patient is asked to strain or cough. This is not advisable in children because the procedure is too painful and rarely yields any useful information.
- Unlike umbilical hernias, inguinal hernias in children are potentially serious. IH requires repair as soon as possible because of the risk of strangulation. Urgent referral is required if the child is < 6 months of age.
- Inguinal hernia in girls is far less common than in boys. A lump in the inguinal area may contain an ovary or, rarely, a testicle. The latter suggests testicular feminisation, which is confirmed by chromosomal analysis showing 46 XY.

Penile swelling

Core messages

➤ Swelling of the penis, often with inflammation and pain, may occur in association with nappy rash or forceful attempt to retract the foreskin. Other common causes are balanitis (inflammation of the glans) and posthitis (inflammation of the prepuce). Balano-posthitis refers to inflammation of both sites. Priapism, a non-erotic, unwanted, persistent erection, is a relatively frequent complication in children with sickle-cell anaemia (SCA). Trauma is another important cause of priapism, which may be high-flow due to an arteriovenous shunt or low-flow when there is obstruction to the venous outflow.

➤ The oedema of nephrotic syndrome (NS) or Henoch–Schönlein purpura (HSP) accumulates in dependent sites and often causes penile and scrotal swelling. It is easy to differentiate balanitis from oedema: the later lacks redness and other inflammatory signs.

➤ Practically all cases of penile swelling require immediate medical attention, and most require referral. Causes are shown in Box 11.3.

BOX 11.3 Common causes of penile swelling

Penile causes
- Balanitis
- Trauma
- Paraphimosis
- Penile torsion
- Tumour (including carcinoma)
- Epidermal inclusion cyst
- Condom-induced allergy (latex allergy)

Systemic causes
- Priapism
- Generalised oedema (e.g. nephrotic syndrome, Henoch–Schönlein purpura)
- Congenital lymphoedema
- Drugs (cocaine, serotonin re-uptake inhibitors)

PRACTICE POINTS

- The foreskin is normally non-retractile and attached to the glans in neonates. It becomes retractile in about 40% by age 1 year, 90% by age 4 years and 95% by age 15 years. Attempts to forcefully retract the foreskin (e.g. for cleansing) is dangerous; this can lead to balanitis or paraphimosis (*see* Box 11.4 for management of balanitis).
- Cases of paraphimosis (a retracted foreskin behind the corona glans penis which can not be reduced) require immediate attention if ischaemia of the glans is to be prevented. Firm manual compression, with EMLA cream and gauze, will usually reduce the constriction.
- Balanitis, the most common cause of penile inflammation, may result from allergy, seborrhoeic dermatitis, insect bites or from any erosion of the skin allowing bacteria (usually staphylococci) to invade. Sexually transmitted disease should be considered in sexually active adolescents.

- Although sickle cell anaemia is the most common and well-known cause of priapism, other rarer causes are penile neoplasms, leukaemia (particularly chronic granulocytic leukaemia), cocaine abuse and scorpion bite. Parents of children with SCA should be informed of priapism as a possible complication of SCA and advised to seek immediate medical assistance if it occurs.
- Priapism can lead to ischaemia, erectile dysfunction and impotence in the future. Immediate management of children with priapism includes ice packs, bed rest, emptying the bladder, oral or IV hydration, analgesics. Morphine may be required.
- The oedema in nephrotic syndrome is initially subtle, appearing around the eyes and in the lower legs, but the penile swelling is more recognisable and may be the first initial sign of the disease.

BOX 11.4 Management of balanitis

- Balanitis affects more than 4% of boys and is usually associated with a prepuce which is partly or completely non-retractile
- Mild balanitis causing mild redness and discomfort requires simple analgesics, cleansers or antiseptic solutions and reassurance
- Balanitis with systemic manifestations (e.g. fever) requires systemic antibiotic treatment
- Differentiating between physiological and pathological phimosis is important. Most referrals for phimosis seen in paediatric urological clinics are normal physiological phimosis due to age-related non-retractile foreskin (*see above*, in Practice points)
- Foreskin ballooning is usually a benign condition as long as it is painless with otherwise normal appearance of the penis
- There are conflicting opinions amongst health professionals regarding circumcision. Indications for circumcision requiring referral may include:
  > Severe phimosis with ballooning of the foreskin during micturition
  > Recurrent or persistent balanitis
  > Recurrent urinary tract infections, particularly with a history of balanitis or phimosis
  > Paraphimosis

Scrotal swelling

Core messages

➤ Scrotal swelling is very common in children; it may be acute or chronic, painful or painless. Common causes are shown in Box 11.5.

➤ The two most common painless causes are hydrocele and inguinal hernia. Hydrocele is caused by drainage of peritoneal fluid through a narrow patent processus vaginalis, while IH is due to wide patent processus vaginalis that allows omentum or bowel to pass into the scrotum.

➤ Inguinal hernia is frequently associated with undescended testis, prematurity and connective tissue diseases such as Marfan's syndrome.

The four most common painful causes of scrotal swelling are testicular torsion, torsion of testicular appendage, incarcerated inguinal hernia and epididymitis/orchitis. These cases need urgent evaluation and referral to hospital.

BOX 11.5 Common causes of scrotal swelling

Inside the scrotum
- Idiopathic scrotal oedema (ISO)
- Trauma (scrotal haematoma)

Testicular causes
- Testicular torsion
- Orchitis
- Testicular tumour (e.g. hamartoma)

Supra-testicular
- Torsion of the spermatic cord
- Varicocele
- Epididymitis

Systemic/abdominal
- Generalised oedema, e.g. nephrotic syndrome
- Inguinal hernia
- Hydrocele
- Vasculitis (Henoch–Schönlein purpura, Kawasaki disease)

PRACTICE POINTS

- In a mobile child with hydrocele, the size characteristically increases during the daytime and decreases overnight.
- Epididymitis is the most common cause of scrotal swelling in sexually active young adolescents. This is an ascending infection from the urethra. However, it is important not to miss torsion of the testis. Onset usually gradual in contrast to torsion.
- Idiopathic scrotal oedema (ISO) is usually caused by allergy and may mimic torsion. The scrotum is swollen and red in ISO, there are no symptoms, and the testis characteristically feels normal and not tender. ISO often extends to the groin and perineum. Parents can be reassured that the swelling will disappear in a few days without treatment, leaving some purpuric discolouration.
- Varicocele occurs in about 5% of all adolescent boys and may occasionally cause subfertility.
- Abrupt onset of painful scrotal swelling, sometimes with abdominal pain or vomiting, is usually caused by strangulated hernia or testicular torsion. The onset of pain in torsion of testicular appendix is usually gradual.
- Epididymitis/orchitis may mimic testicular torsion; the inflammation is, however, commonly secondary to viral infection (e.g. mumps) or STD. In addition, the pain is more gradual in epididymitis/orchitis, nausea and vomiting is uncommon, and it is often associated with fever, dysuria and pyuria. If in doubt, refer to avoid infarction of the testis.

Vaginal discharge

Core messages

➤ Vaginal discharge is the most common gynaecological problem in girls.

➤ Physiologically, vaginal discharge occurs in neonatal girls who often experience vaginal bleeding (pseudo-menstruation) as a result of withdrawal of maternal oestrogen. A rise in oestrogen at the onset of puberty causes another physiological discharge (leucorrhoea). Box 11.6 shows the main causes of vaginal discharge.

➤ The most common cause of pathological conditions of vaginal discharge is non-specific vaginal discharge (occurring in up to 70% in girls), which is caused by poor perineal hygiene; tendency of the labia minora to open on squatting, predisposing to infection; and close proximity of the anal orifice to the vagina, allowing transfer of faecal bacteria to the vagina. Other contributory factors include the use of systemic antibiotics and steroids, wearing tight-fitting clothes such as tights, and the use of irritants such as detergents and bubble bath.

➤ Children with vaginal discharge present with pruritis, frequent urination, dysuria, daytime incontinence, sleep disturbance or erythema of the vulva. Knickers are usually stained with discharge.

➤ Sexual abuse is a serious problem; a high index of suspicion is required to make the diagnosis. The parent or carer should be asked sensitively if they have any concerns.

BOX 11.6 Common causes of vaginal discharge

- Physiological:
  - › Neonatal vaginal discharge
  - › Pre-pubertal (leucorrhoea)
- Contact and allergic dermatitis
- Lichen sclerosus
- Lichen planus
- Scabies

- Vulvovaginitis:
  - › Non-specific
  - › Bacterial infection (e.g. *Streptococcus*)
  - › *Candida* infection
  - › STD (including from child abuse)
  - › Foreign body
  - › Threadworms
  - › Child abuse

PRACTICE POINTS

- Physiological discharge and bleeding in neonate girls is usually creamy white and subsides at age 2 weeks. Any discharge or bleeding after 2–3 weeks warrants investigation.
- Non-specific discharge is typically brown or green, has a foetid odour and may be associated with bacterial infection secondary to faecal contamination.
- Threadworm infection typically causes recurrent vulvovaginitis and manifests as nocturnal scratching due to female worms depositing eggs on the perineum.
- Discharge caused by *Candida* infection is rare before puberty but may occur in infancy. Risk factors in later age include systemic use of antibiotics and steroids.
- Child sexual abuse refers to the involvement of children in sexual activities (including fondling, masturbation, penetration), which they do not understand or

give consent to (consent is invalid in young children). Most perpetrators of child sexual abuse are close relatives or friends who typically begin relating to the child during non-sexual activities to gain the child's trust.

- An interview with the child suspected of being sexually abused is the most valuable component of medical evaluation, using the child's words for body parts, drawings and age-appropriate questions. Suspected child sexual abuse should always be referred immediately to social services for further evaluation. A GP without additional training should not attempt this. This should always be done by an expert in consultation with police and social services.

- Child sexual abuse may present with symptoms not related directly to their genitalia. These include sleep disturbance, non-specific behaviour changes, phobias, anorexia, poor school performance and social withdrawal. Later on, victims often present with post-traumatic stress disorder (PTSD). A normal physical examination in a child suspected of receiving child sexual abuse does not exclude such an abuse.

- Clinicians should be aware of local policies and referral routes in cases of suspected child sexual abuse. Referral to child social services should be made urgently; the parents' consent should be sought unless this would be likely to lead to further harm of the child.

- Lichen sclerosus is characterised by a sharply demarcated area of hypopigmentation around the vulva and the perianal area. It is associated with intense itching and bleeds easily with normal toilet activities such as genital wiping.

- Foreign body should always be considered when vaginal discharge has a foul odour. Common objects include clumped toilet tissue or small parts of toys. Examination under general anaesthesia may be indicated.

- UTI is very common in association with vaginal discharge. Unless the UTI and/or threadworms are treated, treatment for vaginal discharge is inadequate and it will likely recur.

Labial adhesions

➤ Approximately 3% of pre-pubertal girls (peak age 13–23 months) have this disorder, which is often asymptomatic.

➤ These adhesions may be mistaken for a possible congenital absence of the vagina.

➤ If the adhesions are partial (usually affecting the posterior part of the labia minora), they are unlikely to cause any problem and it may be best to leave them alone. The adhesions very often resolve spontaneously in 6–12 months (in about 80% of cases).

➤ In cases which persist but are asymptomatic, the natural rise in the female hormone oestrogen that occurs at puberty will usually correct the anomaly.

➤ If the adhesion extends to cover the opening of the urethra, the child is at risk of recurrent UTIs, obstruction of urinary flow and vaginal discharge through pooling of urine in the vagina. The child should be referred for possible surgical separation of the adhesion. Where there is no obstruction, oestrogen creams are indicated (see below).

Treatment

Treatment consists of:

➤ Avoid irritants such as bubble bath and strong soaps.
➤ The nappy area should be as clean and dry as possible. Urine and stools should be removed promptly.
➤ Children should be taught to wipe their bottoms after defecation from front to back.
➤ Topical oestrogen cream (e.g. Gynest containing 0.01% estriol) applied each evening (small pea-size amount squeezed on the index finger and applied on the fused labia) to the adhesions for 2 weeks is effective. This is followed by the use of a lubricating ointment such as petroleum jelly for 1–2 months after the adhesions separate. Can be used for 4 weeks if no or minimal separation obtained. Side-effects include appearance of local pigmentation, prominence of the labia and blood-spotting or slight vaginal bleeding following the treatment. These side-effects are transient and disappear after the treatment has discontinued.

REFERENCES

1. Birmingham Research Unit. Weekly Returns Service. Annual report 2004. London. Royal College of GPs; 2004.
2. Urinary tract infection in children. Diagnosis, treatment and long-term management. Clinical guidelines, August 2007. www.rcog.org.uk

CHAPTER 12

Ear, nose, throat

EARACHES/INFECTION

Core messages

➤ Earache (Otalgia) is a very common reason for seeking medical attention (Box 12.1).

➤ Otitis media (OM) is usually caused by viruses, e.g. adenovirus and influenza. Otitis externa (OE) is mostly caused by *Pseudomonas* and staphylococci.

➤ In contrast to adults, referred pain from outside the ears (extrinsic causes) is common in paediatric patients, occurring via 5 main sources: trigeminal nerve (sensory distribution of the face, teeth, gums); facial nerve (temporomandibular joint or Bell's palsy); glossopharyngeal nerve (tonsils, pharynx); vagus nerve (laryngopharynx or oesophagus) or via the 2nd–3rd cervical vertebrae (cervical spine). In all these cases, patients have a normal otological examination.

➤ Ramsay–Hunt syndrome (auditory herpes zoster) usually presents with severe ear pain. Clues for this syndrome are vesicles on the pinna and in the external auditory canal in the distribution of the sensory branch of the facial nerve.

BOX 12.1 Causes of otalgia

- Infective acute otitis media (AOM)
- Infective otitis externa
- Referred pain (toothache, tonsillopharyngitis)
- Foreign body
- Eustachian tube dysfunction
- Infected eczematous dermatitis
- Mastoiditis
- Temporomandibular arthritis
- Ramsay–Hunt syndrome (herpes zoster oticus)

Diagnosis of otitis media

(*See* Box 12.2.)

BOX 12.2 Diagnostic features of acute otitis media

- History of or the presence of an upper respiratory tract infection
- Acute onset of symptoms and signs
- Discomfort affecting normal activity and sleep
- Fever occurs in 30–50%
- Red, cloudy and/or bulging tympanic membrane (TM) with decreased mobility*
- Middle-ear structures are frequently obscured
- Discharging ear

* Motility of the TM can be assessed using both positive and negative pressure by examination with a pneumatic otoscope.

Management
(*See* Box 12.3.)

BOX 12.3 Therapeutic guidelines for otitis media (OM) and acute otitis media (AOM)

- Appropriate analgesia
- Antibiotics are not routinely indicated in OM
- Antibiotics for AOM are indicated if there is:
  - ❯ Fever >38.6°C
  - ❯ Ill-looking appearance
  - ❯ Signs of impending perforation
  - ❯ No improvement of symptoms, particularly persistent fever, after 48 hours

- Choices of antibiotics include:
  - ❯ Amoxicillin*
  - ❯ Macrolides, e.g. azithromycin* (rather than clarithromycin or erythromycin)
  - ❯ Co-amoxiclav
  - ❯ Cephalosporin
- Decongestant, antihistamine and steroids are of no value

* First-line antibiotic treatment.

🔖 RED FLAGS

- The tympanic membrane of a crying baby is often red on inspection but without bulging or obscuring of the middle-ear structures; do not misdiagnose OM.
- The presence of otalgia in the absence of otological findings indicates the need for a thorough examination to determine the source of referred pain.
- Bloody discharge may follow direct trauma; a foreign body in the ear canal and, rarely, cancer should be excluded.
- A child with suppuration in the middle ear or mastoid is at risk of developing subdural or extradural abscess, meningitis and brain abscess. Persistent fever with little or no response to antibiotic therapy, severe otal-

gia and persistent headache, vomiting, lethargy or irritability, and tender mastoid area on pressing all require immediate referral.

- Children with recurrent OM should undergo baseline immune evaluation, e.g. full blood count (FBC) and immunoglobulins.
- In Ramsay–Hunt syndrome, the associated hearing loss and facial palsy may be permanent (in about 50% of cases).

Criteria for referral
➤ Persisting hearing problems for >3 months following an episode of OM
➤ Recurrent OM, e.g. >6 episodes within 12 months
➤ Persistent otorrhoea
➤ Concern about OM complications, e.g. mastoiditis, meningitis, etc

Management of otitis media with effusion (OME)[1]
(Also known as glue ear or chronic serous otitis media.)

Initial assessment
➤ OME is a middle-ear effusion without symptoms of inflammation or infection, such as fever or pain.
➤ Features, which may suggest OME are:
  ➢ Recurrent OM, URTIs, frequent nasal obstruction
  ➢ Hearing impairment, which is usually mild (20–30 dB)
  ➢ Delayed speech and language development
  ➢ Behaviour problems, particularly inattention, lack of concentration or intolerance to loud sounds
  ➢ Complaints of fullness in the ear, mild earache and tinnitus.
➤ Diagnosis can be confirmed by the following:
  ➢ Otoscopic examination: dullness of the tympanic membrane (TM) with loss of the light reflex. The TM may be yellow or blue and is usually retracted, its mobility impaired, opaque-appearing and non-erythematous (unless the child is crying)
  ➢ Hearing testing, e.g. picture vocabulary test or distraction test
  ➢ Tympanometry. This is very useful, particularly if the TM cannot be visualised.
➤ Following suppurative OM, effusion will be present in:
  ➢ 80% of cases at 2 weeks
  ➢ 40% of cases at 1 month
  ➢ 20% of cases at 2 months
  ➢ 10% of cases at 3 months.

Initial treatment
➤ Watchful waiting is indicated if the effusion has persisted for <3 months and the child is not significantly symptomatic.
➤ Review after 3 months.
➤ There is no evidence to support the use of the following: antibiotics, topical or systemic antihistamines, topical or systemic decongestants, topical or systemic steroids, homeopathy, or dietary modification, e.g. probiotics.[1]

When to refer
➤ Hearing impairment persistent, for >3 months.
➤ Any hearing impairment which is causing speech delay.
➤ Significant hearing loss after 3 months often requires myringotomy with insertion of grommets to improve middle-ear ventilation.
➤ In cases of persistence of OME despite tympanostomy tubes, adenoidectomy irrespective of adenoid size may benefit some children. Adenoidectomy is more strongly indicated in cases where the adenoid hypertrophy is causing symptoms, e.g. snoring and restlessness at night.

Surgical intervention should be considered for:
➤ Persistent bilateral OME documented for >3 months with a hearing loss in the better ear of 25–30 dB or more, averaged over the 0.5, 1, 2 and 4 kHz frequencies.

🏴 RED FLAGS

- Children with Down's syndrome and those with cleft palate are particularly susceptible to OME, which often occurs at an early age and is likely to be persistent. Early and regular evaluation, including referral to an ENT specialist, is required.
- Deep retraction pockets in the tympanic membrane may lead to permanent structural damage and cholesteatoma, which can be prevented by an early insertion of grommets.

Grommets
➤ Although surgery (insertion of grommets, adenoidectomy, or both) results in short-term hearing gain (about 12 dB improvement in hearing), evidence for its long-term benefits is lacking. Box 12.4 provides some tips for children with grommets.

BOX 12.4 Practice tips for children with grommets

- After insertion of grommets, 13% of children develop otorrhoea through the tube even though it is properly placed and patent. Otorrhoea persists in 5% at 1 year
- Grommets should fall out in 6–9 months and the perforation should heal spontaneously
- Persistent perforation occurs in <1% of cases and surgery may be required later
- Surface swimming is allowed without earplugs, but if diving or using water chutes, well-fitting silicone rubber earplugs (or a plug made with cotton wool and smeared with Vaseline) should be worn. Bath water is much worse than swimming-pool water because of the higher concentration of bacteria from the rest of the body and irritant soap

---

➤ It is common for the child's ear to ooze or bleed for 1 or 2 days postoperatively. Some earache is also common. Infection following grommet insertion commonly presents with otorrhoea and requires antibiotic treatment.
➤ A hearing test in 6–8 weeks is recommended.
➤ Otoscopy should be performed at 4–6 months in primary care to ensure that the grommets are still in situ and to check for any problems.

➤ Referral back to ENT is indicated for:
  ➣ Recurrent otalgia
  ➣ Recurrent symptoms suggestive of OME, especially parental concerns of recurrence of hearing loss
  ➣ Perforation or significant retraction of the TM
  ➣ Suspected cholesteatoma: sac-like structure of white, shiny and greasy tissue granulation in the atticoantral part of the eardrum accompanied by a foul-smelling discharge
  ➣ Retained grommet after >2 years.

RED FLAG

- Cholesteatoma should be recognised because a delay may lead to invasion and destruction of the mastoid bone and spread to the intracranial cavity. Urgent referral to ENT specialists is required.

Management of otitis externa

Diagnosis

➤ OE is usually due to water contamination following swimming or to dermatitis of the external canal, and to use of cotton buds.
➤ Pain is the predominant symptom; elicit pre-auricular tenderness.
➤ Examination includes oedema, erythema, otorrhoea and tender pre-auricular lymph node.
➤ A swab of the discharge should be taken if there is incomplete response to initial treatment.

Initial management

➤ Oral analgesics (paracetamol or ibuprofen).
➤ Topical antibiotic preparations containing neomycin, polymyxin or gentamicin.
➤ Keep ear dry.
➤ During and after an episode of acute OE, children should not swim and the ears should be protected from water during bathing.
➤ Consider ear toilet when the acute inflammation subsides. An insertion of an ear wick may be necessary if the ear canal is very oedematous.

When to refer

➤ Severe ear pain not relieved by analgesics.
➤ Cellulitis beyond the ear canal (child usually requires IV antibiotics).

PRACTICE POINTS

- While AOM is more common in infants and toddlers, OE is more common in older children and adolescents.
- OE, also called swimmer's ear, tends to recur in children who swim. Instillation of 2% acetic acid (vinegar) immediately after swimming is effective in preventing this.

🏳 **RED FLAGS**

- Signs of cholesteatoma should not be misdiagnosed as OE.
- Some topical otic preparations (neomycin, colistin, polymyxin), used to treat OE, can cause contact dermatitis which manifests as erythema, vesiculation and oedema.

EAR SYRINGING

Core messages

➤ Cerumen (ear wax) provides protection for the ear canal and needs to be removed only if there are symptoms of pain or discomfort, hearing impairment or interference with a proper view of the TM.

➤ Young children, cognitively impaired children (e.g. with Down's syndrome), those wearing hearing aids and those with anatomically deformed ear canal are at high risk for impacted ear wax.

➤ Irrigation of the ear canal gently with warm water (see next section) is effective provided that the eardrum is intact, there are no signs of OE and no history of previous ear surgery or unilateral deafness.

➤ Cerumenolytic agents and wax softeners include sterile saline solution, olive oil, almond oil or sodium bicarbonate ear drops. There is no significant difference in efficacy between them.

➤ The child should lie down with the affected ear uppermost for 5–10 minutes after ear drops have been installed.

➤ If the ear wax is impacted, ear drops should be used twice daily for a few days before syringing or micro-suction.

Syringing

Equipment required:

➤ Auroscope
➤ Tissue
➤ Towel
➤ Propulse ear syringe
➤ Noots tank

Procedure

➤ Explain procedure to child and parent. Ask the child to indicate any discomfort.
➤ Ensure that a softening agent, e.g. olive oil, has been used for at least 5 days prior to the procedure, and that the ear wax is soft.
➤ Use the largest speculum on the auroscope that will fit into the ear.
➤ Gently pull the pinna upwards and backwards to straighten the canal.
➤ Protect the child with a towel.
➤ Ask the child (if old enough) or the parent to support the Noots tank.
➤ After the wax has been removed, perform a final check to ensure that the canal is clear and there has been no damage to the eardrum.
➤ Discuss prevention, especially not using cotton buds.

HEARING LOSS

Core messages

➤ Severe hearing loss is usually caused by a lesion in the cochlea or the auditory nerve and its central connections (sensorineural hearing loss, SNHL). Varying degrees of conductive hearing loss is very common, mainly as a result of otitis media with effusion (OME). Severe persistent OME may cause a significant delay in language acquisition.

➤ The diagnosis of high-frequency hearing loss is often difficult to make and thus made late. As most consonant sounds are middle- or high-pitched, the child appears to hear well but is poor at understanding what is said. Only a mumble of unclear sounds are heard. The child is often regarded as 'slow'.

➤ It is estimated that 1–2 newborns per 1000 live births have varying degrees of bilateral SNHL, and 90% of them have no family history of deafness (Table 12.1).

➤ The most common neonatal screening is otoacoustic emissions (OAEs). Babies who do not pass on OAEs should be screened using auditory brainstem response (ABR). More information is obtained on www.hearing.screening.nhs.uk

➤ Box 12.5 lists the main risk factors for hearing impairment.

TABLE 12.1 Degrees of hearing loss

<25 dB	Normal hearing
25–35 dB	Mild hearing loss
40–60 dB	Moderate hearing loss
60–90 dB	Severe hearing loss
>90 dB	Profound hearing loss

BOX 12.5 Risk factors for hearing loss

- Family history of deafness
- Parental smoking (risk factor for OME)
- Low birthweight, particularly <1500 g
- Use of ototoxic drugs, e.g. gentamicin
- Craniofacial malformations
- The presence of pre-auricular pit or tag
- Severe perinatal asphyxia
- Severe jaundice, bilirubin > 400 μmol/L
- Congenital infections, e.g. toxoplasmosis, rubella
- History of CNS infection, e.g. meningitis
- Recurrent or persistent OME for >3 months
- Trauma associated with loss of consciousness
- Down's syndrome, cleft palate, Turner's syndrome

Detection of hearing impairment

➤ This should begin as early as possible. Parental concerns usually precede medical detection and diagnosis of hearing impairment by 6–12 months. Primary-care physicians are in a unique position to respond to these concerns, and identify whether the child's speech and language development is delayed (Table 12.2).

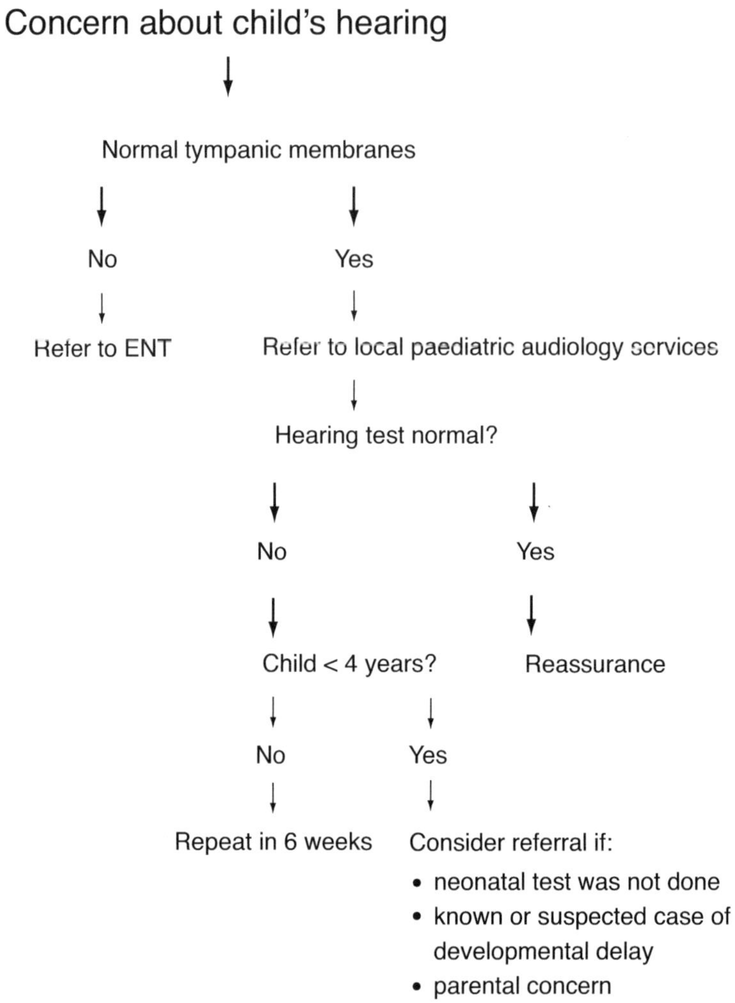

Concern about child's hearing

↓

Normal tympanic membranes

↓   ↓

No   Yes

↓   ↓

Refer to ENT   Refer to local paediatric audiology services

↓

Hearing test normal?

↓   ↓

No   Yes

↓   ↓

Child < 4 years?   Reassurance

↓   ↓

No   Yes

↓   ↓

Repeat in 6 weeks   Consider referral if:
- neonatal test was not done
- known or suspected case of developmental delay
- parental concern

FIGURE 12.1 Referral pathway for hearing impairment

BOX 12.6 Management of hearing loss

Conductive
- See sections on OME and grommets, above

Sensorineural
- Medical examination, full developmental assessment and possible investigation
- Ophthalmic examination, as eye problems may co-exist
- Genetic counselling (hereditary hearing loss, syndromes)
- Assessment for special educational needs
- Hearing-aid provision
- Support by deaf societies such as the National Deaf Children's Society and the Royal National Institute for the Deaf

➤ In the high-risk category for hearing loss or if children are significantly slow in achieving the developmental milestones shown in Table 12.2, hearing tests should be considered (Table 12.3).

➤ Figure 12.1 shows summary points for children suspected of hearing loss.

TABLE 12.2 Developmental milestones related to hearing ability at ages 0–24 months

Age (months)	Normal developmental milestones
0–1	Startles, blinks or quiets briefly to loud sounds (bell)
2–4	Coos, increases vocalisation when spoken to, quiets to mother's voice, laughs
5–6	Shows excitement at voices, localises the sounds presented in a horizontal plane, vocalising 'ah-goo'
7–12	Imitates sounds, responds to name when called, can say 'mama' or 'dada' (non-specifically) aged 9 months
	One word with meaning (10 months)
15	Four or five words
18	Should follow simple spoken directions
21	20–50 words, combines two words
24	At least 50 words, 3-word sentences

TABLE 12.3 Hearing tests

Age	Test	Comments
Birth	Otoacoustic emission (OAE)	Quick, simple and sensitive test; can detect low hearing loss. Test routinely performed in all neonates whilst in hospital
	Brainstem-evoked potential (BSEP)	Too time-consuming for universal screening. BSEP is useful if the baby fails a second testing with OAE
> 3 years	Pure tone audiometry	Best diagnostic test at all ages once cooperation is possible. Children are referred to ENT specialist if thresholds > 25 dB hearing loss
Any age	Tympanometry	Used to assess the flexibility of the TM

Management

(*See* Box 12.6.)

Full explanation of the nature of the hearing loss to parents and teachers is helpful and leads to better cooperation and more-effective communication.

NOSE

Persistent nasal discharge/blocked nose

Core messages

➤ By far the most common causes of persistent nasal discharge or blockage are viral infectious rhinitis, allergic rhinitis and adenoidal hypertrophy.

➤ In neonates and young infants, blocked nose (snuffles) is common due to the presence of mucus in a narrowed nasal passage. It is loud during feeding and sleep, and disappears at age 4–5 months. Parents should be reassured, provided the baby is well and thriving. Nasal malformations such as congenital narrowing of the nasal passage, choanal atresia (incidence 1 in 7000 live births) and stenosis have to be considered in the differential diagnosis, particularly if the symptoms are persistent.

➤ Although the vast majority of causes are benign and self-limiting, serious conditions include nasopharyngeal tumours, encephalocele and foreign body. In these conditions, discharge is usually purulent, foul-smelling with or without blood, and unilateral.

➤ It is easy for the clinician to diagnose polyps clinically: in contrast to the highly vascularised pink turbinate tissue, nasal polyps are grey, shiny, grape-looking masses present between the nasal turbinates and the septum, and not tender.

Causes of nasal discharge/blocked nose are provided in Table 12.4.

TABLE 12.4 Summary of the causes of persistent nasal discharge/blockage

Causes	Diagnosis	Comments
Congenital	Baby snuffles	Caused by mucus in a narrowed nasal passage. It becomes loud during feeding, disappears at age 4–5 months
Infection	Viral rhinitis	Extremely common; discharge is at first watery, may become viscous and green in colour
	Bacterial rhinitis	Rare. Typically, cold symptoms, previously present, worsen with facial pain, fever and green discharge
Allergy	Seasonal	Pollen, grass, weeds, moulds spores. History is diagnostic
	Perennial	House dust mite, animal dander
Obstruction	Adenoid hypertrophy	Symptoms include nasal congestion, snoring, mouth breathing, sleep disturbance, recurrent otitis media
	Foreign body	Often presenting as purulent unilateral nasal discharge, sometimes bloody, nasal pain
	Nasal polyposis	Associated with cystic fibrosis, persistent discharge from allergy or inflammation

Evaluation of a child with persistent nasal symptoms
Symptoms
(Acute: ≤7 days; persistent: ≥7 days)
➤ Itchy nose
➤ Sneezing
➤ Watery nasal discharge
➤ Itchy, watery eyes (70% of patients with allergic rhinitis have ocular symptoms)

Signs
➤ Pale and swollen mucosa
➤ Nasal polyosis
➤ Creases across the nose (allergic salute)
➤ Darkened areas under the lower eyelids

Degree of severity

Mild
➤ Normal sleep
➤ No impaired daily activities
➤ Normal school attendance
➤ No troublesome symptoms

Moderate–severe
➤ Abnormal sleep
➤ Impaired daily activities
➤ Absence from school
➤ Troublesome symptoms

Referral may be considered if:
➤ there is no rapid solution and symptoms persist
➤ foreign body or polyps are suspected

When to refer for allergy testing
➤ Patients with significantly discomforting or disabling symptoms that are not controlled by medications and allergy avoidance

Management
➤ Non-sedating antihistamine is indicated in cases of allergic rhinitis.
➤ Decongestants are of no benefit, particularly in young children.
➤ Vitamin C in a dose of 0.2 mg to 2000 mg has a modest but consistent effect in reduction of common cold symptoms when taken during the illness.[2]
➤ Antibiotics may have a mild or modest benefit in older children. Around 8 children must be treated in order to achieve 1 additional cure. Antibiotics may be considered in cases of associated systemic manifestations such as fever or suspected sinusitis.
➤ Antiviral agents: benefit from antivirals has not been demonstrated.

For mild intermittent symptoms of allergic rhinitis
➤ Avoidance of allergens
➤ Non-sedating antihistamine

For moderate persistent symptoms
➤ Intranasal steroid added to non-sedating antihistamine

Severe persistent symptoms
➤ Short course of oral steroids
➤ Non-sedating antihistamine
➤ Antibiotics as above
➤ Consider referral

Acute nose bleed (epistaxis)

Initial work-up

(*See* Fig 12.2.)

➤ Initial assessment for signs of shock and the need for resuscitation
➤ History and physical examination
➤ Rule out blood dyscrasia:
   ➢ Past medical and family history
   ➢ Spontaneous bruising or bleeding
   ➢ Consider FBC and coagulation screen with PT and PTT

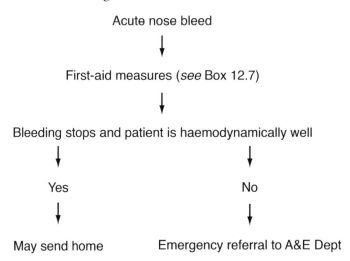

FIGURE 12.2 Summary of management of epistaxis

BOX 12.7 First-aid measures for treating acute nose bleed

- Sit patient down
- Lean patient forward to avoid blood trickling into pharynx
- Pinch the cartilaginous part of the nose gently for about 5–10 minutes, repeat the procedure if re-bleed occurs
- If the bleeding persists, consider referral for possible:
  › anterior nasal pack, which may need to be inserted by an experienced doctor
  › local application of a solution of oxymetazoline, xylometazoline or ephedrine
  › cauterisation

OBSTRUCTIVE SLEEP APNOEA (OSA)

Initial work-up

➤ Prevalence about 1%; peak age 2–5 years, coinciding with normal lymphoid hyperplasia and frequent upper respiratory tract infections. Predisposing conditions are shown in Box 12.8.
➤ Symptoms include snoring/apnoea, and chronic mouth-breathing observed by the parents.

➤ Sleep disturbance characterised by labour respiration, restlessness and waking at night, unusual sleep positions to maintain a patent upper airway.
➤ Daytime somnolence, impaired daytime and school performance.
➤ In severe cases: right-sided heart failure, arrhythmia, developmental delay.

Assessment

➤ Physical examination during wakefulness may be entirely normal. Diagnosis of OSA is not excluded by normal physical examination when the history suggests otherwise.
➤ Enlarged tonsils and adenoids are the commonest cause.
➤ Exclude other causes (*see* Box 12.8).

Treatment

➤ Medications (e.g. nasal decongestants or topical steroids) have limited value.
➤ Because adenotonsillar enlargement is the most common cause of OSA, adenotonsillectomy is indicated.

Refer when:

➤ There is witnessed sleep apnoea
➤ Sleep disturbance persists, >3 months
➤ There is chronic snoring and/or mouth-breathing.

Further investigation includes polysomnography with oxygen saturation monitoring and/or MRI.

BOX 12.8 Conditions predisposing to OSA

- Adenotonsillar hyperplasia
- Down's syndrome
- Congenital craniofacial abnormalities:
  › Small nasopharynx
  › Micrognathia
  › Macroglossia
- Obesity
- Persistent nasal obstruction
- Neuromuscular diseases

SORE THROAT

Core messages

➤ Upper respiratory tract infections (URTIs) are the most common illness and the most common medical reason for school absence in children. An infection rate of 6–8 infections a year is normal. A higher incidence is found in infants and children who attend nursery and whose siblings attend nursery or school.
➤ Viruses are by far the most common causes of URTIs, and more than 200 viruses can cause URTIs. Acute tonsillopharyngitis with exudates is usually of viral origin. Antibiotics are therefore not indicated for the majority of cases (Box 12.9).
➤ Group A beta-haemolytic streptococci (GAHS) is the only common bacterial causative agent. Viral and bacterial tonsillopharyngitis have overlapping features, and clinically they are often indistinguishable from each other.
➤ The main indication for antibiotic therapy of bacterial pharyngitis is not only to treat

the symptoms but also to prevent complications, e.g. peritonsillar abscess, rheumatic fever (RF) and glomerulonephritis (GN). Penicillin is the antibiotic of choice for suspected bacterial tonsillopharyngitis (Box 12.10).

➤ Acute tonsillopharyngitis is uncommon in children younger than 1 year of age, peaks at the age of 4–7 years and continues throughout later childhood.

➤ Asymptomatic colonisation with group A streptococci occurs in 10–20% of normal school-aged children. They are not at risk of developing RF or GN, and do not require antibiotic treatment.

➤ While herpetic stomatitis (caused by herpesvirus) has lesions on the gingiva, in herpangina (caused by coxsackie virus) there are discrete punctuate vesicles, surrounded by erythematous rings on the soft palate, anterior pillars and uvula.

Causes

Causes of sore throat are given in Box 12.9.

BOX 12.9 Causes of sore throat

Viral

Viral URTI (including tonsillopharyngitis), glandular fever, herpetic gingivostomatitis, herpangina, immunodeficiency (e.g. HIV infection)

Bacterial

Bacterial tonsillitis, scarlet fever, retropharyngeal or peritonsillar abscess

Fungal

Oropharyngeal thrush

Others

Leucopenia neutropenia, psychogenic causes, aphthous ulceration

---

BOX 12.10 Features which favour a bacterial cause of sore throat and may need antibiotics

● Absence of URTI symptoms (no runny nose or cough)
● Unwell or ill-looking patient
● Patient aged 5–15 years
● Tonsillar enlargement with diffuse redness, exudates
● Redness of the pharynx and tonsillar pillars, with petechial spots on the soft palate
● Enlarged and tender anterior cervical lymph nodes
● High fever, temperatures > 39.0°C

Laboratory testing

(Laboratory testing is not required in the majority of cases.)

➤ FBC may show leucocytosis in bacterial infection, lymphocytosis in glandular fever; C-reactive protein (CRP).

➤ Rapid antigen testing for GAHS is more commonly used in the USA and has sensitivity and specificity of up to >90%. PCR-based tests (polymerase chain reaction) are now available and are equivalent or superior to culture. A throat swab to culture group A streptococci may be useful, but the result will take 24–48 hours to arrive.

➤ An anti-streptolysin O-titre (ASO titre) with a 4-fold increase in 1–2 weeks is the only diagnostic test for streptococcal infection because of the colonisation that commonly occurs.

➤ Monospot is useful to diagnose glandular fever (sensitivity 90%; specificity 95%). Immunoglobulin M (IgM) for Epstein–Barr virus (EBV) is positive in almost 100% of cases. PCR for detection of EBV is now commonly used to aid diagnosis.

RED FLAGS

- Beware that agranulocytosis may present with sore throat as the first sign of the disease.
- Many systemic diseases (e.g. Crohn's disease) manifest as ulcers in the oral cavity, which present as sore throat. Look for an underlying disease with any unexplained mouth ulcers, especially if severe, prolonged or multiple.
- Consider immunosuppression, e.g. HIV, in any child older than a neonate who has *Candida* infection.
- When there is a membranous exudate on the tonsils, mononucleosis is likely. Ampicillin-related antibiotics, including co-amoxiclav, should not be used because of the risk of severe rash in the presence of glandular fever.

Management

Table 12.5 summarises management of sore throat.

TABLE 12.5 Management of sore throat

Category	Medication	Comments
Beneficial	Adequate hydration	Frequent intake of liquids
	Analgesics (paracetamol or ibuprofen)	Paracetamol as first line of treatment; ibuprofen should not be given if there are signs of dehydration
	Saline nose drops	Drops can loosen nasal secretions and help with sneezing
	Antibiotics	If symptoms and signs suggest bacterial cause (*see* Box 12.10)
Frequently used remedies but with insufficient evidence of their benefits	Antihistamine Decongestants Lozenges Gargles Water vaporiser Expectorants Cough suppressants Vitamin C[2]	There are hundreds of over-the-counter medications for treating the common cold. Although it is tempting to turn to medications, unless the child is very ill it is best to avoid most of them

TONSILLECTOMY

➤ Tonsillectomy is one of the most frequently performed surgical procedures in the UK, particularly in children. It accounts for about 20% of all operations performed by otolaryngologists.

➤ Studies have not shown a clear clinical benefit of tonsillectomy in children. A Cochrane review showed only a modest benefit of tonsillectomy/adenotonsillectomy in the treatment of recurrent tonsillitis.[3]

➤ Tonsillectomy in children < 2–3 years old is generally performed for obstructive sleep apnoea.

➤ Some tips for evaluating for tonsillectomy are given in Box 12.11.

BOX 12.11 Top tips for evaluating for tonsillectomy

- Large tonsil size alone without symptoms of obstruction is not an indication for tonsillectomy. Enlarged size without infection is common
- Watchful waiting is more appropriate than tonsillectomy for children with mild and recurrent sore throats
- Tonsillectomy may be considered for:
  - ❯ 7 or more documented, clinically significant episodes of tonsillitis which have prevented normal functioning in the preceding year
  - ❯ Exclusion of tumour
  - ❯ Peri-tonsillar abscess
  - ❯ Obstructive sleep apnoea
- Patients should be made aware that postoperatively:
  - ❯ They are likely to have pain for up to 6 days following tonsillectomy
  - ❯ Minor complications such as haemorrhage may occur (in about 4% of patients)
  - ❯ Anti-emetic drugs are likely to be needed to prevent postoperative nausea and vomiting

---

STRIDOR AND HOARSENESS

Core messages

➤ Stridor and hoarseness commonly occur subsequent to an acute upper airway obstruction in association with a viral URTI (causing croup or laryngotracheobronchitis) or without it (causing spasmodic croup). Symptoms are usually mild and transient and recovery within a few days is expected. Persistent hoarseness suggests cord paralysis or tumours (Box 12.12).

➤ Croup is mostly caused by viruses; the parainfluenza type B are the major pathogens. Bacterial causes are rare: *Mycoplasma pneumoniae* can cause croup, *Staphylococcus aureus* bacterial tracheitis and *Haemophilus influenzae* type B epiglottitis.

➤ Croup is characterised by an URTI followed by abrupt onset of barking cough, inspiratory stridor, hoarseness and varying degrees of respiratory distress. Degrees of severity are shown in Table 12.6.

➤ Persistent stridor commencing in the first few weeks of life is usually caused by laryngomalacia as a result of collapse of the supraglottic structure during inspiration. A child with laryngomalacia has a normal cry and no cough.

BOX 12.12 Acute and persistent causes of stridor

Acute
- Laryngotracheobronchitis (viral croup)
- Spasmodic croup
- Angioedema
- Overuse of the voice (excessive crying)
- Epiglottitis
- Infectious mononucleosis
- Bacterial tracheitis
- Aspiration of foreign body
- Hypocalcaemic tetany
- Retropharyngeal or peritonsillar abscess
- Measles croup
- Diphtheria

Persistent
- Laryngomalacia
- Tumour, e.g. papilloma, haemangioma, nodule
- Laryngeal web
- Hypothyroidism
- Recurrent laryngeal nerve palsy (postoperative)
- Vascular ring

TABLE 12.6 Assessment of severity of croup

	Mild croup; can be managed at home	Severe croup; refer immediately to hospital
Mental status	Normal	Agitated or exhausted
Severity of stridor	Mild	Severe
Ability to talk	Yes	Difficult
Respiratory rate, pulse rate	Normal	Increased
Fever	Absent or low-grade	Temperature >39.0°C
Accessory muscle use	No	Yes
Air entry	Normal	Decreased
Level of consciousness	Normal	Drowsy

Recommended investigations (for persistent stridor)

(Most cases of acute hoarseness and stridor do not need any investigation.)

➤ Thyroid function test (TFT) to exclude hypothyroidism
➤ Serum calcium to confirm hypocalcaemia
➤ Chest X-ray may diagnose vascular ring or aspiration. An upper-airway X-ray to evaluate possible retropharyngeal or peritonsillar abscess may be performed
➤ Direct laryngoscopy to diagnose laryngeal node (post-ventilation), haemangiomas and unilateral or bilateral paralysis of the vocal cord
➤ CT or MRI of the head to diagnose Chiari's malformation

PRACTICE POINTS

- In neonates: laryngeal injury may occur subsequent to birth trauma, and results in unilateral vocal cord paralysis (usually left side) producing hoarseness with mild stridor. Bilateral paralysis of the vocal cord causes, in addition, dyspnoea. The prognosis of post-ventilation aphonia/hoarseness is good and recovery is expected.

- Nocturnal onset of acute stridor with barking cough and hoarse voice is almost certainly croup, viral or spasmodic. The prognosis is excellent. Only about 1–2% of children with viral croup have severe symptoms requiring intensive care and intubation.
- A child with croup who rapidly becomes unwell with high fever may have developed an extension of the infection into the respiratory tract, or bacterial tracheitis as a complication of the viral croup, or may have bacterial epiglottitis.
- In epiglottitis the voice is actually not hoarse, but muffled because vocal cords are not affected. Ask about Haemophilus influenzae B (HiB) vaccination.
- The most important aspect of acute stridor is to differentiate between a life-threatening illness such as epiglottitis or foreign body, and a relatively harmless croup caused by a viral infection.
- Laryngomalacia is the most common cause of persistent stridor during infancy. It is caused by a soft-tissue laxity above the vocal cords, which collapses during inspiration. Parents can be reassured that recovery will occur at age 12–18 months, often even earlier. Once the diagnosis of laryngomalacia is made, direct examination of the larynx is not indicated unless there are atypical features such as associated feeding problems or worsening stridor.

RED FLAGS

- In cases of viral croup or epiglottitis, throat inspection, including the use of a tongue depressor, may result in sudden cardiorespiratory arrest and therefore should be omitted.
- Symptoms of laryngotracheobronchitis do not usually continue for more than a few days. Persistent symptoms require laryngoscopy to detect the cause.
- A young child (6 months to 2 years old) with sudden choking, coughing with or without stridor or hoarseness should be suspected of having foreign body.
- In severe allergic reaction, sudden onset of angioedema of the subglottic areas may occur, causing sudden stridor and respiratory distress. Adrenaline injection is life-saving.
- Stridor may be caused by papilloma, which is the most common tumour of the larynx. Although it is usually benign and often regresses at the time of puberty, it can extend into the lower airways and lungs, causing a serious disease.
- Do not diagnose laryngomalacia if there are signs of respiratory distress, apnoea or cyanotic episodes, or failure to thrive.

BOX 12.13 Therapeutic tips in stridor

- Most afebrile or febrile children with mild symptoms of croup can usually be managed at home
- Patients should be disturbed as little as possible
- Monitoring the patient is important, including respiratory rate and pulse rate: increases in these may be the first signs of hypoxia
- The use of steam from a shower in a closed bathroom or steam from a vaporiser is helpful and may terminate the laryngeal spasm within a few minutes
- Steroids reduce inflammatory oedema, and are given as:
  > dexamethasone 0.3 mg/kg/dose by mouth or by injection before transfer to hospital
  > budesonide inhalation 2 mg as a single dose or in 2 divided doses separated by 30 minutes; dose may be repeated after 12 hours if necessary

---

SWALLOWING DIFFICULTY (DYSPHAGIA)

Core messages

➤ Swallowing is a complex mechanism involving some 50 muscle pairs to bring swallowed material to the stomach.

➤ Swallowing is developed as early as 20 weeks of gestation and is established at 33–34 weeks of gestation.

➤ Dysphagia is defined as a difficulty in swallowing and is categorised by location into impaired transfer of fluids or food from the oral cavity to the oesophagus (*pre-oesophageal dysphagia*) or from the oesophagus to the stomach (*oesophageal dysphagia*).

➤ Causes of pre-oesophageal dysphagia include myasthenia gravis and pseudo-bulbar palsy. Causes of oesophageal dysphagia include stricture and oesophagitis.

➤ Dysphagia may include pain during swallowing (odynophagia), food sticking in the throat, feeling of a lump in the throat, chest pain or discomfort during swallowing, or regurgitation through the mouth or nose. In infants dysphagia may manifest as low interest in food, body stiffness or vomiting during feeding, unusual lengthy feeding, coughing or gagging during feeding.

BOX 12.14 Causes of dysphagia

Pre-oesophageal
- Neuromuscular (e.g. myasthenia gravis, bulbar palsy)
- Globus hystericus

- Plummer–Vinson syndrome (iron-deficiency)

Oesophageal
- Tonsillitis, tonsillar abscess, epiglottitis
- Oesophagitis (gastro-oesophageal reflux)
- Vascular ring
- Oesophageal foreign body

- Achalasia
- Lower oesophageal ring (Schatzki's ring)
- Oesophageal diverticulum (pharyngeal or oesophageal)
- Drugs (potassium chloride, quinidine)

Recommended investigations

➤ Chest X-ray for possible vascular ring
➤ Barium meal to detect causes of dysphagia, including external compression
➤ Oesophagoscopy to identify structural abnormalities

PRACTICE POINTS

- A young patient who complains of having a lump in the throat or neck that is unrelated to swallowing is likely to have globus hystericus. This usually occurs in association with anxiety, stress or grief.
- An untreated severe iron-deficiency anaemia can cause a thin mucosal membrane that grows across the lumen of the oesophagus.
- Achalasia is a neurogenic oesophageal disorder of unknown aetiology which is characterised by absence of peristalsis during swallowing. This can be demonstrated by barium meal.
- Unless the cause of the swallowing difficulty is easily established and acute (e.g. tonsillitis), the patient should be referred.
- It is important to treat gastro-oesophageal reflux before oesophagitis and stricture develop.
- Infants with swallowing difficulty who are fed by mouth are at high risk of aspiration, which leads to recurrent aspiration pneumonia.
- Children with cerebral palsy who are at risk of aspiration may be referred to a paediatric neurologist and surgeon for consideration of gastrostomy.
- Although accidentally ingested cleaning solutions are the most common agents causing oesophageal stricture, certain drugs such as potassium chloride, tetracycline and quinidine can cause stricture if temporarily lodged in the oesophagus.

SINUSITIS

Initial work-up

➤ History and physical examination are consistent with sinusitis (Box 12.15).
➤ Most cases of sinusitis are caused by viral infection, which usually clears up sponta-neously. It needs to be differentiated from bacterial infection (Table 12.7). Antibiotic therapy or X-ray is not usually needed.
➤ Sinus X-ray and CT scan of the mucosa may show thickening, air–fluid levels and sinus opacification, but these findings often do not distinguish between viral and bacterial sinusitis. Therefore, the findings have to be interpreted along with the clin-ical data.

Initial treatment

➤ Saline irrigation or nasal spray, analgesics. There is little evidence to support the use of decongestants, increased room humidity and steam vaporiser.
➤ A broad-spectrum antibiotic for 2 weeks should be used for bacterial sinusitis.

Referral

➤ Persistent or worsening symptoms despite antibiotic therapy.

➤ Urgent referral in case of complication such as severe pain, ocular symptoms.

BOX 12.15 Typical symptoms and signs of sinusitis

Common

- Maxillary or frontal pain
- Other symptoms of URTI, including cough

- Rhinorrhoea (clear or purulent)
- Associated signs of otitis media
- Fever

Rare

- Decreased sense of smell
- Headaches (more common in adults)

- Facial pain, tenderness (more common in adults)

TABLE 12.7 Symptoms and signs differentiating viral and bacterial sinusitis

	Viral sinusitis	Bacterial sinusitis
Persistent symptoms	< 7 days	> 7 days
Fever	None or low-grade	Temperature > 39.0°C
Severity of symptoms	Mild	Severe
Worsening symptoms	No	Yes

LYMPHADENOPATHY AND NECK MASS

Core messages

➤ Lumps in the neck are common and are usually benign. Their causes are shown in Box 12.16.

➤ Of the many lumps found in the neck, cervical lymphadenopathy is the most common physical finding. It is usually reactive to a viral infection, causing small (<1 cm), non-tender (sometimes tender if the infection is acute), mobile lymph nodes, considered normal in children. A review in 2 weeks is advisable.

➤ Lymph nodes are not considered enlarged until their diameter exceeds 1 cm for cervical and axillary lymph nodes and 1.5 cm for inguinal lymph nodes.

➤ About one-third of neonates have palpable lymph nodes, usually smaller than 1 cm in diameter. They are commonly present in the inguinal area (due to the prevalence of infection of the nappy area), but may also be noted in the cervical or axillary region.

➤ Generalised lymphadenopathy indicates involvement of enlarged lymph nodes in more than 2 node regions.

➤ Pathological lymphadenopathy is suggested by abnormally large lymph nodes, tenderness, lymph nodes matted together or fixed to the skin or underlying structures, or localised in the supra-clavicular area.

BOX 12.16 Causes of lymphadenopathy and neck lump

Lymph nodes
- Infections:
  - > Reactive lymphadenitis due to local infection
  - > Tuberculosis lymphadenitis
  - > Mononucleosis
  - > Kawasaki disease

- Autoimmune diseases:
  - > Rheumatoid arthritis
  - > Systemic lupus erythematosus (SLE)
- Malignancy (e.g. lymphoma)
- Lymphangioma (cystic hygroma)

Neck cyst
- Dermoid cyst
- Thyroglossal cyst

- Branchial cyst

Others
- Sternomastoid tumour
- Goitre

- Pharyngeal pouch

Recommended investigations

➤ Chest X-ray is the first-line investigation in suspected cases of tuberculosis (TB) or lymphoma.

➤ FBC: leucocytosis suggests infection; atypical lymphocytes for mononucleosis; leucopenia for SLE; anaemia suggests chronic infection or lymphoma.

➤ LFTs: abnormal in EBV, cytomegalovirus.

➤ Monospot test or immunoglobulin G (IgG) for EBV.

➤ Tuberculin skin test for suspected TB adenitis.

PRACTICE POINTS

- The size of the neck mass needs to be documented, to monitor progress.
- Reactive lymphadenopathy is the most common cause of lumps in the neck. Parents usually fear the possibility of cancer and need to be reassured. Parents should also be told that reactive lymphadenopathy may last months or years, and may enlarge again in response to another viral infection.
- Reactive lymphadenopathy should be differentiated from TB lymphadenitis. The latter is suspected if the lymphadenopathy is associated with persistent or unexplained fever, night sweats, anorexia or weight loss, or if the mass does not undergo spontaneous regression to its normal size within 6–8 weeks. If biopsy is required, there is a small risk of fistula.
- Thyroglossal cyst, which develops from remnant thyroglossal duct, is painless and localised in the midline, but becomes enlarged and tender if infected. The pathognomonic sign is its vertical movement on swallowing or tongue protrusion.
- The usual branchial cyst looks like an insignificant-looking papule on the side of the neck, off-centre (in contrast to thyroglossal cyst).
- The commonest cause of acquired goitre in children is Hashimoto thyroiditis, with normal thyroid function tests (TFTs) or TFTs suggestive of hypothyroidism.

- Generalised lymphadenopathy suggests either systemic infection (e.g. AIDS, mononucleosis, toxoplasmosis), autoimmune disease (e.g. rheumatoid arthritis) or malignancy (e.g. leukaemia).
- Lymphoma is often associated with B-symptoms which manifest as fever, weight loss and night sweating
- Juvenile idiopathic arthritis often presents with generalised lymphadenopathy (Still's disease) in association with fever, rash and hepatosplenomegaly.

RED FLAGS

- Detection of neck mass(es) greater than 1 cm in diameter, which are matted or fixed to the underlying structures, require referral urgently within 2 weeks to a paediatric specialist.
- A thyroglossal cyst (midline cyst) should never be excised before confirming that there is other functional thyroid tissue elsewhere.

REFERENCES

1. NICE guidelines, 2008. CG60: Surgical management of OME. www.nice.org.uk/CG060
2. Vitamin C for preventing and treating the common cold. www.summaries.cochrane.org/CD000980
3. Burton MJ, Isaacson G, Rosenfield RM. Extracts from the Cochrane Library: Tonsillectomy for chronic/recurrent acute tonsillitis. Otolaryngology Head Neck Surg 2009; **140**(1): 15–8.

CHAPTER 13

Ophthalmology

INTRODUCTION

Primary-care physicians play a crucial role in the management of eye problems in children, in particular in vision screening which is a vital part of routine care. Essential equipment includes:

➤ an interesting toy, preferably red, for fixation
➤ an eye chart
➤ a blue light
➤ a Wood's lamp
➤ fluorescein strips
➤ an ophthalmoscope.

THE ACUTE RED EYE

Core messages

➤ Acutely red eye is a common presenting complaint in primary care and is caused by a variety of conditions (Box 13.1). GPs should be able to diagnose most causes of acutely red eye (Table 13.1) and decide if urgent referral is indicated.
➤ Assessment of the red eyes should undertake the following steps:
  ➤ Detailed history, which includes presence or absence of pain, itching, discharge (watery or pus), loss of vision and ocular trauma.
  ➤ Careful inspection of the eyes for distribution of redness and swelling, and source and appearance of any discharge. Visual acuity in infants and young children is tested by the ability to fixate and follow a target. A Snellen chart can be used at about 5 or 6 years of age. Eversion is performed in a cooperative child, particularly if a foreign body is suspected.
  ➤ Fluorescein stain may be used to assess corneal injury (especially if the eye is painful and the child is old enough to tolerate its application).

BOX 13.1 Causes of acutely red eyes

Conjunctiva
- Viral conjunctivitis
- Bacterial conjunctivitis (*Chlamydia* or gonococcal)
- Chemical conjunctivitis (e.g. use of silver nitrate for prophylaxis or household cleaning substances)
- Allergic conjunctivitis
- Conjunctivitis associated with systemic diseases
- Haemorrhagic conjunctivitis (caused e.g. by picornavirus)
- Subconjunctival haemorrhage

Sclera

- Episcleritis
- Diffuse scleritis
- Nodular scleritis
- Necrotising scleritis

Cornea

- Viral or bacterial keratitis
- Syphilitic interstitial keratitis
- Epidemic keratoconjunctivitis

Uvea

- Acute uveitis (e.g. associated with rheumatoid arthritis)
- Glaucoma

Lacrimal gland

- Lacrimal duct obstruction
- Dacryocystitis

Any part of the eye

- Trauma (including foreign body)

TABLE 13.1 Description of painless and painful causes of acutely red eyes

Condition	Description
Red eye with little or no pain	
Ophthalmia neonatorum	This form of conjunctivitis, occurring in the first 28 days of life, is the most common eye disease of newborns. The presence of pus from an eye swab suggests the diagnosis (*see* Chapter 1). It is no longer a notifiable disease
Conjunctivitis	Gritty or itchy discomfort; normal visual acuity unless keratitis co-exists, photophobia is uncommon. Causes include: • Viral conjunctivitis: redness of the entire conjunctiva, watery discharge; usually caused by adenovirus and often associated with a viral upper respiratory tract infection (Fig 13.1) • Bacterial conjunctivitis: has usually a rapid onset, often caused by staphylococci, with redness maximal at the inferior conjunctiva and purulent discharge. • *Chlamydia* is the most common cause of neonatal conjunctivitis in the UK. Gonococcal conjunctivitis presents in the first few days of life with a rapidly progressive profuse purulent discharge with lid oedema. The cornea is rapidly affected leading to ulceration. (*See* Chapter 1) • Allergic conjunctivitis: is usually seasonal with bilateral significant itching, runny nose, swollen lids and positive family history of atopy
Subconjunctival haemorrhage (hyposphagma)	This may result from injury, inflammation, severe straining (e.g. during delivery), or coughing. The condition may appear alarming but it is self-limiting, and requires no treatment
Acute painful red eye	
Keratitis	There is circumcorneal redness, foreign body sensation and photophobia. Possible cause: contact lens wear or infection with herpes simplex

(*continued*)

Condition	Description
Anterior uveitis	Blurred vision with reduced visual acuity; photophobia; pain on accommodation; and lacrimation. Associated with autoimmune diseases, e.g. pauci-articular rheumatoid arthritis
Episcleritis/scleritis	Episcleritis and diffuse scleritis (90% of all cases of scleritis) are usually benign. The condition frequently accompanies rheumatoid arthritis. Episcleritis is a fairly benign self-limiting condition with localised redness and inflammation of part of the lateral sclera
Acute glaucoma	Severely painful, photophobia and decreased visual acuity. Signs include hazy cornea; corneal enlargement in neonates
Trauma	Usually painful with corneal abrasion. Fluorescein eye drops reveal a corneal abrasion or ulcer

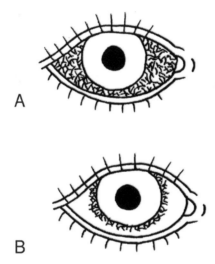

FIGURE 13.1 A: Diffuse redness of the conjunctiva seen in viral conjunctivitis. B: Circumcorneal redness seen in anterior uveitis and corneal ulcer

PRACTICE POINTS

- Episcleral and retinal haemorrhages in neonates are common during vaginal delivery. Although these are alarming to parents and clinicians, they are harmless and disappear within 2 weeks.
- At birth the nasolacrimal duct is often blocked, causing watering eyes (epiphora), sticky eyes and recurrent conjunctivitis. The onset is slow. Eyes typically glued together by sticky discharge after sleeping. Diagnosis is made by the history or by refluxing discharge with a pressure over the lacrimal sac. This resolves spontaneously in over 95% of cases over the first few months. The child should

be referred for probing of the nasolacrimal duct if this persists beyond 1 year of age.

- Ophthalmia neonatorum can be potentially blinding, and requires urgent diagnosis and treatment (*see* also Table 13.1). Once principally caused by gonococcal infection, the most common cause is now *Chlamydia* or staphylococci. The topical antimicrobial agent silver nitrate may cause chemical conjunctivitis, but this is rare nowadays.
- The most common cause of acutely red eyes is viral conjunctivitis, which is highly contagious. Its management is given in Box 13.2.
- Bilateral redness of the eyes often suggests a viral, bacterial or allergic conjunctivitis, while unilateral redness suggests foreign body (FB). FB may be detected by everting the upper lid to check for concealed FBs.
- Epidemic keratoconjunctivitis is common and highly infectious, often caused by adenovirus type 8. Symptoms include itching, blurred vision and photophobia. Signs are oedema and follicles of the conjunctiva with pre-auricular lymphadenopathy. It tends to resolve spontaneously within 1–3 weeks.
- Steroids should never be prescribed unless herpes infection has been excluded. Referral to an ophthalmologist is indicated if the diagnosis is unclear.
- Orbital cellulitis presents as involving swelling of both eyelids. This must be differentiated from rhabdomyosarcoma, which is usually associated with a rapidly developing proptosis. Some cases present with a slowly developing eyelid and conjunctival oedema.

BOX 13.2 Summary of management of conjunctivitis

Viral
- Self-limiting, give antibiotics only for secondary bacterial infection (see above for symptoms suggestive of viral cause)
- Cold compresses may help the discomfort
- Strict hygiene standards must be maintained, including frequent washing of hands

Bacterial
- Eye swab (particularly in severe cases or in treatment failure)
- Frequent installation of antibiotic drops (1 drop at least every 2 hours; for less-severe infection 3–4 times daily is generally sufficient; drops are more practical than ointments), such as chloramphenicol or fusidic acid. Systemic antibiotics may be required for severe cases
- Frequent eyelid cleaning with cotton wool and warm water

Allergic
- Opticrom (sodium cromoglycate 4% drops; 1–2 qds) to be used preferably before the allergy season begins
- Oral antihistamine if other allergic symptoms exist

Referral

Referral to an ophthalmologist is indicated:
➤ In all cases of acutely red eyes except for nasolacrimal duct obstruction, viral, mild bacterial or allergic conjunctivitis
➤ If the diagnosis of the red eye is unclear
➤ If conjunctivitis fails to settle within 5–7 days
➤ If trauma is more than mild or there is evidence of penetrating injury
➤ If there is associated eye tenderness, or reduced visual acuity
➤ If the eye is associated with proptosis
➤ If there are associated systemic manifestations.

SQUINTS (STRABISMUS)

Core messages

➤ Strabismus, or squint, is a common ophthalmic problem affecting 4–5% of children younger than 6 years of age. It may be constant or intermittent, manifest or latent, unilateral or bilateral. The main causes are listed in Box 13.3.
➤ Strabismus may be either *congenital* (better termed 'infantile', as this allows inclusion of cases of strabismus developed within the first few months of life) or *acquired*. The most important and serious cause of strabismus is retinoblastoma.
➤ Strabismus is divided into *non-paralytic* and *paralytic*. Non-paralytic strabismus includes convergent squint, also known as esotropia; divergent squint, also known as exotropia; upward squint (hyperdeviation) and downward squint (hypodeviation).
➤ Paralytic strabismus may be secondary to absence, hypoplasia or palsy of:
  ➢ oculomotor (3rd cranial) nerve, which is characterised by exophoria, hypodeviation, ptosis and possibly dilated pupil
  ➢ trochlear (4th cranial) nerve, which is characterised by hyperdeviation and elevation in eye adduction
  ➢ abducens (6th cranial) nerve, which is characterised by esophoria and causing a lateral rectus palsy.
➤ Paralytic strabismus may also be due to myogenic causes (e.g. myopathy or myositis) and lesions at the neuromuscular junction (e.g. myasthenia gravis).

BOX 13.3 Main causes of squint

- Pseudo-squint due to broad epicanthic folds
- Congenital (infantile) strabismus
- Refractive errors (myopia, hyperopia, strabismus), including accommodative strabismus
- Paralytic strabismus due to cranial nerve palsy, and to neuromuscular disorders
- Tumours
- Migraine ophthalmoplegia (transient)
- Möbius syndrome

How to examine for squints

Eye movements

➤ Child is asked to (or attracted to) look at an object/toy, which is moved in an 'H' pattern at a distance of 30 cm. Paralytic squint can easily be detected.

Corneal light reflex

➤ Useful for children who are not cooperative (below the age of 3 years). A light source is held between the examiner and the child, at 25 cm from the child. The light's reflection is seen in the centre of the child's pupil in healthy eyes and in children with pseudo-strabismus (Fig 13.2 and Fig 13.3 – *see* Plate section).

Cover test

➤ For children who are cooperative with reasonably good vision in each eye. While the child looks at a distant object, the examiner covers each of the child's eyes and watches for movement of the eye which has been left uncovered.
  ➣ If no movement occurs, the eye has no squint.
  ➣ If the uncovered eye makes a re-fixation movement, manifest squint is present.
  ➣ If the cover test is normal (i.e. absence of a manifest squint), each eye is then covered and uncovered. If the just-uncovered eye makes a re-fixation movement, latent squint is present.

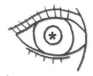 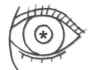 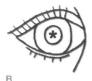 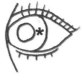

A   B

FIGURE 13.2 A: Normal corneal light reflexes on both pupils. B: In esotropia of the left eye, the light lies on the lateral aspect of the cornea with the eye also deviated medially

PRACTICE POINTS

● Pseudo-strabismus is a common cause of referral to ophthalmology. It is usually caused by epicanthic folds or a broad, flat nasal bridge. Normal eye alignment can be shown by the normal corneal light reflexes.
● Up to the age of 6 months, intermittent strabismus is normal, occurring particularly as outward deviation in about two-thirds of neonates. After the age of 6 months, any degree of strabismus needs to be referred for refractive correction with spectacles and occlusion therapy. Intervention within 6–12 months of life will increase the chances of normal vision.
● Accommodative strabismus usually manifests at 2–4 years of age. It is a convergent strabismus occurring during accommodation (focusing), caused mainly by hyperopia (far-sightedness). Amblyopia occurs in the majority of cases if untreated.
● An injury to one of the three ocular nerves (3rd, 4th and 6th) will cause strabismus, the angle of which will vary according to the direction of gaze.
● Features differentiating non-paralytic from paralytic squints are shown in Table 13.2.
● Recent onset of a paralytic ocular muscle usually presents with double vision that increases when looking in the direction of the affected ocular muscle.

- When a child presents with a head tilt, it is vital to examine eye movement. A 4th ocular nerve palsy causes a contralateral head tilt, i.e. a head tilt to the right caused by left-sided nerve palsy; and vice versa. Conversely, a 6th nerve palsy causes head-tilting on the same side as the palsy. The reason for the tilt is to avoid diplopia.
- In a child with any ocular disorder, including strabismus, assessment of visual acuity is essential. Untreated squint results in amblyopia with permanent visual impairment.
- Ophthalmoplegic migraine is a rare condition characterised by headaches and ipsilateral (to same side as the headache) oculomotor nerve palsy. It is most common in older children and young adults, and is transient with full recovery between attacks.
- Retinoblastoma, with an incidence of 1 in 20 000 births, is the most important cause of acquired strabismus. The tumour also presents with unilateral or bilateral leucocoria (a white pupil) or uncommonly as a red eye. Retinoblastoma is most curable if diagnosed early; death is inevitable if untreated.
- Möbius syndrome is rare; it is characterised by paretic facial muscles (expressionless face, impaired sucking and smiling), inability to move the eyes from side to side, and associated limb and chest-wall defects.

TABLE 13.2 Differential diagnosis between non-paralytic and paralytic squint

	Non-paralytic squint	Paralytic squint
Onset	Slow	Rapid
Diplopia	Absent	Present
Eye movement	Normal	Limited in direction of action of the paralytic muscle
Head posture	Normal	Often tilted
Symptoms (e.g. nausea, vomiting and headache)	Absent	Usually present

Referral
➤ All cases with strabismus require referral after the age of 6 months, or even earlier in case of large-angle strabismus.
➤ Diagnosis of pseudo-squint should be established (observation and corneal light reflex) to avoid unnecessary referral.
➤ The first episode of ophthalmoplegic migraine may also require referral to establish the diagnosis, but recurrent episodes may not require this.

NYSTAGMUS
➤ This is rhythmical oscillation of one or both eyes, which is commonly associated with visual defects.
➤ Associated visual defects include congenital abnormalities such as cataract, optic atrophy or albinism. An acquired form of nystagmus may be caused by a CNS tumour, which requires immediate referral.

➤ Spasmus nutans is an acquired form of nystagmus which consists of a pendular type of nystagmus, head-nodding and torticollis.

PROPTOSIS (EXOPHTHALMOS)

Core messages

➤ Proptosis, also known as exophthalmos or protrusion of the eyes, is a forward displacement of the eye which may have a variety of causes (Table 13.3). Practically all causes are serious and require urgent referral.

TABLE 13.3 Main causes of proptosis

Cause	Examples
Shallow orbit	Crouzon's syndrome
CNS anomaly	Orbital encephalocele
Infection	Orbital cellulitis
Tumour/cyst	Orbital capillary haemangioma
	Lymphangioma
	Lacrimal gland cyst/tumour
	Optic nerve glioma, meningioma (involving sphenoid wing), metastatic neuroblastoma
	Deep dermoid cyst
	Juvenile xanthogranuloma, Wegener's granulomatosis
	Histiocytosis (eosinophilic granuloma)
	Sarcoidosis (granulomatosis disease)
	Fibrous dysplasia
Haemorrhage	Trauma
Endocrine	Graves' disease (thyroid orbitopathy)

Recommended investigations

(Usually performed in hospital.)

➤ FBC: leucocytosis in inflammatory disease, differential count for suspected leukaemia
➤ TFTs for suspected hyperthyroidism
➤ Tumour markers in urine (VMA (vanillylmandelic acid) and HVA (homovanillic acid))elevated in neuroblastoma in 95% of cases
➤ Orbital and renal ultrasound for metastatic neuroblastoma
➤ CT (or MRI) for any suspected cranial tumour

PRACTICE POINTS

● Urgent referral of all cases of proptosis is essential.
● Orbital capillary haemangioma (strawberry naevus) is the most common orbital tumour in children, often affecting the upper lid. The tumour has a rapid growth during the first 6 months of life and regresses spontaneously at 4–6 years of age.
● Assessment of a child with proptosis should include assessment of visual acuity, ocular muscle movement, measuring of proptosis, pupillary size, reaction to light, fundi, and systemic examination.

- Optic gliomas are usually benign, often asymptomatic, and commonly present with visual disturbance. Optic gliomas are associated with neurofibromatosis type 1. Unilateral glioma typically presents with afferent pupillary defect. A light source on the affected eye produces pupil dilation (instead of constriction), while the unaffected eye produces bilateral pupil constriction.
- Proptosis caused by Graves' disease may occur in older children. Complications, e.g. optic neuropathy, corneal problems and extraocular muscular involvement, are significantly less likely in children than in adults.
- Neuroblastoma, the most common solid tumour of childhood, metastasises frequently into the orbit. Horner's syndrome (with or without orbital ecchymoses) is another presentation. The tumour arises from the adrenal glands, cervical sympathetic chain or mediastinum.
- A proptotic eye not adequately protected by the lids is at risk of keratopathy, strabismus, diplopia and decreased visual acuity.
- Orbital cellulitis, commonly caused by paranasal sinusitis, first manifests as a red swelling of the eyelid. Prompt treatment with IV antibiotics at this stage dramatically improves the outcome. Complications include extension of the infection into the cranial cavity, causing meningitis, cavernous sinus thrombosis and epidural, subdural or brain abscess. Admission to hospital is urgently required.

ACUTE LOSS OF VISION

Core messages

➤ Acute visual loss is a frightening experience not only for children but also for the parents. Urgent referral is required.

➤ Conditions causing visual impairment are uncommon (about 2–5 cases per 10 000 births).

➤ Visual loss is due to abnormalities either within the ocular structures or within neural visual pathways in the CNS. Causes are listed in Box 13.4.

➤ Visual loss within the eyes is easy to detect, e.g. corneal opacity, cataract or optic atrophy.

➤ Most causes of cortical visual loss occur in children with neurodisability which may follow asphyxia at birth with or without seizures, and development of spasticity or hypotonia. Rarely, cortical visual loss occurs as an isolated neurological phenomenon.

➤ Eye examination should be included in the 6-week check (Box 13.5).

BOX 13.4 Main causes of acute loss of vision

Ocular causes
- Eye trauma
- Retinal detachment
- Optic neuritis

- Glaucoma, uveitis, keratitis, trachoma
- Macular degeneration
- Retinal migraine

CNS causes
- Migraine
- Intracranial haemorrhage
- Raised intracranial pressure (optic glioma, posterior fossa tumour)
- Occipital lobe seizures

- Cortical blindness
- Amaurosis fugax
- Infection (meningitis, congenital varicella)
- Stroke
- Familial transient visual loss

Systemic causes
- Thromboembolic phenomenon
- Drugs (e.g. gentamicin)
- Collagen diseases (e.g. rheumatoid arthritis)
- Conversion symptom (hysteria)

- Postprandial transient visual loss (after heavy meal)
- TORCH infection
- HIV infection

BOX 13.5 Examination of the eyes at 6-week check

- Parental concerns about vision should always be taken seriously
- General inspection may detect abnormalities, e.g. nystagmus. Unilateral corneal enlargement suggests congenital glaucoma
- Intermittent squints are normal in infants at this age, particularly when they are tired. If intermittent squints are detected, a review in 6 weeks should be arranged
- Ophthalmoscope (held at 20–25 cm from the baby's eye) is used to elicit the red reflex (dark spots in the red reflex may be due to cataracts). See Fig 13.4
- Visual acuity is likely to be normal if the baby blinks or turns the head towards the light source

---

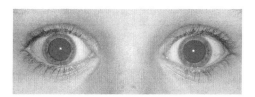

FIGURE 13.4 Bilateral stippled red reflexes which may indicate a mild cataract

Recommended investigations

(Usually performed in secondary care.)

➤ Electrophysiological testing with electroretinography (ERG) for retinal causes of visual impairment

➤ MRI of the eye and head for suspected tumour

➤ EEG for cases with seizures

➤ TORCH screening test (IgM for cytomegalovirus (CMV), herpes simplex, rubella), urine for rubella virus isolation, as indicated clinically

➤ HIV DNA detected by PCR (polymerase chain reaction), if clinically indicated

PRACTICE POINTS

- GPs should be able to detect most eye abnormalities using examination techniques which include eye movement, pupillary reflex, visual fields and visual acuity. The last is tested using:
  - An object (bright-coloured toy) for infants during first few months of life, to assess the child's ability to fixate and follow. Fixation to a midline object can be achieved in the first 2–6 weeks, past midline by 1–3 months, and the child can follow an object 180° by 35 months of age.
  - Various cards with common pictures are used for a child 2–4 years of age. The child is asked to name each picture close to the examiner and at a distance.
  - A Snellen chart for older children.
- If the outcome of the visual assessment is inconclusive, referral for an orthoptic assessment should be made.
- Detection of visual impairment in children is essential to prevent delay in treatment. Treatable conditions include cataract, retinopathy of prematurity (ROP), glaucoma and retinoblastoma. Many of these conditions have genetic implications.
- The most common cause of transient visual loss in children is during the visual aura of a classic migraine. Aura is defined as a recurrent disorder that develops over 5–29 minutes and lasts for < 1 hour (see also the migraine section in Chapter 14).
- Nystagmus is commonly associated with visual defects, including congenital cataract, optic atrophy or albinism, or acquired by CNS tumours.
- Transient monocular visual loss lasting 1–5 minutes is usually referred to as amaurosis fugax, resulting from cerebral ischemia. While migraine aura may present with flashes of light (photopsia), amaurosis fugax presents as a blackout or a curtain across the vision.
- Occipital seizures (e.g. benign partial epilepsy with occipital paroxysms) are not rare; visual symptoms are prominent and include amaurosis, multi-coloured illusions or hallucinations and eye deviation, followed by hemiclonic seizures or automatisms. EEG is usually diagnostic.
- Leukocoria (white pupil reflex) is usually a sign of serious diseases such as retinoblastoma, cataract or persistent hyperplastic primary vitreous. Untreated or delayed treatment of cataract leads to a permanent vision loss. Urgent referral is required.
- Some systemically administered medications, e.g. steroids, may cause cataracts. Steroids may also cause glaucoma.
- Before diagnosing migraine or amaurosis as a possible loss of vision, remember that thromboembolic events may occur in predisposing conditions such as polycythaemia, sickle-cell anaemia or homocystinuria.
- While papilloedema is a cardinal sign of increased intracranial pressure (ICP), in

infants separation of the cranial sutures and bulging of the anterior fontanelle decompresses the ICP. This means that the ICP may not be raised so that papilloedema may not be seen.

Referral
All children with acute loss of vision should be referred to an ophthalmologist.

DIPLOPIA (DOUBLE VISION)
Core messages
➤ Diplopia, simultaneous perception of two images of a single object, is less common in children than in adults mainly because of the lower incidence of strokes and other intracranial lesions.
➤ The most common cause of diplopia in children is misalignment of the visual axes, occurring particularly in association with disorders affecting the cranial nerves (3rd, 4th and 6th) innervating the 6 ocular muscles.
➤ Other causes involve mechanical interference with ocular motion or disorder of neuromuscular transmission (Box 13.6).
➤ Diplopia is either binocular or monocular.
   ➢ Binocular diplopia arises as a result of the misalignment of the two eyes to each other (e.g. in strabismus). This diplopia can be corrected by covering either eye.
   ➢ Monocular diplopia is caused by abnormality in the cornea (e.g. severe astigmatism), in the lens (e.g. cataract, dislocated lens) or in the vitreous humour (e.g. vitreous cysts). Monocular diplopia persists in one eye despite covering the other eye.
➤ Diplopia can be the first manifestation of many systemic muscular or neurological disorders; some are of serious nature and diplopia warrants prompt evaluation.
➤ A detailed history and examination will establish the likely cause of diplopia in the majority of cases.

BOX 13.6 Causes of diplopia

Ocular causes
- Physiological
- Strabismus (particularly paralytic)
- Post-surgery for refractive errors
- Intraocular diseases (e.g. dislocated lens)
- Trauma
- Retinoblastoma
- Sarcoidosis

CNS causes
- Increased intracranial pressure
- Ophthalmoplegic migraine
- Basilar artery migraine
- Stroke

Systemic causes
- Myasthenia gravis
- Drugs (e.g. antiepileptics)
- Thyroid ophthalmopathy
- Conversion symptom (hysteria)
- Möbius syndrome

Recommended investigations

(Usually performed in secondary care.)

➤ TFTs for suspected cases of hyperthyroidism

➤ A chest X-ray for suggested cases of sarcoidosis to show bilateral hilar lymphadenopathy

➤ MRI of the head may show tumour, areas of infarction or even arterial aneurysm

➤ Anti-acetylcholine antibodies in plasma and electromyelography (EMG) for suspected myasthenia gravis

---

PRACTICE POINTS

- Common causes of diplopia are strabismus and posterior fossa tumour. However, the brain of a young child often learns how to suppress the image of the weaker, misaligned eye. Therefore diplopia may not be the presenting feature in these conditions. Head-tilting may occur instead.
- Differentiating monocular from binocular diplopia is simple: covering each eye will correct binocular diplopia, while monocular diplopia will persist in the affected eye.
- Migraine may present as a transient 3rd nerve palsy on the same side as the headache (ophthalmoplegic migraine).
- When a child presents with diplopia and ptosis, 3rd nerve palsy is likely. However, Horner's syndrome is another possibility; this presents as a small pupil and reduced sweating on the affected side, which will help to differentiate the conditions.
- The 6th nerve has a long intracranial course so is susceptible to damage from a cranial tumour. Therefore, an acquired 6th nerve palsy is usually an ominous sign requiring urgent referral.
- Diplopia may be the first complaint in children with lens dislocation, including those with Marfan's syndrome or homocystinuria (malar flush, neurodisability, thromboembolic events).
- A typical basilar artery migraine (e.g. diplopia, vertigo, ataxia and headache) should be differentiated from an intracranial tumour. Urgent CT or MRI is often needed, particularly if it is the first episode.
- Although adolescents with hysteria may present with diplopia, this diagnosis should be one of exclusion.

Referral

Referral to secondary care is usually required for all pathological causes of diplopia.

DISORDERS OF THE EYELID

➤ Eyelid disorders are common in children and range from benign, self-resolving to serious malignant processes (Box 13.7). Therefore a complete ophthalmic and systemic examination is required.

➤ Congenital ptosis (drooping eyelid) is usually due to developmental dystrophy of the levator muscle, often associated with strabismus (in about 30% of cases), and amblyopia. Examples are Marcus–Gunn jaw-winking phenomenon and Möbius syndrome.

➤ Disorders of the eyelid are important to clinicians because of their association with systemic diseases such as myasthenia gravis, myotonic dystrophy, botulism and Horner's syndrome.

BOX 13.7 Main abnormalities of the eyelid

- Epicanthic, telecanthic and epicanthic inversus folds
- Congenital ptosis (e.g. Marcus–Gunn jaw-winking)
- Acquired ptosis (myasthenia gravis, muscular dystrophy, e.g. myotonic dystrophy or facioscapulohumeral dystrophy)
- Coloboma (may be associated with Goldenhar syndrome)
- Tumour (haemangioma, dermoid cyst)
- Congenital ectropion
- Tumour/cyst (e.g. haemangioma)
- Acute blepharitis (eyelash inflammation by skin bacteria)
- Congenital entropion
- Meibomian cyst
- Stye or hordeolum which is an abscess, usually harmless
- Chalazion (inflammation of the Meibomian cyst)
- Sparse or absent eyebrows (ectodermal dysplasia, alopecia)
- Lash abnormalities
- Eyebrow abnormalities

Recommended investigations

(Usually performed in secondary care.)

➤ A chest X-ray and CT scan in cases of suspected myasthenia gravis for evidence of enlarged thymus and thymoma
➤ Creatinine phosphokinase (CPK) in blood for muscular diseases
➤ ECG for suspected muscular dystrophy and myopathies
➤ Anti-acetylcholine antibodies in plasma for suspected myasthenia gravis
➤ EMG may be diagnostic in cases of myasthenia gravis and myotonic dystrophy

PRACTICE POINTS

- Epicanthic folds are present in most infants and young children and become less apparent with peaking of the nasal bridge as the child gets older. They may be associated with many syndromes and chromosomal abnormalities.
- Telecanthus (increased width between the medial canthi) and epicanthus inversus (epicanthic folds originating from the lower lid) are other anomalies. The latter is often inherited as autosomal dominant; females may be infertile.
- Children with ptosis commonly raise the eyebrows or lift the chin in an attempt to maintain binocular vision.
- In Marcus–Gunn jaw-winking (5% of all cases with ptosis), the upper lid rises as the jaw opens (e.g. during sucking or chewing). This synkinesis (simultaneous movement) occurs as a result of anomalous connection between the 3rd and 5th cranial nerves.

- Eyebrow abnormalities include sparse or absent eyebrows (e.g. alopecia, ectodermal dysplasia) and eyebrows joining together medially (e.g. Waardenburg's syndrome, Cornelia de Lang syndrome).
- Children with ptosis should be referred for ophthalmic opinion and surgery, particularly if they have abnormal head posture, amblyopia (lazy eyes), abnormal visual field and if the ptosis is cosmetically unacceptable.
- Entropion (inward turning of the lid margin and lashes) can cause corneal damage. Infants commonly present with irritability. Larsen's syndrome (multiple joint dislocations, cleft palate, and neurodisability) has to be excluded. Urgent consultation with an ophthalmologist is required.
- Patients with ectropion (outward turning of the lid margin) are at risk of exposure to keratopathy, overflow of tears and conjunctivitis. This may occur in association with facial palsy resulting from weakness of the orbicularis muscle. Again, urgent ophthalmic consultation is required.
- All cases of myasthenia gravis require referral to hospital for consideration of edrophonium (Tensilon) test to confirm the diagnosis. Prior to the test, the ptosis and strabismus are measured. Facilities for cardiopulmonary resuscitation should be available.

Referral

Referral to an ophthalmological specialist is required for all cases with eyelid disorders except clear and benign cases, e.g. epicanthic folds or chalazion.

CHAPTER 14

Neurology

CONGENITAL ANOMALIES OF THE CENTRAL NERVOUS SYSTEM (CNS)

Anencephaly

This anomaly occurs when the cephalic end of the neural tube fails to close, usually between the 23rd and 26th days of pregnancy, resulting in the absence of a major portion of the brain, skull and scalp. Affected infants are either stillborn or die within a few days of birth. The incidence is approximately 1 : 1000 live births; risk of recurrence is 4%.

Macrocephaly

Macrocephaly is a large head defined as a head circumference (HC) more than 2 standard deviations (i.e. > 98th centile on a growth chart) above average for age and sex. The condition is common and is usually familial, inherited as autosomal dominant (familial macrocephaly), but may be due to rare causes including Sotos syndrome, achondroplasia, neurofibromatosis and metabolic storage disorder. Familial macrocephaly can be diagnosed if:

➤ The child has a high HC (> 2 standard deviations above the mean) during the first year of life. The HC follows a consistent centile line as the child grows.
➤ The child is asymptomatic with no evidence of a syndrome or increased intracranial pressure (ICP).
➤ There is a positive family history of macrocephaly.
➤ A cranial ultrasound scan is normal (MRI may be requested if the anterior fontanelle has closed).

The condition is usually benign and parents can be reassured. A small percentage of children may develop developmental delay. The HC should be monitored regularly.

Microcephaly

➤ Small head defined as HC > 3 standard deviations below the mean for age and sex.
➤ There is often a genetic cause.
➤ May be associated with chromosomal abnormalities such as Down's syndrome, or secondary to intrauterine infection (e.g. cytomegalovirus) or drugs (fetal alcohol syndrome).

Hydrocephalus

This is characterised by an HC measurement that crosses the centile lines upwards, together with features of increased ICP.

➤ **In infants:** tense, full or bulging fontanelle (beware that the fontanelle may become

full when the baby cries), sutures widely separated with prominent skull veins and downward gaze of the eyes, irritability, poor feeding, vomiting and high-pitched cry.
➤ **In toddlers:** as above, with the addition of headaches, regression of cognitive skills.
➤ **In older children:** as above, with the addition of changes of vision, personality and behaviour. Slow cognitive deterioration may occur.

The condition needs to be differentiated from macrocephaly which is a much more common cause of head enlargement (see above). Children with hydrocephalus who have been treated with a shunt are at high risk of developing complications (Table 14.1).

TABLE 14.1 Symptoms and signs of shunt complications

Complication	Symptoms and signs
Shunt malfunction/obstruction	Are those of hydrocephalus itself?
Under-drainage	Are those of hydrocephalus itself?
Over-drainage	Are those of subdural haematoma caused by a collapsed ventricle and tears of blood vessels?
Local infection	Inflammatory changes of the skin around the shunt entry
Systemic infection	Septicaemia, mainly caused by *Staphylococcus epidermidis* causing fever, and other features of infection

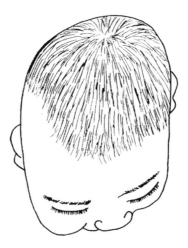

FIGURE 14.1 Plagiocephaly in the right occipital area causing forehead protrusion on the same side

Plagiocephaly
➤ This common condition is usually caused by a preferential sleeping position and is characterised by flattening of one side or the whole of the baby's occiput (Fig 14.1).
➤ The greatest deformity usually occurs in the first 3 months of life. The incidence has increased dramatically because of the 'Back to Sleep' campaign to reduce the incidence of sudden infant death syndrome.

➤ Plagiocephaly is more common in pre-term infants, infants with hypotonicity and in those with developmental delay.
➤ Its importance is entirely cosmetic, and the shape of the head will usually correct itself by 12–18 months of age.
➤ The diagnosis of plagiocephaly is clinical and a skull X-ray to confirm the patency of the skull sutures is usually unnecessary.
➤ Characteristic signs (best detected when standing behind the infant and looking from above) include:
  ➣ The head-flattening is associated with compensatory ipsilateral protrusion or bulge of the forehead
  ➣ Elevation of the ipsilateral orbit and eyebrow
  ➣ Anteriorly positioned ipsilateral ear
  ➣ Separation of the skull suture with no palpable bony ridges.

Management includes:
➤ Parents need reassurance because they are often concerned with the cosmetic appearance of their child's head. The parents can be told that slow improvement will continue and the deformity does not interfere with brain development.
➤ Alteration of the sleeping position encouraging babies to look in a different direction to the head-flattening to see their parents, siblings, bright-coloured toys or mobiles. This can be achieved with a rolled-up towel under the mattress.
➤ The more time babies spend in the prone position, the earlier is the correction of the head shape. So playing with the baby on his or her stomach will accelerate the natural improvement.
➤ Helmet and bands – the use of these is controversial and generally not supported by good evidence.

Craniosynostosis
Premature fusion of one or more cranial sutures usually results in an abnormal head shape.
➤ The most common form is scaphocephaly caused by premature fusion of the sagittal suture.
➤ Frontal synostosis caused by fusion of the coronal sutures leads to unilateral flattening of the forehead.
➤ Unilateral lambdoid synostosis, due to premature fusion of one lambdoid suture, is an important deformity because of the flattening occiput and the possible difficulty in differentiating it from positional plagiocephaly (see above). Lambdoid synostosis, however:
  ➣ is very rare (incidence 1 in 150 000 neonates), in contrast to the very common plagiocephaly
  ➣ shows a prominent bony ridge on palpation of the occipital suture
  ➣ has a forehead which does not protrude, and the ear is in a normal position.

Spina bifida occulta
This common anomaly results from a midline defect of one or more vertebral bodies. The defect is usually covered by a layer of normal skin, but sometimes it is covered by patches of hair or skin discolouration. The condition is usually asymptomatic.

Meningocele

This is a midline defect in the posterior vertebral arches, usually of the lower lumbar vertebrae, through which meninges protrude. The protrusion is usually covered by normal skin and presents as a fluctuant midline mass. The spinal cord is usually normal.

Meningomyelocele

Spinal cord is exposed through opening of the spine, resulting in partial or complete paralysis of the parts of the body below the spinal opening.

CEREBRAL HAEMORRHAGE (SUBDURAL HAEMATOMA)

Neonates. Premature infants, particularly those with respiratory distress, may develop intra-ventricular haemorrhage during the first few days of life (*see* Chapter 1). Full-term large babies may develop subdural haematoma which results from a tear of the falx, tentorium, or superficial cortical veins. Birth injury and breech deliveries are risk factors. Children usually present with seizures, often focal seizures.

Infants. Symptoms at this age include a decreased level of consciousness, irritability, vomiting, poor feeding and seizures. Hydrocephalus may occur. Most cases are due to child abuse.

Older children. Symptoms include headache, vomiting, excessive drowsiness, motor deficit, focal seizures and personality change. Most cases are due to trauma such as sport injury.

HEADACHE

Core messages

➤ Headache is a very common problem, occurring in about 50% of children aged 7 years and 80% of children aged 15 years.

➤ Although most causes of headaches in children are benign, it is essential to consider an underlying systemic disease. A headache worse in the morning, which increases with stooping or straining, suggests raised ICP.

➤ It is simple to differentiate the two most common causes of headaches: migraine disrupts the child's activity, whereas tension headache does not.

➤ Infants or toddlers with headache may present with irritability, unwillingness to play, crying while holding the head, or vomiting.

➤ Alternating hemiplegia may be the first sign of later migraine. Frequent vasoconstriction causing hemiplegia causes ischaemia, which may lead to cerebral injury and developmental delay later on.

➤ Cluster headache is rare in children; it is characterised by severe, unilateral pain affecting the orbital and supra-orbital areas. Associated features include conjunctival injection, lacrimal and nasal congestion and facial sweating. The pain lasts 15–180 minutes and occurs several times daily in series over weeks or months, separated by remission of months or years.

➤ Benign ICP is characterised by symptoms of raised ICP (e.g. headaches, vomiting, papilloedema) with a normal level of consciousness, CSF and ventricular size (as evident by CT or MRI). Focal neurological signs are absent. An urgent same-day referral to hospital is required to exclude brain tumour.

➤ Basilar migraine (presenting with vertigo, diplopia, blurred vision, ataxia) should be differentiated from posterior fossa tumour and requires referral for further assessment.

➤ Neuro-imaging is not indicated on a routine basis in children with recurrent headaches and normal physical examination. It is indicated with abnormal neurological examination, progressive headaches or co-existing seizure. Common and rare causes of headache are listed in Box 14.1.

BOX 14.1 Causes of headaches

Common
- Common viral infections
- Migraine
- Tension headaches

- Head injury
- Sinusitis

Rare

- Eye strain
- Cluster headaches
- CNS infection (meningitis, brain abscess)

- Increased intracranial pressure (ICP), including benign ICP
- Hypertension

Migraine and tension headaches

Migraine without aura (common migraine)– the most common type of migraine – is defined in Box 14.2. Criteria for diagnosing migraine with aura (classical migraine) are defined in Box 14.3. Guidelines for treatment are given in Box 14.4.

BOX 14.2 Criteria for diagnosing migraine without aura

>5 attacks fulfilling the following criteria:
- Headache lasting 1–72 hours
- At least 1 of the following accompanies headache:
  > Nausea and/or vomiting
  > Photophobia and phonophobia

- Headache has at least 2 of the following 4 criteria:
  > Bilateral or unilateral location
  > Pulsating quality
  > Moderate to severe pain intensity
  > Aggravated by physical activities, e.g. climbing stairs

BOX 14.3 Criteria for diagnosing migraine with aura

At least 2 attacks showing at least 3 of the 4 following criteria:
- One or more reversible aura symptoms
- At least 1 aura develops gradually, >4 minutes
- No aura symptoms lasting >1 hour
- Headache follows aura with a pain-free interval of <1 hour, but may begin before or simultaneously with aura

---

BOX 14.4 Management guidelines for migraine

- Avoid excessive use of analgesics as this may cause analgesic-overuse headache
- Analgesics such as paracetamol, ibuprofen are effective first-line treatment in migraine. 5HT$_1$ agonists such as sumatriptan may be considered as second-line if analgesics are inadequate

	Dose (mg)	Frequency
Paracetamol	15 mg/kg	4- to 6 hourly
Migraleve	1 pink tablet at onset, then yellow tablet 4-hourly (analgesic + anti-emetic)	
Ibuprofen	7.5–10 mg/kg	8-hourly
Sumatriptan*		
Nasal	10–20 mg	Single dose, repeated once after at least 2 hours
Oral	25–50 mg	As above

- Migraine prophylaxis should be considered if the child is missing > 3 days of school in a month and/or having 1–2 attacks/week that interfere with performing of daily activities. The quality of evidence to support the use of drug prophylaxis in paediatric migraine was poor (The Cochrane Library: drugs for preventing migraine headaches in children. Published online 2008); in practice, however, propranolol (first choice), anticonvulsants (topiramate and sodium valproate) and pizotifen may also be used and are superior to placebo. Acupuncture has also been considered for patients with poorly controlled migraine

* 5HT$_1$ agonists such as sumatriptan are recommended as monotherapy and should not be taken concurrently with other therapies for acute migraine.

Tension headache is the second most common type of headache. Box 14.5 and Box 14.6 give diagnostic criteria and treatment guidelines.

BOX 14.5 Diagnostic criteria for tension-type headaches

Several headaches fulfilling the following criteria:
- Headache lasting 30 minutes to 7 days
- At least 2 of the following pain characteristics:
  - ❯ Pressing or tightening (not pulsating)
  - ❯ Mild or moderate intensity
  - ❯ Bilateral location
  - ❯ No aggravation by physical activities
- Both of the following:
  - ❯ No nausea or vomiting
  - ❯ No photophobia or phonophobia
- No evidence of structural or metabolic disease

BOX 14.6 Therapeutic guidelines for tension headache

- Avoidance of or minimising causes or triggers
- A trial with analgesics is indicated
- Avoid frequent and excessive analgesic consumption
- Medications such as tricyclic antidepressants (e.g. amitriptyline), muscle relaxants, anticonvulsants (topiramate or gabapentin) and serotonin re-uptake inhibitors (fluoxetine) are sometimes used by specialists
- Tranquilisers such as diazepam should not be used because of the side-effects, including risk of dependence
- Relaxation training or biofeedback may help

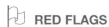 **RED FLAGS**

See Table 14.2.

TABLE 14.2 Features of headache requiring immediate referral

Symptoms	Signs
• Late-night or early-morning headache that progressively worsens over days and weeks	• Skin petechial rash
• Persistent vomiting, or vomiting late at night or early morning	• Papilloedema, pupillary change
• Confusion, extreme irritability	• Neck stiffness
• Extreme drowsiness	• High BP, low pulse rate
• Diplopia, loss of vision	• Ataxia
• Significant change in behaviour, mood or personality	
• Unexplained fever	

Migraine variants

In families with a history of migraine, migraine variants are common and include the items shown in Table 14.3.

TABLE 14.3 Clinical presentation of migraine variants

Abdominal migraine	Episodic abdominal pain, moderate to severe, typically peri-umbilical, often in the absence of headache
	Accompanied nausea with or without vomiting, pallor
	Usually lasts a few hours, range 1–72 hours; is terminated by sleep
	Typical age 4–8 years, very rarely before 2 years
	Strong family history of migraine
Cyclic vomiting	Bouts of vomiting which may lead to dehydration
	Headache may or may not be felt
	Infants are typically affected

(continued)

Ophthalmic migraine	Unilateral eye pain and 3rd nerve palsy with ptosis, papillary dilation and external eye deviation
Basilar artery migraine	Ataxia, vertigo, dysarthria, weakness, syncope, scotoma or transient blindness
Acute confusional state	Change in orientation, personality or behaviour (restless, hyperactive)
	Confusion may last minutes to hours
	May occur after minor head trauma
Benign paroxysmal vertigo of childhood	Sudden unsteadiness with nystagmus and vomiting occurring typically in toddlers (median age 18 months). Child appears frightened and pale
	The spell lasts minutes and often occurs in clusters over several days, then subsides for weeks or months
	Normal neurological examination and vestibular function
	Typically there is a family history of migraine and the child will develop typical migraine in the future
Paroxysmal torticollis of infancy	Recurrent episodes of head tilt associated with pallor, agitation and vomiting
	Typically occurs in infancy; spontaneous remission occurs aged 2–3 years
	If the episode persists, abnormalities in the cervical vertebrae (e.g. dislocation) or posterior fossa tumour should be excluded

TREMOR

Jitteriness, a rhythmic tremor of equal amplitude, is very common in healthy neonates, particularly premature infants and when babies are crying. Box 14.7 shows common and rare causes of tremor. Table 11.4 gives a summary of the three main types of tremor. Tips for diagnosing tremor are provided in Box 14.8, and guidelines as to when to refer patients are given in Box 14.9.

BOX 14.7 Causes of tremor

Common
- Physiological tremor
- Essential tremor (autosomal dominant)
- Anxiety
- Medications (e.g. beta$_2$ agonists for asthma)

Rare
- Cerebral palsy
- Acute confusional state
- Writing tremor
- Hyperthyroidism
- Wilson's disease
- Juvenile Parkinson's disease
- Spinocerebellar ataxia
- Acute intermittent porphyria

TABLE 11.4 The three main types of tremor

Type	Characteristics	Example
Resting	High amplitude, decreases with target-directed movement	Parkinson's disease
		Drugs (neuroleptics, metoclopramide)
Postural	Low amplitude, increases with voluntary movement	Physiological or essential tremor, drug or alcohol withdrawal
Intention	Increases with target-directed movement	Cerebellar diseases, drug-induced

Investigation

➤ Blood glucose, calcium
➤ Urine: for copper and serum ceruloplasmin in suspected Wilson's disease
➤ TFTs for suspected hyperthyroidism
➤ Imaging of the brain for cerebral or cerebellar causes

BOX 14.8 Tips for diagnosing tremor

- Jitteriness in neonates needs to be differentiated from seizure caused by hypoglycaemia or hypocalcaemia. Normal jitteriness has no abnormal gaze or eye movement, bradycardia or tachycardia
- Drug addiction (e.g. cocaine, heroin, amphetamine) among pregnant women has increased steadily over recent years. The result is an increased incidence of neonatal withdrawal syndrome with irritability, jitteriness and occasionally seizures. Obtaining a detailed maternal drug history is essential
- Physiological tremor probably occurs in most individuals when the arms are extended. This is enhanced by anxiety, stress or caffeine. More-subtle tremor can be demonstrated by holding a piece of paper on the outstretched hands
- Essential tremor may be unilateral
- Asthma medications such as beta$_2$ agonists and theophylline, anticonvulsants such as valproate and tricyclic antidepressants may cause tremor. Although tremor caused by salbutamol is benign, parents should be made aware of this at the time the drug is prescribed to avoid parental anxiety
- Tremor needs to be differentiated from tics, which are actually jerks, are non-rhythmic and can affect any muscle. Chorea is usually symmetric, more rapid than tremor, jerky and affects predominately the face
- In any child with progressive or acute tremor, serious conditions such as Wilson's disease, hyperthyroidism, hypoglycaemia, hypocalcaemia, neuroblastoma and pheochromocytoma must be excluded

---

> **BOX 14.9** Refer cases of tremor if
>
> - It is occurring in an awake and alert neonate and when the tremor persists beyond the 2nd week of life
> - It is acute, rapidly progressive or may have an underlying cause such as hypoglycaemia or hypocalcaemia
> - It is causing difficulty in writing or activities in daily life
> - The cause is uncertain
> - There is excessive parental concern

OTHER MOVEMENT DISORDERS

(*See* Table 14.5.)

TABLE 14.5 The main non-tremor movement disorders

Ataxia	Acute cerebellar ataxia, often follows a viral illness
	Ataxia caused by drugs such as phenytoin
	Genetic, e.g. ataxia telangiectasia, Friedrich's ataxia
	Metabolic, e.g. abetalipoproteinaemia
Chorea	Sydenham's chorea as a manifestation of rheumatic fever
	Systemic lupus erythematosus
	Chorea caused by drugs such as phenothiazines and haloperidol (tardive dyskinesia)
	Huntington's chorea
Dystonia	Genetic, e.g. dystonia musculorum deformans
	Cerebral palsy
	Drug-induced, e.g. phenothiazines, haloperidol
Tics	Transient tics, lasting weeks and months
	Tourette syndrome, associated with vocalisation (obscene words), compulsive behaviour and ADHD
Myoclonia	Myoclonic jerks, commonly occurring at sleep onset
	Myoclonic epilepsy

SEIZURES

Core messages

> ➤ Seizures are common in children, occurring in 5–7% of children.
> ➤ The normal organised tonic–clonic seizure patterns seen in older infants and children are not seen in neonates. Seizure patterns in neonates include focal clonic, multi-focal jerks, apnoea eye blinking and jitteriness.
> ➤ In older children, febrile seizure (FS) is the most common cause of seizures, occurring in 3–4% of cases, followed by epilepsy.
> ➤ Epilepsy should not be diagnosed unless seizures recur and they are unprovoked (e.g. by fever or low calcium levels).
> ➤ The term 'seizure' is used in preference to 'convulsion', as some seizures have no abnormal convulsive movements.

➤ Children with newly suspected cases of epilepsy should be referred to a paediatric neurologist, hospital or community paediatrician with an interest in epilepsy, ideally within 4 weeks.

➤ Any seizure has to be differentiated from pseudo-seizure occurring with conversion symptoms. Common and rare causes of seizure are listed in Box 14.10.

BOX 14.10 Main causes of seizure

Common
- Febrile seizure
- Epilepsy (generalised and partial)
- Metabolic

- Infections
- Pseudo-seizure

Rare
- Cerebral haemorrhage
- Intracranial tumours

- Drug-induced
- Mitochondrial disease

INVESTIGATION OF EPILEPSY

Diagnosis of epilepsy, aetiology and classification can often be made on a detailed history alone. Once the diagnosis is established, children are best followed up by paediatric neurologists or paediatricians with an interest in epilepsy. Those children seen initially in the community may undergo some investigations, including those shown in Table 14.6.

TABLE 14.6 Investigation for epileptic seizures

Urine	Clinitest: positive if the urine contains reducing substances. Clinistick is used to detect glucose
	Aminoacids
Blood	**First-line tests** (can be performed in primary care): U&E, glucose, calcium, phosphate and alkaline phosphatase, magnesium, acid–base status
	Second-line tests (usually performed in secondary care): ammonia, lactate, metabolic screens, chromosomal analysis if there is evidence of dysmorphic features
EEG	Will help establish whether the seizures are epileptic or non-epileptic. Interictal EEG has a range of diagnostic sensitivities between 25% and 55%. It is useful for: • Confirming a diagnosis such as focus in partial epilepsy or 3-second spikes and waves in absence seizures, or hypsarrhythmia pattern in West's syndrome • Classification, i.e. does the patient have generalised or partial epilepsy? • Showing evidence of photosensitivity • Prognosis • Choice of treatment
Imaging	Cranial ultrasound performed when the anterior fontanelle is open (it closes between 9 and 18 months of age).
	Neuroimaging with CT and MRI (images provided by MRI are far superior to those obtained by CT)
Radio-isotope scanning	SPECT (single-photon emission tomography) and PET (positron emission tomography) are used in selected cases prior to surgery

Management of seizures in primary care

Epilepsy clinic

➤ Although GPs and primary-care teams can provide excellent services for children with epilepsy, there is a limit to what these services can offer. There are difficulties which GPs face if they alone manage patients with epilepsy, including lack of expertise and time. Therefore there is a need for referral to a paediatric outpatient clinic or epilepsy clinic.

➤ For the majority of parents, the educational, social and psychological needs of their children with epilepsy are at least as important as establishing the correct diagnosis of epilepsy and controlling the disease with anti-epilepsy drugs (AEDs). Ideally, the various problems of epileptic children are managed by a multidisciplinary team within a specialist clinic (epilepsy clinic). The team should include the following:
  ➢ neurologist, hospital or community paediatrician with an interest in the subject
  ➢ specialist nurse
  ➢ clinical psychologist
  ➢ social worker.

➤ The purposes of the clinic are to:
  ➢ Form a close link between hospital and community services, including GP practices and various related departments
  ➢ Establish the diagnosis of epilepsy (clinical and initiating investigation)
  ➢ Provide information about epilepsy, triggers of seizure, first aid during a seizure, purpose and duration of medication
  ➢ Initiate treatment
  ➢ Provide psychological, educational and social support
  ➢ Arrange follow-up appointments.

➤ The epilepsy specialist nurse plays a pivotal role in providing a close link with epileptic children and their families. A nurse is an ideal person for establishing a link with affected families, offering valuable information and visiting the epileptic child at home. She also has an important role in ensuring a better compliance with medication and addressing any adverse family dynamics, misinformation or stigmatisation.

Treatment of seizures

(*See* Fig 14.2.)

Pre-hospital treatment

Airway
Breathing
Circulation
Check blood glucose

↓

Buccal midazolam 0.5 mg/kg
or
Rectal diazepam 0.5 mg/kg

↓

Call the ambulance

FIGURE 14.2 Emergency treatment of seizure in primary care

Management of epilepsy

It is not usually recommended to start an anti-epileptic drug after a single seizure. Once there have been recurrent seizures and before AEDs are prescribed, the following conditions should be met:

➤ The diagnosis of epilepsy has been established beyond doubt (*see* Table 14.8 below).
➤ The child and the parents should receive full information about the effects of the drugs and their side-effects.
➤ The child's wishes regarding whether to take an AED should be taken into consideration.

The objective of seizure treatment is to achieve complete or near-complete seizure control. Table 14.7 shows the main AEDs used for children with newly diagnosed epilepsy. For years, phenobarbitone and phenytoin were considered first-line drugs, but these are rarely used nowadays except phenobarbitone for neonates with seizures and phenytoin for status epilepticus.

TABLE 14.7 Common anticonvulsants with 1st and 2nd choice in treatment of epilepsy

Seizure type	First-line drug	Second-line drug
Generalised	Sodium valproate	Carbamazepine
(e.g. tonic–clonic)	Lamotrigine	
Myoclonic	Sodium valproate	Lamotrigine, clobazam
Absence seizure	Sodium valproate	Lamotrigine, clobazam
Partial	Carbamazepine	Gabapentin, topiramate
Infantile spasms	Vigabatrin	Prednisolone, valproate

Febrile seizure (FS)

Core messages

➤ Febrile seizure is the most common form of seizure in children, occurring in 3–4% of children. Criteria for diagnosis are shown in Box 14.11.
➤ Febrile seizure is divided into *simple* (80%) and *complex* (20%). The latter have focal features and/or are prolonged (>10 minutes) and/or are repeated in the same episode.
➤ Viral infections, particularly human herpesvirus 6, precipitate most febrile seizures.
➤ Bacterial illnesses are infrequently implicated in the precipitation of febrile seizure, except malaria, *Shigella* and *Salmonella*. Bacteraemia occurs in about 2% of cases.
➤ About one-third of children with febrile seizure will have at least one recurrence.
➤ Recurrent febrile seizures are more likely if the child is younger than 1 year at the time of the first febrile seizure, the fever provoking the first febrile seizure was relatively low, and there is a family history of febrile seizure.
➤ Routine brain imaging and EEG are not indicated following a febrile seizure.
➤ The risk of epilepsy following febrile seizures is 7% at 25 years of age.
➤ Regular prophylactic medication to prevent recurrent FSs is not recommended.
➤ The prognosis for a child with recurrent FSs is generally good. Development is unaffected.

BOX 14.11 Criteria for diagnosing simple febrile seizure

- Age 6 months to 6 years
- No focal or prolonged (<10 minutes) seizures
- Presence of fever with temperature > 38.0°C
- No subsequent paralysis
- Family and/or own history of febrile seizure (not always present)

 RED FLAGS

Bacterial meningitis rarely precipitates febrile seizure. It can be differentiated by the following:

- Children with meningitis were usually unwell with headaches, drowsiness and vomiting before the onset of seizure. Children with febrile seizure were well before the onset of seizure.
- The seizures in meningitis are usually complex.
- The child with meningitis does not show signs of recovery following seizure, in contrast to that with febrile seizure.
- In there is any doubt, lumbar puncture should be performed to exclude meningitis.

TABLE 14.8 Conditions mimicking seizures

Simple faint	Condition is rare before 10 years of age; usually precipitated by pain, fear and particularly by prolonged periods of standing in a warm environment
	May be associated with brief tonic contraction, abnormal movements, upward deviation of the eyes and even urinary incontinence
Breath-holding attacks	Diagnosis of breath-holding spells is easy from the history: both types (cyanotic and pallid) are triggered by upsetting or painful events
	Cyanosis always appears first before seizure
	(*See* also Chapter 3)
Benign myoclonus of early infancy	Brief bursts of myoclonic jerks, occurring mainly while the infant is awake
	There is no impaired consciousness, alteration of facial colour or abnormal eye movements
	Child's development and EEG are normal
Benign sleep myoclonus of infancy	Intermittent myoclonic jerks during sleep, starting from a few days of life and ceasing usually by 3–6 months of age
	The jerks do not involve the face and do not wake the child
Benign paroxysmal vertigo	*See* Table 14.3 and the section on sleep disorders, below
Long Q–T syndrome	Characterised by sudden loss of consciousness in association with exercise or emotional or stressful experience
	(*See* Chapter 10)
Narcolepsy	See section on sleep disorders, below

Night terrors	*See* section on sleep disorders, below
Pseudo-seizure	Characterised by:
	• Age 10–18 years, especially in females
	• Bizarre 'seizure' with pelvic thrusting and rolling movements; cessation is usually sudden
	• Post-ictal drowsiness or confusion is unusual
	• Absence of cyanosis, tongue biting or injury
	• Video recording of the event is useful and often diagnostic
	• Normal EEG showing often excess of muscle artifacts
	• Normal serum prolactin (raised in true epilepsy)

Indications for referring children with seizures

(*See* Box 14.12.)

BOX 14.12 Indications for referring children with seizures

- First seizure, febrile or afebrile. Routine referral if there are no concerning features
- Recurrent seizures (epilepsy)
- Urgent referral to A&E for seizures:
  - ❯ with focal neurological signs, severe, multiple, prolonged seizure
  - ❯ where there is excessive parental concerns
  - ❯ if unwell child; or abnormal neurological signs

Prognosis

➤ The prognosis of children with epilepsy is generally good.

➤ In children with febrile seizure, death or persistent motor deficit following simple seizures is unusual. Febrile seizures associated with increased intellectual deficits are more likely in children with:
  - ➣ pre-existing neurological or developmental abnormalities and
  - ➣ in those who develop subsequent afebrile seizures.

➤ In children whose anticonvulsant therapy has been withdrawn after prolonged control, about 30% will experience recurrence of seizures; of these 85% will relapse within 5 years of drug withdrawal.

➤ Factors associated with increased risk of relapse are:
  - ➣ long duration of epilepsy before control
  - ➣ pre-existing neurological deficits
  - ➣ abnormal EEG before anticonvulsants were discontinued
  - ➣ early onset of seizure below 2 years of age.

In conclusion, the neurologically normal child who has not had many seizures before control and whose EEG is normal or slightly abnormal is at low risk of seizure recurrence on stopping medications after 2 years.

Mortality

Mortality due to epilepsy is a significant concern. It is 2–4 times more common than for children without epilepsy. This risk is highest among children and young adults. Death in a child with epilepsy may be due to the following:

➤ Underlying cause, such as neuro-degenerative disorder
➤ Accident during epileptic seizure (trauma, drowning, aspiration, suffocation)
➤ Status epilepticus
➤ Suicide
➤ Sudden death in epilepsy (SUDEP), defined as sudden, unexpected, non-traumatic and non-drowning death in an individual with epilepsy in which autopsy does not reveal an anatomical or toxicological cause for the death. SUDEP causes about 500 deaths each year in the UK. Criteria for SUDEP are:
  ➤ Patient has epilepsy, i.e. recurrent and unprovoked seizures
  ➤ Patient died unexpectedly while in reasonable health
  ➤ Death occurred suddenly within minutes
  ➤ Death occurred without suspicious circumstances
  ➤ Death was not due to direct result of seizure or status epilepticus
  ➤ An obvious medical cause could not be determined at autopsy.

Certain factors known to be associated with an increased risk of mortality include:

➤ Symptomatic epilepsy (e.g. cerebral malformation, developmental delay)
➤ Uncontrolled generalised tonic–clonic seizures
➤ Patients with sleep seizures
➤ Poor compliance with AEDs
➤ Sudden and frequent changes to AEDs
➤ Lack of sleep or food, presence of stress, excess alcohol intake
➤ Seizure occurrence when alone or living alone.

Minimising the risk of mortality includes:

➤ Identifying those with poorly controlled epilepsy and ensuring they have access to specialised centres. A referral to epilepsy specialists for a review is important.
➤ Offering continued education/information about epilepsy. AEDs should always be taken as prescribed and the child should never run out of medications. Patients are to be advised to take missed doses of AEDs as soon as they remember. Encourage patients to keep seizure diaries.
➤ Referring patient to epilepsy specialist nurse (e.g. for counselling and education).
➤ Recommending lifestyle changes including:
  ➤ Use a shower instead of the bath
  ➤ Swimming should be supervised
  ➤ Ensure regular sleep and avoid fatigue
  ➤ Avoid recreational drugs, excessive alcohol.

Useful sources of information

➤ Epilepsy Action
  (British Epilepsy Association, BEA)
  New Anstey House
  Gate Way Drive

Yeadon, Leeds LS19 7XY
Helpline: 0808 800 5050
email: epilepsy@epilepsy.org.uk
www.epilepsy.org.uk
BEA provides information, advice and practical support plus downloadable
leaflets in many languages.
➤ The National Society for Epilepsy
Chesham Lane, Chalfont St Peter
Buckinghamshire SL9 0RJ
www.epilepsysociety.org.uk
Helpline: 01494 601 400
➤ Young Epilepsy
(National Centre for Young People with Epilepsy)
Helpline: 01342 831342
email: info@youngepilepsy.org.uk
www.ncype.org.uk
➤ Benefit Enquiry Line, Department for Work and Pensions (DWP)
Freephone: 0800 882 200
➤ Epilepsy Association of Scotland
Helpline: 0808 800 2200
www.epilepsyscotland.org.uk
➤ The Welsh Epilepsy Association
Helpline: 08457 413 774

NEUROMUSCULAR WEAKNESS

Core messages

➤ Weakness is a decreased ability to voluntarily and actively move muscles against resistance. Its causes are shown in Box 14.13.
➤ An upper motor neurone (UMN) lesion may manifest as cognitive deficiency or
mental deficit, decreased muscle power (palsy and not paralysis), increased muscle
tone = spasticity, hyperactive reflexes, myoclonus and intact sensation.
➤ A lower motor neurone (LMN) lesion may manifest as normal intellect, markedly
reduced muscle power (paralysis), reduced muscle tone and reflexes, and fasciculation (present with anterior horn cell disease).
➤ Weakness must be differentiated from hypotonia, fatigue and ataxia.
➤ Unilateral facial palsy in a neonate is usually due to forceps delivery and has an
almost 100% spontaneous recovery rate. The facial asymmetry is not apparent until
the child is crying. The spontaneous recovery rate of an older child with the acquired
form of Bell's palsy is about 80%.
➤ Möbius syndrome is characterised by facial weakness, drooling, dysphagia, dys-
arthria and bilateral weakness of the abducens nerve causing inability for eye
abduction.

BOX 14.13 Causes of neuromuscular weakness

- Cerebral and spinal cord injuries
- Muscular dystrophies (e.g. Duchenne's, myotonic)
- Bell's palsy
- Migrainous hemiplegia
- Neuropathies (e.g. Guillain–Barré syndrome)
- Neuromuscular junction diseases (e.g. myasthenia gravis)
- Congenital myopathies (e.g. central core disease)
- Metabolic myopathies
- Cerebral or spinal tumour
- Botulism
- Poliomyelitis
- Möbius syndrome (weakness of the facial muscles)
- Periodic paralysis (hyper- and hypokalaemic)
- Drugs (e.g. steroids)
- Motor neurone disease
- Transient myelitis
- Familial dysautonomia (Riley–Day syndrome)

PRACTICE POINTS

- Examination of a child with weakness should always begin with observation, including the head (shape and size), face (for dysmorphism), eyes (for strabismus, ophthalmoplegia), skin and muscles (for any lesion, atrophy, hypertrophy, fasciculation), gait (waddling, ataxic) and whether there is difficulty in arising from the floor.
- Proximal muscle weakness (shoulders and hips) indicates a myopathy, while distal weakness (hands) a neuropathy. Myotonic dystrophy is an exception, with weakness affecting the hands.
- Bell's palsy may be caused by herpes simplex virus, mainly type 1. Combined treatment with corticosteroids (1 mg/kg/day for 7 days) and oral aciclovir (100–200 mg 5 times daily for 5 days) may improve the chance of the recovery rate to >90% if this treatment is performed within 3 days of disease onset.
- Hypotonia may exist without weakness, e.g. in children with Down's syndrome, whereby muscles have reduced muscle tone but movements are preserved. A normal anti-gravity power excludes limb weakness.
- Some children, such as those with leucodystrophies, usually have both UMN and LMN lesions. Thus, localising a single lesion may not be possible.
- Because specific therapy is available for many neuromuscular diseases and because of genetic and prognostic implications, accurate diagnosis with the help of investigation is essential. These children require referral to hospital for further assessment if neuromuscular weakness is suspected.
- Walking is defined as an achievement of 6 steps. Inability to walk by the age of 18 months may indicate a neuromuscular disease. CPK should be checked to exclude muscular dystrophy.
- Children with periodic paralysis are normal between episodes. These episodes become more frequent, eventually causing permanent weakness.

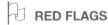 **RED FLAGS**

- In Lyme disease, caused by the spirochete *Borrelia burgdorferi*, facial palsy is common and may be the initial or only manifestation of the disease.
- Agenesis of the depressor angularis oris muscle is a congenital defect due to underdevelopment of the muscle controlling the lip. It should not be mistaken as facial palsy. The anomaly is permanent.

STIFF NECK

Core messages

➤ Stiff neck is a common presentation to both emergency and primary-care clinicians. The symptom is extremely important because of the possibility of meningitis and other serious bacterial infections such as pneumonia.

➤ Meningism is an important symptom and always requires emergency evaluation. It is characterised by the presence of neck stiffness when the neck is flexed.

➤ In infants, stiff neck is often caused by shortening of the sternomastoid muscle with swelling (sternomastoid tumour). In older children, an important cause is torticollis (wry neck), which is characterised by holding the neck tilted to one side with the chin rotated in the opposite direction. This responds to physiotherapy.

➤ The most common cause of meningism is meningeal irritation (meningitis, cerebral haemorrhage), but some cases may not have demonstrable meningeal infection (Box 14.14).

➤ In contrast to torticollis and lymphadenitis, a child with meningism is usually ill-looking with fever.

BOX 14.14 Common and rare causes of neck stiffness

Common

- Meningitis
- Pneumonia (upper lobe pneumonia)
- Viral upper respiratory tract infection with cervical lymphadenitis

- Acute torticollis (cervical muscle trauma)
- Muscular torticollis (sternomastoid tumour)
- Neck injury (whiplash injury)

Rare

- Klippel–Feil syndrome
- Sandifer syndrome (gastro-oesophageal reflux)
- Visual defects (nystagmus, superior oblique paresis)
- Dystonic drug reaction
- Hysteria

- Cervical spine infection
- Rheumatoid arthritis
- Polymyalgia rheumatica
- Intracranial haemorrhage
- Retropharyngeal abscess
- Spasmus nutans
- Pterygium colli

DIAGNOSTIC TIPS

- Torticollis resulting from sternomastoid tumour is asymptomatic in the first few days of life. At 10–20 days, a mass is frequently felt in the muscle. The mass gradually disappears and the fibrous tissue contracts, causing limited head motion and torticollis.
- Those infants with a stiff neck but no history of birth trauma and no palpable mass should have anterioposterior and lateral spine X-rays to exclude structural abnormalities before starting physiotherapy.
- Neck stiffness is a cardinal sign of meningeal irritation, however it is often absent in neonates and small infants with meningitis.
- Other causes of neck pain include lymphadenitis, acute pharyngitis and sleeping awkwardly.
- Children with torticollis and dystonic drug reaction look well despite the stiff neck, in contrast to those with meningitis or pneumonia.
- A child with Klippel–Feil malformation (short neck, fusion of the cervical vertebrae) has a high rate of renal malformations (40%).
- Any child with meningism should be considered as a case of meningitis until proven otherwise.
- Even if pneumonia is diagnosed, a child with meningism requires a lumbar puncture to confirm or exclude meningitis.

RED FLAGS

- Drug history is of paramount importance to confirm a rare case of dystonic drug reaction (oculogyric crisis, especially with metoclopramide).
- The skin of a child with meningism should be carefully searched for any rash or petechiae in case of meningococcal disease.
- Meningitis, particularly meningococcal septicaemia, may initially mimic a virus-like illness. Within a few hours the disease can rapidly progress to septic shock, hypotension, disseminated intravascular coagulation and death.

ACUTE CONFUSIONAL STATE (ACS)

Core messages

➤ ACS is a sudden alteration in mental state leading to an inappropriate interaction with people and environment.

➤ It is characterised by an acute and dramatic onset of disorientation, impaired concentration and subtle motor signs such as tremor.

➤ In older children, disorientation for time is striking.

➤ In the absence of a relevant medical history (such as sickle-cell anaemia or medication), the differential diagnosis can be quite difficult and challenging to clinicians. Box 14.15 lists causes of ACS.

➤ A child presenting with ACS should be regarded as a medical emergency. Referral to hospital is urgently required.

BOX 14.15 Common and rare causes of ACS

Common
- Migraine
- Side-effect of medication (e.g. antihistamine, anti-epilepsy drug)
- Encephalitis/encephalopathy

- Non-convulsive status epilepticus (NCSE)
- Psychosis
- Head injury
- Hypoglycaemia

Rare
- Brain tumour
- Systemic lupus erythematosus
- Brain haemorrhage
- Metabolic disorder

- HIV infection
- Malignant hypertension
- Cerebral venous sinus thrombosis
- Carbon monoxide poisoning

DIAGNOSTIC TIPS

- Diagnosis of the first episode of acute confusional migraine is often difficult; drug abuse such as that of amphetamine, cocaine and ecstasy, or encephalitis and non-convulsive status epilepticus (NCSE) need to be considered. Family history of migraine, severe headache or visual symptoms prior to the confusion may suggest the diagnosis.
- Minor trauma can occasionally trigger a major ACS grossly disproportionate to the degree of trauma.
- A confusional state of migraine often lasts several minutes to hours. It may be the first presentation before being replaced by typical migraine attacks.
- Symptoms of psychosis include delusion, hallucination and paranoid ideation. The role of clinicians is to exclude a medical cause. An urgent referral to psychiatric services is required after excluding a serious organic cause.
- Patients with systemic lupus erythematosus (SLE) can present with serious psychiatric illness. Personality changes, depression and psychosis are prominent in SLE. Laboratory testing for SLE is urgently required.

Management tips

➤ The first step in evaluating any child with psychosis is to take a full drug history, including illicit drugs. Cocaine, amphetamine and ecstasy are the commonest causes.
➤ Treatment of ACS is directed at the underlying problem, including withdrawal of any offending toxin and drugs and correcting metabolic errors as soon as possible.

SLEEP DISORDERS

Core messages

➤ Children require sufficient sleep, although they vary in their requirement. Sleep duration is age-dependent. In each 24 hours, young infants need on average 14 hours of sleep, which is almost evenly distributed during the day and night. Children aged 6–12 years require about 10–11 hours of sleep and teens about 9 hours.
➤ Small infants often have transient apnoea episodes at night, which are harmless.

Referral to hospital is not required if these episodes are not associated with cyanosis or bradycardia.

➤ It is almost normal that infants awake several times at night. The prevalence is around 30% among infants. Older children (4–12 years) commonly present with bedtime resistance. Insufficient night sleep is likely to affect the child's mood and behaviour during the day, leading to school problems such as reduced attention span, aggressiveness and poor performance.

➤ Parasomnia refers to disruptive sleep-related disorders occurring during non-rapid eye movement (NREM) sleep, and include sleep-walking, sleep terrors and confusional arousal. Those disorders occurring during REM sleep include absent sleep paralysis. Hypersomnia, or excessive sleep, includes narcolepsy.

➤ Nightmares are differentiated from night terrors by easy recall of the event in nightmares. Parents of children with night terrors are often woken by a piercing scream, the child looks flushed, frightened and agitated, and is not easily aroused. The child can not recall the event next morning.

➤ In contrast to narcolepsy, Kleine–Levin syndrome is rare. It is characterised by long and recurrent hypersomnia, hyperphagia and sometimes hypersexuality.

Causes of sleep disorders are listed in Box 14.16.

BOX 14.16 Common and rare causes of sleep disorders

Common
- Insomnia caused by illness, pain or itching
- Insomnia due to improper sleep routines
- Anxiety

- Parasomnia (e.g. nightmares)
- Hypersomnia (e.g. narcolepsy)
- Obstructive sleep apnoea syndrome (OSAS)

Rare
- Side-effects of drugs (methylphenidate, caffeine)

- Kleine–Levin syndrome

RED FLAGS

- Sleep-walking occurs occasionally in 20–40% of children, and frequently in 3–4%; the typical age is 4–8 years. Serious accidents may occur during sleep-walking. Securing the environment is essential, including securing windows and installing locks or alarms on outside doors.
- Beware of several sleep-related epileptic seizures (Table 14.9). Autonomic symptoms and secondary generalisation may occur in these sleep-related epilepsies and may mimic 'sleep disturbance'.
- Beware nocturnal frontal-lobe epilepsy (NFLE), which may mimic night terrors. A child with NFLE has a variety of motor features and vocalisation. EEG may help in establishing diagnosis.

TABLE 14.9 Some types of epilepsy which predominately occur at night and may mimic sleep disturbance such as night terror

Diagnosis	Distinguishing features
Benign sleep myoclonus	Face is never involved, facial colour is normal
	Cessation at age 3–6 months
	EEG is normal
Juvenile myoclonic epilepsy (5–10% of all epilepsies)	Bilateral single or multiple myoclonic jerks, predominately the arms, occurring when drowsy or shortly after awakening
	EEG is usually diagnostic
Benign partial epilepsy with centrotemporal spikes (rolandic) (10–15% of all epilepsies)	Unilateral paraesthesiae followed by tonic and/or clonic seizure involving the tongue, lips, cheek, pharynx and occasionally the arm, occurring during sleep or awakening
	EEG is usually diagnostic
Benign occipital epilepsy	Partial epilepsy with onset (mainly nocturnal) of vomiting, pallor, sweating, tonic eye deviations and visual hallucinations
Nocturnal frontal-lobe epilepsy	Presents with motor features (kicking, hitting, thrashing, cycling and scissoring of the legs) and vocalisation (shouting, grunting, screaming, and coughing). Seizures are usually brief and multiple, in contrast to night terrors which usually are longer and occur only once at night
	EEG helps in establishing diagnosis

Management tips
➤ Most children with various sleep disorders grow out of them in later childhood. The parents should be reassured and adequate explanation given.
➤ Regular and adequate sleep routines increase the amount of deep NREM sleep.
➤ Parents of children with bedtime resistance are advised to:
  ➣ Set regular bedtimes and morning waking times and stick to these
  ➣ Calm children down before bedtime; read a story to them
  ➣ Withdraw from the bedroom and ignore the child's protestation. Should the child wander out of the bedroom, tell him or her firmly to return, and if this fails, physically carry the child back to the bedroom with minimal affective contact, several times if necessary
  ➣ Reward the child with praise or stickers in the morning if the night-time behaviour has been good or improved.
➤ Although many parents and clinicians often turn to medication to treat children's insomnia, it is far more important to search for any underlying cause (e.g. anxiety), which needs to be treated first.
➤ Obstructive sleep apnoea syndrome (OSAS), which manifests as snoring and frequent cessation of sleep, is an important cause of insomnia. Children with Down's syndrome, triangular chin and long soft palate are at risk of having OSAS. The child may need tonsillectomy and/or adenoidectomy.
➤ During sleep-walking, parents should not try to wake or restrain the child. Telling the child about the event is unnecessary. If episodes are frequent, scheduled awakening may help: the child is gently and briefly woken 15–30 minutes before the episode is due, and this is repeated for a month.

Narcolepsy

Narcolepsy is a lifelong problem mostly caused by a lack of a neurotransmitter (hypocretin). Cataplexy is characterised by sudden loss of muscle tone following laughter, excitement or a sudden startle. Criteria for diagnosis of narcolepsy are:

➤ Excessive daytime sleepiness
➤ Paroxysmal episodes of irresistible daytime sleep, anywhere at any time
➤ Patients are easily aroused to an alert state
➤ Positive results of all-night polysomnography, followed by multiple sleep latency test performed during the day
➤ Associated often with:
  ➢ sudden, transient muscle loss (cataplexy) triggered by emotion
  ➢ disturbed nocturnal sleep
  ➢ hallucination and sleep paralysis.

Management includes:

➤ Psychosocial support
➤ Short, regular naps at times when the patient feels sleepiest
➤ Regular exercise
➤ Avoiding certain activities such as swimming
➤ Regular follow-up
➤ CNS stimulants for narcolepsy such as:
  ➢ Modafinil
  ➢ Methylphenidate
  ➢ The tricyclic antidepressant clomipramine
➤ Sodium oxybate is licensed for the treatment of cataplexy.

PRACTICE POINTS

- Narcolepsy may occasionally be mistaken for complex partial seizure. The above diagnostic criteria should readily establish the correct diagnosis.
- Cataplexy may also be mistaken for atonic seizure. Cataplexy is always precipitated by laughter, excitement or a sudden startle.

CHAPTER 15

Endocrinology

DISORDERS OF HEIGHT

The most common paediatric endocrine complaints seen in general practice are those related to height (short stature), weight (overweight or underweight), sexual maturity (premature or delayed puberty), diabetes and thyroid disorders. Growth monitoring in developing countries is primarily aimed at detecting malnutrition. In the UK, the major purpose of growth monitoring is early detection of various growth disorders (Box 15.1), such as Turner's syndrome, growth hormone deficiency and coeliac disease.[1]

Short stature

Core messages

➤ Measuring a baseline length at the 6-week check is recommended if an abnormality in the history or physical examination is suspected.

➤ Measuring the height of both parents is essential in evaluating a child with short stature and predicting the ultimate height of the child.

➤ In children younger than 24 months, recumbent length is significantly greater than standing height.

➤ Children's annual height increase varies according to their age (Table 15.1).

➤ Short stature is defined as a height < the 3rd centile for age and gender. A length < the 0.4 centile will identify very short children who are more likely to have skeletal or endocrine abnormalities. The World Health Organization (WHO) 9-centile growth charts showing the 0.4 and the 99.6 centiles, should be used. These charts are available at: www.rcpch.ac.uk/growthcharts

➤ Children's growth is like that of trees: they grow faster in spring and summer, therefore growth velocity should be measured for 1 year.

➤ The term 'short stature' is often confused with growth failure. 'Short' is defined as having a height < the 3rd centile, while 'growth failure' is defined as a growth rate < 5 cm/year.

TABLE 15.1 Average annual height increase

Age (years)	Height increase (cm)
0–1	23–28
1–3	7.5–13
3 to puberty	5–7
During puberty	8–9 (girls); 10–10.5 (boys)

BOX 15.1 Causes of short stature

- Familial short stature
- Constitutional delay
- Malnutrition
- Small for gestational age (SGA)
- Chronic disease (e.g. inflammatory bowel disease, coeliac disease)
- Skeletal abnormalities (e.g. achondroplasia)
- Chromosomal (e.g. Turner's syndrome)
- Endocrine (e.g. hypothyroidism, growth hormone deficiency, poorly controlled diabetes)
- Emotional deprivation

Recommended investigations

➤ Full blood count (FBC) for anaemia

➤ Blood glucose for growth hormone deficiency. (Growth hormone deficiency causes increased sensitivity to insulin)

➤ Thyroid function tests (TFTs): T4 and thyroid-stimulating hormone (TSH) for hypothyroidism

➤ Coeliac screen

➤ Plasma gonadotropin levels: elevated in Turner's syndrome

➤ Karyotyping in girls to exclude Turner's syndrome

➤ Bone age (estimated by a wrist X-ray) to differentiate familial short stature from constitutional delay

➤ Ultrasound scan of the heart, kidney and ovaries for Turner's syndrome

---

BOX 15.2 Characteristic features of a child with GH deficiency

- Normal length and weight at birth
- Appear younger than chronological age (infantile)
- The bridge of the nose is depressed and saddle-shaped
- Delayed tooth eruption
- High-pitched voice
- Genitalia are underdeveloped for the child's age

PRACTICE POINTS

- Endocrine diseases as a cause of short stature are rare and account for no more than 5% of causes.
- The three most common causes of short stature worldwide are familial, constitutional delay and malnutrition.
- Children with familial short stature are normal children who have short parents, normal growth rate and bone age, and enter puberty at a normal age. Their ultimate height is related to their parental height.
- Children with constitutional delay have normal growth rate but delayed onset of puberty and bone age. Because of delayed bone age, they have more time to grow and usually achieve a normal adult height.
- Growth hormone (GH) is a major counter-regulatory hormone to insulin; therefore

children with growth hormone deficiency may present with hypoglycaemia, particularly during fasting or mild illness.

- In GH deficiency, the weight/height ratio is increased while it is decreased in chronic disease (e.g. inflammatory bowel disease).
- Early identification of short stature associated with hormonal deficiencies is essential because early treatment improves the outcome for adult height. The vast majority of short children do not have GH deficiency (Box 15.2).
- Turner's syndrome should always be considered when pubertal delay is combined with short stature. Signs may be subtle, as individuals can achieve normal adrenarche (growth of axillary and/or pubic hair) and few have breast development (10–20%).

Referral

When to refer children with short stature:
- Child's height is causing serious concern to the parents.
- Child's height is significantly shorter than expected from parental heights.
- Length or height measurement is below the 0.4 centile.
- Child's height is crossing centile lines downwards between 3 years and puberty.
- Any growth velocity < 4 cm/year.
- Children who were born as small for gestational age (SGA) and who remain short after the age of 3 years. Referral is needed for further diagnostic tests and to decide whether growth hormone treatment is indicated.
- Short stature associated with weight loss, diarrhoea, poor appetite or headaches.
- Any child with short stature and evidence of hypoglycaemia.

Referral should include:
- Serial measurement of height and weight for at least 6 months unless children are under the 0.4 centile.
- Wrist X-ray for bone age.

Excessive height

Core messages

- Children with height > the 99.6th centile are regarded as having excessive height.
- Growth is influenced by hereditary, genetic, illness, nutritional, medication, hormonal and psychological factors.
- A child's potential height usually ranges between the averages of the parents' heights. Hereditary and genetic factors are responsible for most excessive height.
- Marfan's syndrome should be considered in any child with excessive height.
- Girls report concern to their GPs about their height at an earlier age than boys. Society perceives tall and slender girls as beautiful, but excessive height as less acceptable than in boys.
- Growth hormone excess causes gigantism and acromegaly. Other conditions associated with an excessive GH secretion include McCune–Albright syndrome (incidence of gigantism 15–20%), neurofibromatosis type 1, familial somatotropinoma (autosomal dominant) and multiple endocrine neoplasia (Box 15.3).

BOX 15.3 Main causes of children with excessive height

- Hereditary/genetic
- Obesity
- Klinefelter's syndrome
- Pituitary gigantism
- Marfan's syndrome
- Sotos syndrome
- Precocious puberty

- Neurofibromatosis type 1
- Beckwith–Wiedemann syndrome
- Homocystinuria
- Hypogonadism
- Familial somatotropinoma
- Multiple endocrine neoplasia

Recommended investigations

(Majority of tests performed in secondary care.)

➤ Serial growth measurements plotted on WHO 9-centile charts and this should be done in primary care prior to referral
➤ Urine for homocystine: increased in homocystinuria
➤ Insulin growth factor 1 (IGF-1) and GH in blood: elevated in pituitary gigantism and acromegaly
➤ Plasma levels of follicle-stimulating hormone (FSH), luteinising hormone (LH) for Klinefelter's syndrome
➤ Karyotyping for Klinefelter's syndrome
➤ Skeletal X-ray for a child with precocious puberty if Klinefelter's syndrome is suspected; wrist X-ray for other causes of precocious puberty
➤ Echocardiography for Marfan's syndrome to exclude aortic aneurysm
➤ Cranial MRI for suspected pituitary tall stature to exclude adenoma

PRACTICE POINTS

- Over 50% of obese children have a height in the 70–99th centile range.
- Children with Klinefelter's syndrome (incidence 1 : 600 of newborn males) have at least one additional X chromosome. More than 90% of boys with this syndrome remain undiagnosed. Children present with:
  - ○ Difficulties in learning, speech, reading and writing, behaviour problems such as aggressiveness, excessive shyness and antisocial acts.
  - ○ Gynaecomastia (in about 80%) in adolescence. They are at increased risk of malignancy including breast cancer, mediastinal tumours and leukaemia.
  - ○ Infertility with diminished pubic hair and small testes.
- Tall stature may be caused by precocious puberty. The skin should be examined for café-au-lait patches to exclude McCune–Albright syndrome.
- Children with excessive height are at risk of developing orthopaedic problems such as kyphosis or scoliosis, and secondary psychiatric problems.
- Marfan's syndrome is an autosomal-dominant inherited disorder with an incidence of about 1 : 10 000 births. Patients are at risk of early death because of progressive aortic dilation. Arachnodactyly (long, thin fingers) and lens dislocation are important clues. Referral to a paediatrician and ophthalmologist is important.

Referral

Referral should be considered for all cases with excessive height which are not caused by hereditary/genetic factors or obesity. Referral should include serial measurements of height and weight for at least 6 months unless the height is > the 99.4 centile.

DELAYED PUBERTY (DP)

Core messages

➤ Menarche occurs at the median age of 13 years and usually begins 2–3 years after the start of breast enlargement (thelarche). Penile and scrotal enlargement usually occurs 1 year after testicular enlargement which occurs at an average age of 12–13 years.

➤ Delayed puberty is arbitrarily defined as delay in pubertal changes beyond 14 years of age in girls and 16 years of age in boys. The definition includes those children who do not complete their puberty within 5 years from its start.

➤ The cause of delayed puberty in the vast majority of boys and in most girls is constitutional (Box 15.4).

➤ Delayed puberty is usually associated with delayed growth and velocity for chronological age. The exceptions to this are boys with Klinefelter's syndrome who are tall with long arms and legs, having normal adrenarche but small testes.

➤ Puberty can easily be assessed by bone age (wrist X-ray):
  ➣ If bone age is within 1 year of chronological age, puberty either has not or has just started
  ➣ If bone age is > 1 year in advance of chronological age, this indicates that the child is in puberty.

BOX 15.4 Main causes of delayed puberty

- Constitutional
- Chronic diseases (malnutrition, Crohn's disease, coeliac disease, cystic fibrosis, anorexia nervosa)
- Intensive physical exercise
- Chromosomal (Turner's, Noonan's, Klinefelter's syndromes)
- Polycystic ovarian syndrome (PCOS)
- CNS tumour (craniopharyngioma, meningioma, prolactinoma)
- Prader–Willi syndrome
- Irradiation of the gonads, chemotherapy
- Following bone marrow transplantation
- Androgen insensitivity syndrome (testicular feminisation syndrome)

Recommended investigations

➤ FBC and C-reactive protein (CRP) (anaemia with high CRP suggests Crohn's disease)
➤ Screening blood tests for coeliac disease
➤ Hormonal assay: levels of FSH/LH, gonadotropin-releasing hormone (GnRH), oestrogen, testosterone, prolactin, GH, 17-hydroxyprogesterone and dehydroepiandrosterone (DHEA) assay if indicated
➤ Gastrointestinal investigation for suspected Crohn's disease if indicated
➤ TFTs for suspected thyroid disorders
➤ Karyotyping for suspected cases of Turner's syndrome (X0) and Klinefelter's syndrome (XXY)
➤ Wrist X-ray for bone age

➤ Pelvic ultrasound scan to detect ovarian cysts, tumour or ovarian dysgenesis (Turner's syndrome); testicular ultrasound for tumour

PRACTICE POINTS

- The cause of DP can be established in most cases by detailed history and examination, including growth measurement.
- Tanner charts or testicular development are available at: http://en.wikipedia.org/wiki/tanner_scale
- The principal cause of delayed puberty in boys is constitutional.
- Girls have more-frequent pathological causes, e.g. anorexia nervosa, chronic diseases, intensive exercise or chromosomal abnormalities.
- If constitutional delayed puberty is diagnosed, children can be reassured that they will achieve normal puberty later.
- Turner's syndrome is the commonest cause of delayed puberty with short stature in girls. Mean adult height is 143–144 cm. Girls with this syndrome develop normal pubic and axillary hair at the appropriate age; thelarche and menstruation are unusual.

Conditions requiring referral

➤ If the diagnosis of delayed puberty is uncertain or unclear.

➤ If pathological conditions (see list above) are suspected.

➤ All girls with an inguinal hernia should undergo pelvic ultrasound before herniotomy to exclude androgen insensitivity syndrome.

➤ In girls with otherwise normal sexual maturation but delayed menarche and galactorrhoea, prolactinoma is likely. Urgent prolactin level and MRI of the brain should be considered.

➤ Hormonal treatment for short stature is indicated if it is causing distress or school under-performance. Boys with constitutional DP may be treated with oxandrolone if aged > 11.5 years and testosterone if aged >13.5 years, and girls with ethinyl oestradiol.

➤ Girls with Turner's syndrome may require growth hormone. Many girls achieve heights of greater than 150 cm with early treatment.

PRECOCIOUS PUBERTY (PP)

Core messages

➤ Normal sexual development in girls begins with breast development, followed by the appearance of pubic hair, axillary hair, onset of menstruation, acne and adult body odour. In boys, it begins with testicular enlargement followed by enlargement of the penis, the appearance of pubic hair, deep voice, acne and adult body odour.

➤ In many normal girls, thelarche is asymmetric and the breast nodule may be tender and sensitive to friction.

➤ Precocious puberty is defined as puberty occurring at <8 years of age in girls or <9 years of age in boys. Puberty nowadays starts earlier than in previous generations.

➤ The causes of precocious puberty (Box 15.5) are best divided into *central* (hypothalamic), *peripheral* (adrenal, gonadal) and *idiopathic* causes. In more than 90% of girls and 50% of boys, the cause of precocious puberty is idiopathic, i.e. there is no identifiable cause.

➤ Central and peripheral precocious puberty can be differentiated by the absence of breast or testicular enlargement in peripheral causes, which usually present with the appearance of pubic and axillary hair.

➤ PP is often a cause of adverse effects on social behaviour and psychological development. In addition, the associated early growth spurt can cause rapid bone maturation but linear growth ceases early, resulting in short stature.

➤ Partial precocious puberty (PPP) is either an isolated breast development (precocious thelarche) or sexual hair appearance (precocious adrenarche) without other signs of puberty. The condition is usually benign.

BOX 15.5 Main causes of precocious puberty (PP)

Central (hypothalamic or true precocious puberty)
- Identifiable causes (e.g. hamartoma, pineal teratoma, irradiation of the brain, birth injury, hydrocephalus)
- Idiopathic

Peripheral (precocious pseudo-puberty)
- Gonadal (e.g. ovarian cysts, McCune–Albright syndrome)
- Adrenal (e.g. congenital adrenal hyperplasia, tumour)
- Familial PP in males
- Iatrogenic (external sources of sex hormones)
- Mediastinal teratoma
- Partial precocious puberty (PPP), e.g. premature thelarche

Recommended investigations

(Usually performed in secondary care.)

➤ Hormonal assay of GnRH, LH, FSH and sex hormones

➤ Serum level of 17-hydroxyprogesterone, DHEA, cortisol and aldosterone in cases of suspected congenital adrenal hyperplasia (CAH)

➤ Wrist X-ray to assess bone maturation and puberty: if bone age is within 1 year of chronological age, puberty either has not or has just started; bone age in advance of 1 year indicates the child is in puberty

➤ Pelvic ultrasound scan and adrenal visualisation for CAH

➤ CT scan or MRI of the head for all cases suspected of central causes of PP

➤ Skeletal survey for bony fibrous dysplasia for a child with PP and hyperpigmented spots

---

PRACTICE POINTS

- Cerebral injury during the neonatal period or hydrocephalus may cause PP or delayed puberty.
- Precocious thelarche can occur in toddlers; however, the nipple is characteristically pale, immature, thin and transparent and not associated with development of any other secondary sexual characteristics.

- In any child with PP, a careful search of the skin is essential: café-au-lait maculae with a smooth border suggest neurofibromatosis type 1, while larger café-au-lait patches with an irregular outline is consistent with McCune–Albright syndrome (polyostotic fibrous dysplasia of bone, and ovarian cysts).
- Hypothyroidism may cause PP and is associated with short stature and reduced growth velocity and bone age on a wrist X-ray.
- Growth acceleration and advanced bone age favour true PP against PPP.
- Children with a hypothalamic lesion may present with symptoms of diabetes insipidus, including polydipsia, polyuria, hyperthermia, obesity or loss of weight, or inappropriate crying or laughter.
- PP or PPP may put girls at higher risk of sexual abuse and psychological trauma from teasing and bullying.
- Full investigation, including imaging of the CNS and abdomen, should be carried out for all children with PP who have progressive signs of puberty, under the age of 6 years, if there are neurological signs or if the diagnosis is uncertain.
- In a child with central PP, hypothalamic hamartoma is probably the most common identifiable lesion.

Indications for referral

Any child with true precocious puberty or partial precocious puberty.

EXCESSIVE HAIR

Core messages

➤ Hair growth in excess of what is expected for age, sex and ethnicity is termed hirsuitism or hypertrichosis.

➤ While hypertrichosis indicates non-androgenic, excessive vellus hair growth in areas not usually hairy, hirsuitism is an androgen-dependent male pattern of hair growth usually in women.

➤ The most common cause of hypertrichosis or hirsuitism is racial or familial, frequent in people from the Mediterranean area and the Indian subcontinent. In the UK, the most common cause is polycystic ovarian syndrome (PCOS), which is associated with obesity, anovulation (resulting in irregular menstruation, amenorrhoea and infertility) and excessive androgen production (resulting in acne, hirsuitism, alopecia and insulin resistance).

➤ Polycystic ovaries are characterised by a large number of cysts (these are underdeveloped follicles) that are each smaller than 8 mm. Many women with polycystic ovaries have no PCOS, and some women with this syndrome have normal ovaries on ultrasound scan.

➤ Successful weight reduction in patients with PCOS is the most effective method of treating this condition, including restoring normal ovulation.

➤ The most important endocrine causes of excessive hair are congenital adrenal hyperplasia (CAH) and Cushing's syndrome (Box 15.6).

BOX 15.6 Causes of excessive hair growth

- Racial and familial hypertrichosis or hirsuitism
- Drugs (e.g. steroids, phenytoin, cyclosporine, minoxidil)
- Endocrine causes (e.g. Cushing's syndrome, congenital adrenal hyperplasia, adrenal tumour)
- Polycystic ovarian syndrome (PCOS)
- Malnutrition, including anorexia nervosa

- Congenital hypertrichosis
- Hyperprolactinaemia
- Cornelia de Lange syndrome
- Porphyria cutanae tarda
- Sertoli–Leydig cell tumour
- Granulosa-thecal cell tumour
- Idiopathic hirsuitism
- Paraneoplastic syndrome

Recommended investigations

(Usually performed in secondary care.)

➤ Serum testosterone, DHEAS, LH, FSH: raised in PCOS and tumour. Serum 17-hydroxyprogesterone, DHEA to diagnose CAH, serum prolactin for hyperprolactinaemia

➤ TFTs for thyroid diseases

➤ Pelvic ultrasound for determining uterus and ovaries in masculine signs of CAH, identification of multicystic ovaries (pearl necklace) in PCOS and detecting ovarian and adrenal tumours

➤ MRI is often required, particularly if hormonal studies have been inconclusive, and for pituitary adenoma, adrenal and ovarian cysts or tumours

PRACTICE POINTS

- In CAH, masculinisation in female neonates manifests as an enlarged clitoris resembling a penis, and labial fusion. These signs may be mistaken as cryptorchidism and hypospadias.
- The diagnosis of PCOS has to be considered in any adolescent female who presents with amenorrhoea, menstrual irregularities or acanthosis nigricans (a hyperpigmented area which may also be associated with internal malignancy).
- PCOS is associated with the metabolic syndrome of obesity, insulin resistance and type II diabetes.

Conditions requiring referral

➤ Hirsuitism causing disfigurement and/or psychological trauma.

➤ Hirsuitism in pre-pubertal children as this may be an important sign of precocious puberty.

➤ Children with PCOS presenting at the time of puberty with menstrual disturbances, overweight and hirsuitism. Androgen excess may cause deepening voice, acne and masculinisation.

➤ Any acute and/or severe hirsuitism to exclude tumour of the ovary or adrenal cortex.

Management

➤ Management is directed at the underlying cause.

➤ No treatment is indicated for the idiopathic cause if the patient is not concerned about the cosmetic appearance.

➤ Weight reduction is important if overweight.

➤ Plucking is discouraged, as it may result in irritation, folliculitis and scarring.

➤ Available treatments by specialists include electrolysis, thermolysis (diathermia) and laser epilation.

NECK LUMPS AND THYROID DISEASES

Midline neck lumps include those listed in Box 15.7.

BOX 15.7 Causes of neck lumps near the midline

- Goitre
  - › Congenital goitre
  - › Iodine-deficiency goitre
  - › Thyroiditis
  - › Drug-induced goitre (e.g. lithium)
  - › Hyperthyroid goitre
- Ectopic thyroid tissue
- Thyroglossal cyst
- Cystic hygroma
- Branchial cyst (usually off-centre on the neck)
- Dermoid cyst
- Pharyngeal pouch

Recommended investigations

➤ Thyroid function tests: TSH and T4

➤ Auto-antibodies, including anti-thyroid antibodies

➤ Ultrasound

➤ Radioisotope thyroid scan

PRACTICE POINTS

- The neonatal screening programme for congenital hypothyroidism is well established and cost effective.
- Screening TFTs should be performed for those at increased risk of hypothyroidism (Fig 15.1 and Box 15.8).
- The most common cause of acquired hypothyroidism is Hashimoto's thyroiditis, which usually affects adolescents who present with diffusely enlarged, firm and non-tender goitre, cold intolerance, loss of energy, increased sleepiness and growth deceleration.
- Thyroglossal cysts develop from a remnant thyroglossal duct and are usually painless unless infected. They characteristically move upward on swallowing and tongue protrusion (Fig 15.2).
- A branchial cyst appears as an insignificant-looking papule on the side of the neck.

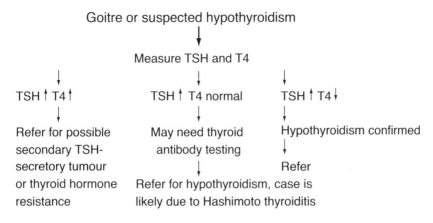

Goitre or suspected hypothyroidism
↓
Measure TSH and T4

↓	↓	↓
TSH ↑ T4 ↑	TSH ↑ T4 normal	TSH ↑ T4 ↓
↓	↓	↓
Refer for possible secondary TSH-secretory tumour or thyroid hormone resistance	May need thyroid antibody testing ↓ Refer for hypothyroidism, case is likely due to Hashimoto thyroiditis	Hypothyroidism confirmed ↓ Refer

FIGURE 15.1 Interpretation of thyroid function tests

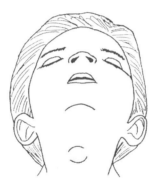

FIGURE 15.2 Thyroglossal cyst usually presents as a painless and smooth midline lump

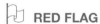 **RED FLAG**

- Excision of a midline cyst should never be considered before ensuring that it is not a thyroid mass.

BOX 15.8 Conditions associated with increased risk of hypothyroidism

- Family history of thyroid diseases
- Down's and Turner's syndromes
- Previous neck irradiation or surgery
- Taking thyrogenic drugs such as amiodarone, lithium, interferon-alpha
- Goitre

- Type 1 diabetes
- Children with autoimmune diseases
- Individual known to be thyroid-antibody positive
- Radioactive iodine or surgery for hyperthyroidism

POLYURIA

Core messages

➤ Polyuria is defined as urine output $> 2 \text{ L/m}^2/24$ hours.

➤ Although causes of polyuria are numerous (Box 15.9), the most common causes are diabetes mellitus, diabetes insipidus, defects of renal tubular transport ability (renal tubular acidosis, RTA) and compulsive drinking (primary polydipsia). Diabetes has usually a short history and is easily diagnosed. A differential diagnosis of these conditions is shown in Table 15.2.

➤ Diabetes insipidus (DI) is caused by deficiency of anti-diuretic hormone (ADH). It may be caused by pituitary tumour (central diabetes insipidus) or the kidneys being unresponsive to the ADH (nephrogenic diabetes insipidus.

➤ Polyuria must be differentiated from more-common complaints of frequency of a small volume of urine. This may require measurement of fluid intake and urine output over 24 hours.

BOX 15.9 Causes of polyuria

- Diabetes mellitus
- Diabetes insipidus
- Compulsive drinking
- Renal tubular acidosis
- Metabolic polyuria (e.g. potassium deficiency)

- Sickle-cell anaemia
- Hypercalcaemia
- Chronic renal failure
- Drugs (diuretics, lithium, chlortetracycline)
- Barter's syndrome

TABLE 15.2 Differential diagnosis between diabetes insipidus (DI), renal tubular acidosis and compulsive drinking

	DI	Renal tubular acidosis	Compulsive drinking
Failure to thrive	Possible	Yes	No
Signs of dehydration	Present	Present	No
Improved polyuria on fluid restriction*	No	No	Yes
Nocturnal polydipsia and polyuria	Yes	Yes	No
Low urine specific gravity	Yes	Yes	No
Systemic acidosis, low serum bicarbonate and potassium, hyperchloraemia, glycosuria	No	Yes	No

* Fluid restriction tests should be carried out in secondary care.

Recommended investigations

➤ Urinalysis for glycosuria and ketones in diabetes mellitus (DM). Specific gravity: low in DI

➤ Blood glucose to confirm DM; acid balance and ketones for diabetic ketoacidosis (DKA)

➤ Osmolality of serum and urine; urine specific gravity

➤ FBC: anaemia is a feature of chronic renal failure and sickle-cell anaemia

➤ Urea and electrolytes (U&E): high creatinine in chronic renal failure; low potassium as a cause of polyuria
➤ Serum calcium for hypercalcaemia
➤ ADH level for DI: low in cranial DI and normal in nephrogenic diabetes insipidus
➤ MRI for central causes of DI, such as craniopharyngioma
➤ Water deprivation test to differentiate between central and nephrogenic DI (done in hospital)

PRACTICE POINTS

- Although the history and physical examination may provide clues to the causes of polyuria, the definitive diagnosis rests on the results of blood glucose, osmolality of the urine and serum, and U&E.
- It is essential to determine whether the child has frequent, small urination or polyuria. Mothers are usually good historians. Observation of the child's urine amount by parents and 24-hour urine collection help establish diagnosis.
- Children with compulsive drinking are readily diagnosed by the long history, absence of weight loss or failure to thrive. Low serum osmolality (<280 mOsm/kg) and urine specific gravity <1.005 establishes the diagnosis. A specific gravity greater than 1.005 excludes the diagnosis of diabetes insipidus.
- The fourth most important cause of polyuria is renal tubular acidosis. Children may present with dehydration, failure to thrive, anorexia and vomiting. Investigations show glycosuria, low serum bicarbonate and potassium, and hyperchloraemia.

RED FLAGS

- All cases of polyuria should be referred to a paediatrician for evaluation except where the child has a clear history of excessive drinking and is well and thriving.
- Chronic dehydration during infancy often presents with irritability, poor feeding, failure to gain weight, dehydration and elevated body temperature.
- An unrecognised chronic dehydration, such as that resulting from DI, would lead to hypernatraemia, seizures and brain damage.
- Long-standing polyuria may cause enlarged bladder, mega-ureter and hydronephrosis.

TYPE 1 DIABETES

Diabetes is a chronic auto-immune disease. The prevalence of diagnosed diabetes in the UK is estimated to be 2.23 per 100 males and 1.64 per 100 females.

Of the estimated >1 million people in England and Wales with diabetes, 20% have type 1 diabetes.[2]

Diagnosis

(*See* Box 15.10.)

BOX 15.10 Diagnosis of type 1 diabetes

- History is typically short (a few days to 2–3 weeks) with polyuria, polydipsia, vomiting, weight loss and abdominal pain.
- Less commonly:
  - ❯ Nocturnal enuresis in a previously toilet-trained child
  - ❯ Recurrent pyogenic skin infections
  - ❯ Chronic weight loss
  - ❯ Vaginal candidiasis
- Signs may include:
  - ❯ Diminished level of consciousness
  - ❯ Dehydration (lethargy, dry mouth, reduced skin turgor)
  - ❯ Hyperpnoea with Kussmaul's respiration (sighing)

- Diagnostic criteria of diabetes mellitus:
  - ❯ Fasting blood glucose level of ≥7.0 mmol/L if symptomatic. This should be repeated if asymptomatic
  - ❯ Random blood glucose level of ≥11.1 mmol/L
  - ❯ Glycated haemoglobin (HbA$_{1c}$) of ≥6.5%
- Diagnostic criteria of diabetic ketoacidosis (DKA):
  - ❯ blood glucose >11 mmol/L with venous pH <7.3 or bicarbonate <15 mmol/L

Management

All children with type 1 diabetes should be referred urgently to paediatric services. Older children and adolescents who are not dehydrated or acidotic may be considered as a day-case by a multidisciplinary team (Box 15.11). Indication for hospital management may include:

➤ Young age (<3 years)
➤ Ketoacidosis
➤ Moderate to severe dehydration
➤ Living a long way from hospital and/or no telephone at home
➤ Language or other communication difficulties
➤ Social or emotional difficulties.

BOX 15.11 Management of type 1 diabetes (*see* also NICE Guidelines)[2]

Children and young people with type 1 diabetes should be:
- Offered an integrated package of care by a multidisciplinary paediatric diabetes care team. Those with suspected type 1 diabetes should be referred immediately (same day) to this team
- Involved (with their families) in making decisions regarding care by the care team at the time of diagnosis, including home-based or inpatient management according to clinical needs, family circumstances and wishes, and residential proximity to inpatient services. Home-based care with support from the local paediatric diabetes care team (including 24-hour telephone access for advice) is safe and as effective as inpatient initial management
- Diagnosed on the criteria specified in the 1999 WHO report on the diagnosis of diabetes, available at http://whqlibdoc.who.int/hq/1999/who_ncd_ncs_99.2.pdf
- Informed that the target for long-term glycaemic control is an HbA$_{1c}$ level of <7.5%
- Undergoing height and weight measurement and their BMI calculated at each clinic visit

---

- Treated according to the guidelines published by the British Society for Paediatric Endocrinology and Diabetes when they develop DKA[3]
- Offered access to mental health professionals, as psychological disturbance (e.g. anxiety, depression, behavioural problems) may interfere with management and wellbeing
- Offered screening testing for:
  > coeliac disease at diagnosis and later if there is a clinical suspicion
  > thyroid disease at diagnosis and annually until transfer to adult services
  > retinopathy annually from the age of 12 years
  > microalbuminuria annually from the age of 12 years
  > blood pressure measurements annually from the age of 12 years
  > Annual footcare reviews and checking the injection site at each clinic visit
- Informed that they may experience a partial remission phase (honeymoon period), during which a low dosage of insulin (0.5 units/kg bodyweight) may be sufficient
- Offered the types of insulin (Table 15.3) which suit their individual needs and with the aim of obtaining $HbA_{1c} < 7.5\%$ without disabling hypoglycaemia and maximising quality of life
- Offered testing of their HbA_{1c} levels 2–4 times per year. The optimal pre-prandial blood glucose level is 4–8 mmol/L and post-prandial is <10 mmol/L
- Encouraged to measure their blood glucose > 4 times daily if they have intercurrent illness
- Offered a structured programme of education
- Offered continuous SC insulin infusion (insulin pump) if they experience severe hypoglycaemia, provided that:
  > multiple-dose insulin therapy has failed, and
  > those receiving it have the commitment and competence to use it effectively
- Encouraged to consume daily 5 portions of fruit and vegetables and a bedtime snack, and take regular exercise.

TABLE 15.3 Available types of insulin regimen

Types of insulin	Action		
	Onset	Duration	Types
Rapid-acting	15–30 minutes	2–5 hours	Humalog, Novolog
Short-acting	30–60 minutes	5–8 hours	Humulin, Novolin
Intermediate-acting	1–2 hours	16–35 hours	Isophane, NPH, Lente
Long-acting	1–2 hours	18–26 hours	Glargine*, Ultralente

*Insulin Glargine (Lantus) and Levemir are long-acting human insulin analogues which allow more consistent release of insulin during the day and reduce the risk of severe nocturnal hypoglycaemia. This is recommended by the NICE guidelines for children with type 1 diabetes.[2]

Education points for a child with diabetes should not be less than 3–4 times per year and should cover the following areas:
➤ *Blood glucose (BG) monitoring.* Optimal targets for short-term glycaemic control are a pre-prandial blood glucose (BG) of 4–8 mol/L and a post-prandial BG of <10 mmol/L.

➤ *Education/information.* This includes information available from the NICE website (www.nice.org.uk), Diabetes UK and Patient UK.

➤ *Nutrition.* Nutritional reviews should occur 2–4 weeks post-diagnosis and ongoing at least once a year by a paediatric dietitian experienced in diabetic management. Nutrition should be based on a total energy intake of:

  ➤ Carbohydrate > 50%
  ➤ Protein 10–15%
  ➤ Fat 30–35%.

➤ *Therapeutics,* which include insulin storage, insulin injection techniques and BG measurements. In addition:

  ➤ Children and their families should be informed that insulin should never be omitted even if the child is unable to eat.
  ➤ Insulin is injected in the abdomen, buttock or non-exercising thighs.
  ➤ There is a risk of accidental IM injections (and hence more rapid absorption) especially in lean individuals or in the upper arms. This can be minimised by using a two-finger pinch technique and an injection angle of 45 degrees.
  ➤ Ketones should be tested if BG is >15 mmol/L or if the child is unwell with abdominal pain, rapid breathing, fever or other symptoms.

➤ *Intercurrent illness.* Guidance should be offered for the management of type 1 diabetes during intercurrent illness (sick-day rules). Include the information that such illness can cause high or low blood glucose levels and that it should be monitored more frequently. Rapid- or short-acting insulins should be available for sick-day management.

➤ *Exercise.* Children should be informed that they can participate in all forms of exercise, provided that:

  ➤ Appropriate attention is given to changes in insulin and dietary management. Exercise may necessitate extra carbohydrate intake and insulin reduction.
  ➤ They are aware that exercise-induced hypoglycaemia may occur several hours after exercise.
  ➤ Additional carbohydrate should be consumed if BG levels are <7 mmol/L before exercise is undertaken.

➤ *Identifying and managing complications.*
  Short-term complications include:

  ➤ Hypoglycaemia that can be prevented by maintaining BG > 4 mmol/L.
  ➤ Dental decay, gingivitis and periodentitis are more common if glycaemic control is poor. These can be prevented by regular brushing and flossing of teeth at least twice daily as well as regular dental examination.
  ➤ Lipohypertrophy is common (estimated to occur at 20–30%), and absorption of insulin from these sites is delayed or erratic. This can be minimised by rotating injection sites.

  Long-term complications (e.g. neuropathy, nephropathy and retinopathy) are rare during childhood. HbA_{1c} is the only measure of glycaemic control that has been shown to be associated with long-term complications of diabetes. It should be measured at least twice a year with a target of <7.5%. Low HBA_{1c} may be associated with asymptomatic hypoglycaemia.

➤ *Psychological care.* Children with diabetes have a greater risk of emotional and behavioural problems (e.g. anxiety, depression) and, mainly in girls, eating disorders. They should be offered access to mental health services.

➤ *General advice* for children with type 1 diabetes should include:

➤ Timely and ongoing opportunities to access information about the development, management and effects of type 1 diabetes.

➤ Cause of diabetes, advice on the effect of alcohol on diabetes.

➤ Awareness that good metabolic control reduces the risk of developing short- and long-term complications of diabetes.

➤ Aims of insulin therapy.

➤ The effects of diet on glycaemic control.

➤ Carrying glucose tablets or readily absorbed carbohydrate. Glucagon should be available at home.

➤ Annual immunisation against influenza for children over the age of 6 months, as recommended by the Department of Health.

➤ Wearing some form of identification.

REFERENCES

1. Grote FK, van Dommelen P, Oostdijk W, et al. Developing evidence-based guidelines for referral for short stature. Arch Dis Child 2008; 93: 212–217.
2. NICE guidelines, 2004 (modified Oct 2011). CG15: Diagnosis and management of type 1 diabetes in children, young people and adults. www.nice.org.uk/CG15
3. www.bsped.org.uk. Endorsed Guidelines: Diabetes Guidelines.

CHAPTER 16

Musculoskeletal diseases

COMMON MINOR ORTHOPAEDIC ANOMALIES

Tip-toeing or tip-toe walking

➤ This is usually a normal finding in toddlers up to 2–3 years of age. Examine for full foot contact while standing and normal movement range when the ankle joint is extended.

➤ If tip-toe walking persists beyond 2–3 years of age, the following diagnoses should be considered:

  ➢ Bilateral congenital tendo-achilles contracture or cerebral palsy (spastic diplegia)

  ➢ Unilateral due to cerebral palsy (hemiplegic type)

  ➢ Occasionally seen in Duchenne muscular dystrophy as a compensation to knee extensor weakness.

Intoeing

➤ This is a common anomaly in infants and young children, characterised by feet turning inwards while walking. If severe, it may cause stumbling or tripping.

➤ Intoeing may be due to foot (metatarsus adductus, Fig 16.1), tibial (internal tibial torsion) or femoral anomalies (femoral anteversion).

➤ Metatarsus adductus is more common in first-born children due to the moulding effect of the uterus and is characterised by adducted forefoot and normal hindfoot causing convex lateral border of the foot.

➤ Most affected feet are flexible and the deformity can be passively corrected by active manipulation or stroking the lateral border of the foot. A mild degree of deformity usually requires no treatment.

➤ Some cases where feet correct to the neutral position, but not beyond, may benefit from orthotics.

➤ Rigid feet that do not correct to the neutral position require referral and may be treated with plaster casts.

RED FLAGS

● About 10% of children with intoeing have acetabular dysplasia predisposing to hip dislocation. Therefore careful examination of the hip is essential.

● Treatment of severe intoeing should not be delayed beyond the age of 8 months in order to obtain the best results.

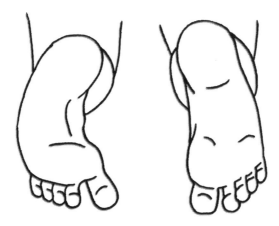

FIGURE 16.1 Intoeing due to metatarsus adductus, more noticeable in the left foot

Flat feet (pes planus)

➤ A common and usually normal anomaly in the early years of childhood due to ligament laxity; significant improvement usually occurs by the age of 6 years.

➤ Flat feet in older children may be secondary to generalised ligament laxity which is often autosomal-dominant inherited and may be idiopathic (Fig 16.2).

➤ Treatment is not required unless the condition is symptomatic, causing pain or abnormal shoe wear. Physical activity, such as walking barefoot at home or over uneven terrain such as a beach, is helpful. There is no evidence to support the use of orthotics. (Gel arch supports may help if the child has aching after standing for long periods.)

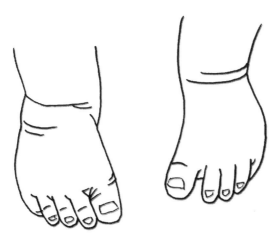

FIGURE 16.2 Bilateral flat feet

Clubfoot (also known as talipes equinovarus)

➤ Incidence of clubfoot is around 1 per 1000 live births. The vast majority of cases are congenital and idiopathic.

➤ Clubfoot is either positional or structural. *Positional clubfoot* can be corrected by manipulation. *Structural clubfoot* is either idiopathic as an isolated abnormality or associated with neuromuscular disorder.
➤ Treatment for structural clubfoot includes manipulation, taping and serial plaster casts and requires referral.

> ⚑ **RED FLAG**
>   ● Clubfoot may be associated with other genetic abnormalities such as congenital heart disease or neural tube defects.

Bowlegs (genu varum)

(*See* Fig 16.3.)
➤ Most cases are physiological (commonly seen at age 1–3 years), resulting from external rotation of the hip combined with internal tibial torsion. Improvement usually occurs by 2 years of age.
➤ Idiopathic tibia vara (Blount's disease, Fig 16.4) is abnormal progressive angulation below the knee. The condition may occur as *infantile* (1–3 years), juvenile (4–10 years) and adolescent (>10 years). The infantile form is the most common form and is related to obesity. Braces are often required; occasionally surgery.
➤ A rare but important cause is rickets.
➤ If Blount's disease or rickets is suspected, this should be investigated with an X–ray and, for rickets, serum calcium, phosphorus, alkaline phosphatase and vitamin D levels.

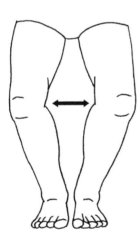

FIGURE 16.3 Bowing of the legs

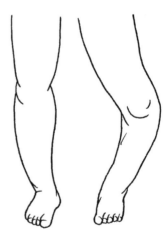

FIGURE 16.4 Tibial bowing (Blount's disease of the left leg)

Knock-knees (Genu valgum)

(*See* Fig 16.5.)

Most cases are physiological (commonly occurring at age 3–5 years). It usually resolves spontaneously at age 5–8 years.

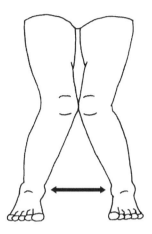

FIGURE 16.5 Knock-knees

Single palmar crease

(*See* Fig 16.6.)

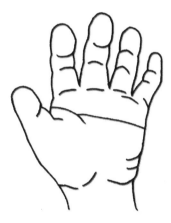

FIGURE 16.6 Single palmar crease

This is often a normal finding on one hand (about 5% of the population) or both hands. It is sometimes associated with syndromes such as Down's syndrome or fetal alcohol syndrome.

Syndactyly

➤ Complete or incomplete webbing between the 2nd and 3rd toe is common and normal in children, requiring no intervention.

➤ However, in syndactyly of the fingers, there may be a shared important neurovascular bundle between the digits. Associated syndromes are numerous. Referral is advisable.

Polydactyly

➤ Extra fingers or toes occur in approximately 2 per 1000 births; about a third of them have positive family history inherited as autosomal recessive.

➤ In most cases (80%), the polydactyly is an isolated finding; in the rest, the condition is associated with numerous syndromes and chromosomal abnormalities.

PAINFUL ARM

Core messages

➤ In children, arm pain usually results from musculoskeletal injuries (sprains, strains, contusion, dislocation and fracture). Box 16.1 lists the main causes.

➤ In the absence of dislocation and fracture, a musculoskeletal pain syndrome (MSPS) can be considered. The pain may affect either part of the arm or the whole upper arm or forearm, often associated with a burning or numbing sensation.

➤ If there is a history suggestive of injury, e.g. sport activity, the diagnosis is evident. A moderate to severe injury is likely to be followed by an inflammatory response which manifests as pain, spasm, reduced arm movement and redness and swelling.

➤ Less-common causes of arm pain include neurovascular and cardiovascular disorders and referred pain from another area such as the neck, chest or abdomen.

BOX 16.1 Main causes of pain in the arm

- Trauma-related:
  - ❯ Pulled elbow (nursemaid's elbow)
  - ❯ Dislocation, fracture
  - ❯ Child abuse
- Non-specific musculoskeletal pain syndrome (MSPS):
  - ❯ Chronic fatigue syndrome (CFS)
  - ❯ Fibromyalgia
  - ❯ Reflex sympathetic dystrophy
- Malignancy (bone tumour)
- Vascular (Raynaud's phenomenon, scurvy)
- Inflammatory:
  - ❯ Myalgia (e.g. viral infection)
  - ❯ Tendonitis and tenosynovitis
  - ❯ Arthritis
  - ❯ Osteomyelitis
  - ❯ Neuritis (neuropathy)
  - ❯ Herpes zoster
- Spinal:
  - ❯ Cervical nerve root compression
  - ❯ Brachial plexus
  - ❯ Spinal abscess

Recommended investigations

High FBC and CRP support the diagnosis of bacterial infection or arthritis

➤ Auto-antibody screen is useful to check for Raynaud's phenomenon

➤ X-ray of the arm excludes fracture or dislocation

➤ Spinal X-ray is indicated if spinal lesions are suspected

➤ Bone scan for suspected osteomyelitis or malignancy

PRACTICE POINTS

- Muscle pain (myalgia) is common in association with many acute conditions, such as viral infection, metabolic disorders, polyneuropathy and myositis.
- Pain in the elbow may be caused by pulled elbow (nursemaid's elbow) caused by someone pulling the child's hand hard (e.g. when stopping the child from falling), causing a subluxation of the radial head.
- MSPS is a diagnosis of exclusion. The pain is poorly localised, and physical examination is normal except for tenderness to light touch over several areas of the arm. Laboratory findings are usually normal.
- Fibromyalgia and reflex sympathetic dystrophy are variant manifestations of MSPS. Although symptoms often overlap with MSPS, they tend to be prolonged and recurrent.
- Fatigue is more prominent than pain in chronic fatigue syndrome (CFS). Although children with MSPS may present with fatigue, this is likely to be mild.
- Children with fibromyalgia may present with symptoms of irritable bowel syndrome (incidence around 50%), migraine or tension headaches (incidence around 50%) or temporomandibular joint dysfunction.
- Growing pains are common and typically:
  - affect the lower limbs
  - pain is episodic, nocturnal and non-articular
  - there is no daytime disability or limp
  - persist for months.
- Children may interpret paraesthesiae and muscle weakness as pain. The presence of paraesthesiae or numbness suggests a neurological condition, e.g. ulnar neuritis.
- Compartment syndrome, though rare in children, affects circulation and function due to increased pressure in a confined space, causing severe pain felt with passive muscle stretching. It requires immediate referral.

RED FLAGS

- With a young child who presents with unexplained pain, the possibility of child abuse, Münchausen by proxy and school phobia should always be considered in the differential diagnosis.
- In any child with trauma, peripheral pulses and capillary refill time (CRT) must be checked.
- Raynaud's phenomenon can present with swelling and pain of the fingers and forearm. If this phenomenon worsens over time and there are associated skin changes, auto-immune diseases such as dermatomyositis, systemic scleroderma or systemic lupus erythematosus should be considered.

PAINFUL LEG AND LIMPING

Core messages

➤ The key to an accurate diagnosis is a careful history, thorough physical and neuro-logical examination, and appropriate radiological and laboratory investigations.

➤ Pain in the leg is common and is caused by many musculoskeletal disorders (Box 16.2). Painful limping is the usual presentation.

➤ These disorders may affect the:

➢ Hip: e.g. transient synovitis, avascular necrosis (Perthes disease) or slipped capi-tal femoral epiphysis

➢ Knee: e.g. avascular necrosis, osteochondritis dissecans or idiopathic adolescent knee pain syndrome

➢ Foot: e.g. poor-fitting shoes, trauma, avascular necrosis of the femoral head or non-articular pain such as growing pains.

BOX 16.2 Causes of painful leg/limping

Limping usually with pain
- Minor muscle strains/sprains/overuse
- Growing pains
- Transient synovitis
- Avascular necrosis of the femoral head (Perthes disease)
- Arthralgia/arthritis (see section on arthritis, below)
- Osteochondritis of the long bone (e.g. in syphilis)

- Fracture (e.g. child abuse)
- Drugs (steroids)
- Malignancy (e.g. leukaemia, lymphoma, bone tumour)
- Sickle-cell anaemia
- Deep venous thrombosis
- Spinal disorders (e.g. sciatica)
- Dermatomyositis
- Polyneuropathy

Limping usually without pain
- As above (except 'growing pains')
- Congenital hip dislocation
- Slipped capital femoral epiphysis

- Cerebral palsy (hemiplegia)
- Psychiatric diseases (e.g. conversion disorder)

Recommended investigations

➤ FBC and CRP are necessary if an infectious aetiology is suspected, e.g. osteomyelitis or septic arthritis

➤ Rheumatoid factor, anti-nuclear antibodies (ANAs), human leucocyte antigen B27 are needed for rheumatological cases

➤ CPK, serum transaminases for muscular diseases

➤ TFTs and growth hormone level in pre-pubertal children with slipped capital fem-oral epiphysis

➤ X-ray of the leg should be considered if the pain persists for >1 week. (Imaging of the bone is normal in the early stages of Perthes disease. The earliest possible radio-logical sign is the 'crescent sign' seen in the frog lateral position)

➤ MRI may be indicated (depending on the X-ray results)

PRACTICE POINTS

- Examination of a child with leg pain should include examination of the shoes for uneven wear or a foreign body, e.g. a nail.
- Patello-femoral crepitations are common and do not indicate serious knee disease.
- Growing pains are non-articular occurring at night for several months. Examination is normal and there is no daytime disability.
- Perthes disease usually presents at age 5–10 years; mean age: 7. Adverse prognosis is related to:
  - ○ delayed diagnosis
  - ○ age at clinical onset – those older than 10 years at diagnosis are very likely to develop early degenerative arthritis in adult life.
- Osgood–Schlatter disease (tibial apophysitis) is a common cause of knee pain in adolescents, particularly those who are active in sport. Typically the pain worsens with exercise, causing limping. There is often swelling and tenderness just below the knee over the tibial tubercle. Pain lasts weeks or months, and usually resolves within 12–24 months.
- Chondromalacia patella (softening of the cartilage on the undersurface of the patella) is also a common cause of chronic knee pain. It mostly occurs in children aged 10–16 years. Pain usually worsens slowly over several months, particularly when going upstairs, squatting or kneeling. Full recovery is slow but normally occurs.
- Transient synovitis presents as sudden onset of limping in a child with recent upper respiratory tract infection. Laboratory and radiological investigations are usually normal.
- Long-term use of steroids can cause osteoporosis, fractures and avascular necrosis.

RED FLAGS

- Many children with hip diseases present with referred knee pain. Examination of both joints is essential.
- In a young child with an unexplained pain, child abuse is always a possibility. Carefully examination of the skin for relevant bruises and for other signs of possible injury is essential. Skeletal survey may be required.
- Slipped capital femoral epiphysis is the most common hip disorder in adolescence. If it occurs before puberty, an endocrine cause such as hypothyroidism or growth hormone deficiency should be excluded.

SPINE

Back pain in children

Core messages

➤ Back pain in young children (<4 years old) is uncommon and has a higher incidence of organic causes (in at least 50%) compared with older children and adults. Cumulative prevalence rises steadily with age, and about 20–45% of young people aged 14–18 years have back pain for longer than 2 weeks. Pupils who carry heavy backpacks (>10% or 15% of their bodyweight) are at high risk of back pain.

➤ Trauma causing muscle or ligament strain that settles in a few weeks is the most common cause. Spondylosis (stress fracture or a defect of the joint between the vertebrae – the interarticularis joints) and spondylolisthesis (forward slipping of one vertebra upon another) are the commonest identifiable causes of low back pain in children and adolescents, often resulting from excessive activities in sport (e.g. gymnastics, dance, high-jump, football).

➤ Rare but serious causes of back pain include infections (e.g. discitis, osteomyelitis), tumours (e.g. osteoid osteoma).

➤ Among other causes of back pain are spinal deformities, particularly Scheuermann's kyphosis (see below) and symptoms of conversion.

PRACTICE POINTS

The spine of a child presenting with back pain should be examined:

● For any midline skin abnormalities such as pigmented naevus or hairy patch
● For any postural deformity, tenderness on palpation of the spine and signs of muscle spasms
● In flexion that increases the strain on the anterior part of the spine, particularly the vertebral bodies and the disk spaces. Pain caused by herniated disk worsens with forward flexion
● In extension that increases the strain on the posterior part of the spine. Pain caused by injury or tumour worsens with extension
● In one-leg extension test (stork test): standing on a single leg with the other leg in flexion at the knee joint and the spine in extension. A positive test involves pain and suggests spondylosis.

RED FLAGS

Serious back pain requiring referral includes:

● Young age, <4 years
● Persistent (> 2 weeks) or increasing pain, disturbing sleep; pain radiating down to the legs
● Functional impairment such as to walking, sport or play
● The presence of systemic signs such as fever, loss of appetite or weight, bladder or intestinal dysfunction
● Abnormal signs on physical examination such as tenderness on palpation or pressing the spine.

Spinal kyphosis

The normal radiological range of kyphosis is 20–40°. Causes of kyphosis include:

➤ *Congenital kyphosis*, caused by congenital malformations of the vertebrae.
➤ *Postural kyphosis*, a common cause of referral from primary care. Typically a complete correction of the kyphosis can be achieved clinically and radiologically on hyperextension of the spine.

➤ *Structural kyphosis*, of which Scheuermann's kyphosis is the most common form affecting 4–8% of the population. The cause is uncertain. It develops in adolescence (typical age 10–15 years) and may become slightly progressive, particularly in boys. The usual presentation is pain (unlikely to be severe) or as a painless kyphosis with compensatory lumbar lordosis and tight hamstrings. Pain typically increases with the length of the deformity. In contrast to postural kyphosis, affected patients cannot actively correct the deformity.

Spinal scoliosis

Scoliosis, defined as a curve of >10°, is divided into:
➤ *Structural scoliosis*, which includes idiopathic scoliosis. This is the most common condition, affecting 2–3% of children, and occurs as an *infantile* (birth to 3 years), *juvenile* (4–10 years) and *adolescent* (>10 years) form. Asymmetry of the posterior chest wall on forward bending should be elicited.
➤ *Non-structural scoliosis.*

Management of kyphosis and scoliosis

➤ There is little evidence that children with mild kyphosis of <60° experience late progression, severe pain or neurological complications. Pre-pubertal patients are managed by an exercise programme, including hyperextension exercises, observation and repeated examination.
➤ Post-pubertal patients with kyphotic curves <70–80° who are otherwise asymptomatic and with acceptable cosmetic appearance of their spine require no treatment. Those with kyphosis >80–90° are likely to be symptomatic and have an unacceptable appearance of the spine; therefore, referral is required for possible surgery.
➤ When examining for scoliosis, the child should be asked to bend forward fully (Fig 16.7). If the curvature does not disappear on this manoeuvre, X-ray of the spine should be requested.

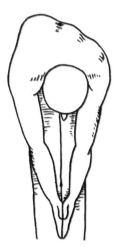

FIGURE 16.7 Scoliosis of the spine may not become apparent unless the patient is asked to bend forward

➤ Scoliosis with curves between 10° and 19° require observation and repeat X-ray after 6 months to check progression. Curves between 20° and 29° may require referral for possible brace (above 25°).

➤ Scoliosis with curves between 20° and 30° usually progresses in pre-pubertal children, but is less likely to do so in post-pubertal ages.

🏳 RED FLAGS

- Patients with spinal deformities require careful examination for the presence of associated neurological abnormalities (such as cerebral palsy and muscular dystrophy) and syndromes.
- The presence of café-au-lait spots (neurofibromatosis type 1), excessive height (Marfan's syndrome), sacral dimple, hairy patches, and foot deformity suggests an underlying cause. Early recognition of such associations and prompt referral are required.
- Persistent or more than occasional complaints of aches in the spine are not normal in patients with kyphosis or scoliosis, and require urgent evaluation.

ARTHRITIS

Core messages

➤ Rheumatic diseases are characterised by an exaggerated autoimmune activity which can be organ-specific (e.g. Hashimoto thyroiditis) or systemic (e.g. juvenile idiopathic arthritis (JIA) and systemic lupus erythematosus (SLE).

➤ Children with arthritis have a better chance of outgrowing their arthritis and have lower complications of disability compared with adults.

BOX 16.3 Types and main causes of arthritis*

Monoarthritis
- Septic arthritis (SA)
- Trauma
- Transient synovitis of the hip
- Monoarthritic juvenile idiopathic arthritis
- Tuberculosis arthritis
- Familial Mediterranean fever (FMF)

Oligoarthritis
- Reactive arthritis (e.g. arthritis of inflammatory bowel disease, e.g. Crohn's disease, ulcerative colitis)
- Oligoarthritic juvenile rheumatoid arthritis (JRA)
- Neoplastic arthritis (leukaemia, lymphoma)
- Juvenile ankylosing spondylitis
- Lyme disease
- Psoriatic arthritis

Polyarthritis
- Viral arthritis (e.g. parvovirus B10)
- Rheumatic fever (RF)
- Polyarthritic JRA
- Collagen disease (e.g. SLE, dermatomyositis)
- Vasculitis (e.g. Kawasaki disease)
- Behcet's disease

* Some types of arthritis (e.g. FMF) may present as mono-, oligo or polyarthritis.

➤ Arthritis may be monoarthritis, oligoarthritis (<5 joints) or polyarthritis (>4 joints). The main causes of arthritis are shown in Box 16.3.

➤ Juvenile idiopathic arthritis and ReA have an auto-immune cause. Reiter's syndrome is a reactive arthritis.

Recommended investigations

➤ FBC, erythrocyte sedimentation rate (ESR), white blood cells (WBCs), platelets

➤ Anti-nuclear antibodies (ANAs)

➤ IgM-rheumatoid factor: usually negative in systemic onset disease but may be positive in polyarthritis. It correlates with disease activity and usually suggests poor prognosis

➤ Ultrasound of the affected joints: very useful in detecting an effusion or assists in aspiration

➤ MRI is very sensitive in differentiating septic arthritis from osteomyelitis and other causes

➤ Bone scan: positive in the majority of cases with septic arthritis

➤ Bone marrow can be diagnostic in suspected neoplastic arthritis

PRACTICE POINTS

- Transient synovitis is common and usually presents with unilateral hip pain and limping and history of a recent upper respiratory tract infection and absence of fever. The differential diagnosis is provided in Box 16.4.
- Systemic-onset juvenile idiopathic arthritis can be diagnosed by intermittent fever (ranging from 39.5°C to 41.2°C), with a daily rise in the evening, then falling to normal in the morning. Fever is usually associated with the occurrence of rash, generalised lymphadenopathy and splenomegaly.
- Rheumatic fever is characterised by migratory arthritis, occurring 2–3 weeks following an untreated group A beta-haemolytic streptococcal pharyngitis. Diagnosis is established by Jones criteria (Box 16.4).
- ANAs are among the most important tests in arthritis: they are positive in nearly 100% of cases of mixed connective tissue diseases (CTD), over 95% of cases in SLE and about 50% of cases in juvenile idiopathic arthritis.
- The principles of management of rheumatic diseases are given in Box 16.5.

BOX 16.4 Differential diagnosis of arthritis in children

Juvenile idiopathic arthritis

- Any arthritis with no known cause which lasts at least 6 weeks in a patient younger than 16 years

Transient synovitis

- This is a common cause of limp in childhood at age 3–7 years
- History of a recent viral upper respiratory tract infection (URTI)
- Acute onset of a limp and hip pain in an otherwise healthy child
- Children typically are afebrile with a limited range of hip motion

- Laboratory findings are usually normal
- It is self-limiting, usually lasting 1–3 weeks

Viral arthritis

- Arthralgias are more common than viral-induced arthritis
- Usually occurs within a week of developing symptoms of a viral infection such as rash; it may precede their onset by a week
- Arthritis is usually symmetrical, self-limiting (may last 2–4 weeks) and bilateral

Rheumatic fever (RF)

- Diagnosis of RF is made when 2 of the major criteria, or 1 major criterion plus 2 minor criteria, are present along with evidence of streptococcal infection
- Major criteria are polyarthritis, carditis, subcutaneous nodules, erythema marginatum and Sydenham's chorea
- Minor criteria are fever, arthralgia, raised CRP or ESR, leucocytosis, ECG showing first-degree heart block, previous episode of RF

Reactive arthritis (including Reiter's syndrome)

- This is an auto-immune arthritis that develops following an infection (occurring 1–3 weeks prior to the onset of arthritis), most commonly a viral URTI or enteric infection (with *Campylobacter*, *Salmonella*, *Shigella* or *Yersinia*)
- Commonly associated with the human leucocyte antigen HLA-B27
- Arthritis typically affects weight-bearing joints (knee and ankle) and is transient, usually lasting less than 6 weeks.

Septic arthritis (SA)

- Septic arthritis is almost always monoarthritis. Joint aspiration is required and shows positive joint fluid culture for bacteria and/or a WBC count in the joint fluid of >50 000 cells/mm^3 (predominately polymorphonuclear cells) with or without positive blood culture (positive in about 50% of cases)
- Septic arthritis is characterised by an abrupt onset of fever and joint pain (fever is usually high, >39.5°C), with severe pain and restricted range of joint movement and refusal to walk

Tuberculosis (TB) arthritis

- Typically mono-arthritis which follows pulmonary TB
- Arthritis is painless, persistent in one joint and unresponsive to conventional treatment

---

BOX 16.5 Principles of management of arthritis

- Management of children with arthritis is complex and challenging. Early referral to a rheumatology team experienced in the care of children with arthritis is important
- The aim of treatment of arthritis is to maintain daily activity, relieve pain, prevent organ damage and disability and avoid drug toxicity
- Medications
  - › Non-steroidal anti-inflammatory drugs (NSAIDs) are used in larger doses and for longer periods for their anti-inflammatory effects rather than for analgesia alone.

Several weeks may elapse before an adequate anti-inflammatory effect has been achieved

> Corticosteroids are a cornerstone of treatment for juvenile idiopathic arthritis, SLE, dermatomyositis and many forms of rheumatic diseases and vasculitis. Long-term use leads to numerous side-effects. Intra-articular injection is particularly useful in patients with juvenile idiopathic arthritis involving one or two joints

> Methotrexate, an analogue of folic acid, plays a central role in the treatment of juvenile idiopathic arthritis and juvenile dermatomyositis. It is usually administered orally in a dose of $10\,mg/m^2$ body surface area once weekly. The low dose of methotrexate causes significantly lower toxicity compared with its use when treating neoplastic diseases

> Etanercept and Infliximab are licensed for the treatment of active juvenile idiopathic arthritis in children aged 4–7 years

● Physical treatment, including physiotherapy, occupational therapy, hydrotherapy and rehabilitation

● Coordination of care with a school nurse, community nurse, social services, community professionals, and others in case of long-term disease

ARTHRALGIA (PAINFUL JOINT)

Core messages

➤ Arthralgia is defined as joint pain not accompanied by obvious clinical signs of arthritis. Every attempt should be made to localise the arthralgia. Once the painful joint is identified, differential diagnosis becomes easy (Box 16.6).

➤ Arthralgia may be generalised involving multiple joints, caused mostly by a viral infection, or involving the hip, knee, ankle or temporomandibular joint.

➤ The best approach to a child with arthralgia and normal examination is to perform

---

BOX 16.6 Main causes of arthralgia

Generalised
● Acute viral infection
● Malignancy (leukaemia, bone tumour)
● Sickle-cell anaemia
● Henoch–Schönlein purpura
● Inflammatory bowel disease (Crohn's disease, ulcerative colitis)
● Rheumatic fever
● Sarcoidosis
● Drugs (e.g. carbimazole)
● Wegener's granulomatosis
● Psychogenic

Hip
● e.g. transient synovitis, Perthes disease, slipped capital femoral epiphysis

Knee
● e.g. chondromalacia, subluxation, osteochondritis, Osgood–Schlatter disease

Ankle
● e.g., sport injury, sprains

careful initial evaluation and inflammatory tests (such as WBC, CRP) followed by periodic monitoring for changes in symptoms or physical findings.

➤ Communication with the parents is vital. They are often concerned that an immediate diagnosis cannot be made. Informing the parents that there is a plan in place to monitor their child's symptoms should help alleviate parental concern.

Recommended investigations

➤ FBC: elevated WBC in bacterial diseases; leucopenia in SLE; CRP

➤ CPK: elevated in dermatomyositis

➤ Hb-electrophoresis and peripheral film for sickle-cell anaemia

➤ Kveim test for suspected sarcoidosis

➤ X-ray: diagnostic for avascular necrosis

➤ Bone scan, e.g. for suspected bone tumour

PRACTICE POINTS

- Arthralgia in association with acute viral illness should be considered as part of myalgia affecting the tissue surrounding the joints.
- Differential diagnosis of arthralgia of the hip includes transient synovitis (typical age 3–7 years, child awakens with severe groin pain causing refusal to walk or limping), Perthes disease or slipped capital femoral epiphysis. The latter affects typically obese short children or those with a rapid growth spurt.
- Painful knee may be caused by traumatic synovitis, haemarthrosis, chondromalacia patella, patellar subluxation or dislocation, synovial plicae, Osgood–Schlatter disease or tumour.
- Patellar subluxation is not uncommon, detected when the knee is in full extension. Displacing the patella laterally often results in the patient pushing away or grabbing the examiner's hand (apprehension sign).
- Painful ankle is often due to sport injury, or referred pain from avascular necrosis of the navicular bone (Köhler's disease) or the metatarsal head (Freiberg's disease).
- Although persistent arthralgia without evidence of arthritis is unusual in juvenile idiopathic arthritis, arthralgia lasting several weeks may occur in the pre-arthritic stage of the disease.
- Wegner's granulomatosis is an uncommon cause of vasculitis mainly affecting the upper and lower respiratory tract. Presentation is usually non-specific and includes fever, myalgia, arthralgia, weight loss, conjunctivitis and uveitis.

⚐ RED FLAGS

- Before diagnosing arthralgia, ensure that there are no signs of arthritis (red, hot and swollen joint) and no obvious clinical evidence of effusion in the joint.
- Knee pain may be a referred pain originating from a diseased hip.
- The finding of haemarthrosis (usually in the knee) is indicative of a serious

injury to ligaments or meniscus or an occult fracture. Urgent referral to orthopaedics is indicated.

MYALGIA (PAINFUL MUSCLES)

Core messages

➤ Acute muscle pain (myalgia) is a very common complaint in association with many infections, mainly viral such as influenza types A and B and coxsackie virus A2 and A9.

➤ Myalgia is often not due to systemic or local spread of the microorganisms, but rather to the interleukin-1 effect, which induces protein breakdown (proteolysis). Amino acids released during proteolysis can be metabolised within the muscle as a direct source of energy and are re-used for the synthesis of new proteins.

➤ Myalgia can also be due to musculoskeletal injury (sprains, strains, overuse, contusions), musculoskeletal pain syndrome (MSPS), myopathic (e.g. dermatomyositis) and neuropathic (Guillain–Barré syndrome) (Box 16.7).

BOX 16.7 Examples of causes of myalgia

- Infection
  - › Many viral infections
  - › Trichinosis
  - › Lyme disease
- Trauma, including child abuse
- Musculoskeletal pain syndrome (MSPS)
  - › Chronic fatigue syndrome (CFS)
  - › Fibromyalgia
- Neural
  - › Acute polyneuropathy (Guillain–Barré-syndrome)

- Metabolic disease
  - › Porphyria
- Drugs
  - › Statins, carbimazole
- Rheumatism/vasculitis/connective tissue disease
  - › Dermatomyositis
  - › Systemic lupus erythematosus (SLE)
  - › Polymyalgia rheumatica
  - › Wegener's granulomatosis
  - › Familial Mediterranean fever (FMF)

Recommended investigations

➤ Urine: proteinuria in SLE and FMF. Urine for porphyrins to confirm porphyria and rhabdomyolysis

➤ FBC may be helpful in showing leucopenia, thrombocytopenia and anaemia in SLE. Eosinophilia in helminthic infection, such as trichinosis and ascaris

➤ CRP is helpful for bacterial infections, CTD, dermatomyositis, and FMF

➤ Auto-antibodies such as ANA are helpful in connective tissue disease

➤ For trichinosis, serological studies (Bentonite flocculation test) and muscle biopsy (showing larvae) will confirm the diagnosis

➤ Ultrasound and/or MRI is helpful in some inflammatory conditions such as dermatomyositis

PRACTICE POINTS

- A child with acute muscular weakness affecting the limb girdle muscles should be suspected of having dermatomyositis until proven otherwise. A peri-orbital rash is an important clue.
- Not all muscle diseases produce pain. Muscle diseases not associated with myalgia include muscular dystrophy and spinal muscular atrophies.
- Diagnostic criteria for FMF are recurring episodes of fever, pain in the abdomen (peritonitis), the chest (pleuritis) or the joints (arthritis) and muscles (myalgia).
- Clinicians should be aware that there are overlapping symptoms between MSPS, fibromyalgia, CFS and reflex sympathetic dystrophy. Fibromyalgia is associated with widespread pain and stiffness in the muscles, sleep disturbance, school absence and fatigue. The condition may need to be differentiated from CFS.

RED FLAGS

- In any child with unexplained muscle pain, child abuse should be considered. Skeletal survey may be needed to confirm.
- Myalgia can be the presenting symptom of some serious diseases including bone tumour.
- Although trichinosis is uncommon in children in the UK, it is common worldwide. Children present with localised myalgia and fever following ingestion of undercooked pork meat. Peri-orbital or facial oedema is very common (80%). Eosinophilia is present in the blood.

CHAPTER 17

Dermatology

ECZEMA
Clinical features
➤ Eczema characteristically begins at 2–3 months of age on the cheeks, often spreading to the rest of the face, neck, wrists and abdomen, and extensor surfaces of the extremities (Fig 17.1 – *see* Plate section). Flexural involvement of the extremities (popliteal and antecubital) occurs later (Fig 17.2 – *see* Plate section). Diagnostic criteria are shown in Box 17.1.

➤ Eczema tends to improve aged 3–5 years. Children are at high risk of developing other atopic conditions such as asthma and hay fever at a later stage.

➤ Seborrhoeic dermatitis (SD) is often difficult to differentiate from eczema. Distinguishing features are shown in Box 17.2.

➤ Secondary infection by staphylococci or *Candida* is prevalent and is the commonest cause of treatment failure.

BOX 17.1 Diagnostic criteria for eczema

● Diagnosis is made by the presence of 3 or more of the following major criteria:
  › History of pruritis, particularly in the skin creases
  › Visible flexural dermatitis involving the skin creases (popliteal and antecubital), later flexural lichenification of the extremities or visible dermatitis on the cheeks and/or extensor areas at <18 months of age (*see* Box 17.3 for degrees of severity)
  › Chronic or chronically relapsing course
  › Individual or family history of atopy (asthma, hay fever, allergic rhinitis, allergic conjunctivitis, atopic dermatitis)
● In addition, 3 or more of the following minor criteria:
  › Dryness of the skin
  › Elevated serum IgE (in about 80%)
  › Early age of onset (<2 years old)
  › Tendency towards skin infection (especially staphylococcal and herpes simplex)
  › Tendency towards hand and foot dermatitis
  › Food allergy (in about 20–30%)

BOX 17.2 Differentiating seborrhoeic dermatitis from eczema

- Seborrhoeic dermatitis is very common and may affect as many as 50% of newborns
- Seborrhoeic dermatitis often begins during the 1st month of life, and usually involves the scalp (cradle cap). The onset of seborrhoeic dermatitis is usually earlier than eczema
- Seborrhoeic dermatitis lesions are typically a greasy, scaly erythematous papular dermatitis
- Pruritus is always present in eczema, in contrast to SD
- Seborrhoeic dermatitis usually disappears by 1 year of age while eczema commonly persists

---

BOX 17.3 The three degrees of eczema severity

Mild

- Areas of dry skin
- Lesions affecting a few areas of the skin
- Infrequent itching

- Undisturbed sleep
- Little impact on daily activities

Moderate

- Areas of dry skin
- Red areas of lesions with or without excoriation

- Frequent itching
- Disturbed sleep

Severe

- Widespread areas of dry skin
- Extensive areas of skin involvement, with bleeding, oozing or cracking or pigmentation

- Incessant itching
- Loss of sleep
- Severe impact on everyday activities

See also NICE guidelines.[1]

Management

➤ Eczema requires long-term management and there is no cure. Emollients and topical steroids are the mainstay of treatment. Treatment of mild and moderate eczema is summarised in Box 17.4.

➤ Treatment is aimed at relieving the symptoms, including particularly the itching. An oral sedating antihistamine is indicated if sleep is disturbed. A non-sedating antihistamine is sometimes required.

➤ Scalp SD responds well to frequent use of medicated shampoo. The scalp needs to be gently massaged for about 5 minutes. Inflamed lesions usually respond promptly to topical steroid therapy.

➤ Emollients should be prescribed in large quantities (250–500 g per month) to encourage generous application.

BOX 17.4 Treatment of eczema

- Bath emollients (e.g. Oilatum)
- Regular use of emollients and soap substitute
- Mild–medium potency topical steroid for affected areas on trunk and limbs (Table 17.1)
- Mild topical steroid for facial eczema (e.g. 0.5–1% hydrocortisone)
- Sedating antihistamine orally if sleep is disturbed

Treatment of moderate eczema

- Emollients and soap substitute (as above)
- Mild and medium topical steroid (as above)
- Consider a short course of potent topical steroid for flares (for 7–14 days)
- Ichthammol as zinc paste (Ichthopaste) and ichthammol bandage for flexures in lichenified eczema
- Consider topical tacrolimus or pimecrolimus (calcineurin inhibitors) if poor response to topical steroids
- If bacterial infection is suspected, the use of a topical antibiotic is of little value unless the area is small; oral flucloxacillin or erythromycin should be used if the infection is widespread
- Skin swabs may be taken if the area of infection is widespread and the skin excoriated
- Antihistamine at night for pruritis

Treatment of severe eczema

- Refer (*see* Box 17.5)

Further advice

- Advise patients to continue their normal diet unless there is a history of reacting to specific foods
- Reassure patient and parents that weak (e.g. hydrocortisone 0.5–1% on the face) and moderate topical steroids for up to 2–3 weeks on the body are safe and effective. The more potent steroids should not be used on the face, genitals or intertriginous areas, or to large areas for prolonged periods
- Advise patient to wear cotton clothing
- Patient should have adequate quantities of emollients (e.g. 1–2 g for severe cases of eczema), soap substitute and bath additives, e.g. 1–2 kg/month

TABLE 17.1 Topical steroid potency

Potency	Examples
Mild	Hydrocortisone 0.5%, 1%
Medium	Betamethasone (Betnovate-RD 0.025%)
	Clobetasone (Eumovate) 0.05%
	Fluocinolone (Synlar 0.01%, 0.025%)
High	Betamethasone (Betnovate-C 0.1%, Diprosone 0.05%)
	Triamcinolone (Aristocort 0.5%)
	Mometasone (Flocon 0.1%)
Highest	Clobetasol (Dermovate 0.05%)

BOX 17.5 Criteria for referral in dermatitis

- Diagnosis is uncertain
- Failure to respond to continuing use of moderately potent steroids
- 1–2 flares/month
- Sleep problem not responding to antihistamine at night
- Associated food allergies
- Recurrent secondary infections or failure of antibiotic treatment
- Severe eczema
- Growth retardation, psychosocial problems such as poor school attendance
- Eczema herpeticum (*see* Red flags)

 RED FLAGS

- Eczema herpeticum (Box 17.6) is a serious infection caused by herpes simplex virus (HSV) which invades eczematous lesions. It can lead to death through dissemination of the virus to the brain and other organs or from secondary staphylococcal or streptococcal infection. Parents of patients with atopic eczema should be offered information on how to recognise it. Urgent referral to hospital is indicated, where it is treated with IV aciclovir and antibiotics.
- A generalised and severe seborrhoeic dermatitis is very common in association with HIV infection.
- Very potent steroid preparations should not be used without specialist advice.

BOX 17.6 Features of eczema herpeticum (Fig 17.3 – *see* Plate section)

- 5–12 days after exposure to the virus (e.g. from a cold-sore virus), multiple, often itchy vesicles develop rapidly over the area of eczema
- Vesicles continue to appear in crops for as long as 7–9 days
- Vesicles often spread to adjoining areas of normal skin
- Systemic reaction includes fever and lethargy

VIRAL WARTS

Core messages

➤ Warts are caused by human papillomaviruses (HPVs), which are transmitted by direct contact and auto-inoculation. HPV is associated with squamous cell carcinoma of the skin and mucous membranes such as the larynx and cervix.

➤ All teenage girls are now offered vaccination against HPV, which consists of three injections given over a period of 12 months. Cervarix is an HPV vaccine aimed at preventing genital warts and cervical cancers. The vaccine does not prevent the virus strain responsible for ordinary warts.

➤ Warts occur in about 10% of children and young people. No single therapy has been proven effective at achieving cure in every patient. Most cases are best left alone. Table 17.2 shows treatment options.

➤ Treatment can remove the warts, but there is a high recurrence rate (50–73%) after treatment.

➤ A Cochrane review identified topical therapy with salicylic acid as safe and effective. The pooled data from RCT demonstrated a cure rate of 73% compared with 48% in the control group.

➤ Cryotherapy is painful and is best avoided in children. In addition, topical treatment is as effective as cryotherapy.

TABLE 17.2 Types of viral warts, and treatment options

Clinical features	Treatment	Tips
Common warts on fingers/dorsum of hands, face (*Verruca vulgaris*)	Leave them alone, or trial with topical salicylic acid (daily application of 15–20% gel)	Usually resistant to treatment, resolve spontaneously in 70% in 2 years Salicylic acid should not be used for children < 2 years of age, if patient has diabetes or impaired peripheral circulation
	Cryotherapy	Painful, potentially scarring; best avoided, particularly for first-line use
Verrucas (plantar warts on sole) (*Verruca plantaris*)	Leave them alone, or salicylic and lactic acid in a collodian basis: Duofilm or Salactol paint containing 16.7% salicylic acid and 16.7% lactic acid	Slow response to treatment May cause allergy; should be avoided in children allergic to elastic adhesive plaster
Plane (flat) warts (*Verruca plana*)	Leave alone or trial with tretinoin 0.025% cream for 4 weeks (specialist use only)	Can cause local irritation
Anogenital warts (*Condylomata acuminata*)	Often asymptomatic and require only simple barrier preparation. If treated: weekly application of 25% podophyllin (not licensed for children)	Very common in sexually active adolescents (40% in the USA)
	Imiquimod (Aldara) cream may be used for genital and peri-anal warts. It is not licensed for children	An immunomodulator. It may cause stricture of the foreskin in male patients

🏳 RED FLAGS

- Genital warts (*Condylomata acuminata*) should not be mistaken for molluscum contagiosum. They are a highly contagious STD. Typical lesions of genital warts are 3–5 mm diameter, flesh-coloured to erythematous papules with slightly verrucous surfaces.
- In patients with persistent and widespread lesions of genital warts, immunodeficiency should be excluded.
- *Condylomata acuminata* are one of the most prevalent STDs in sexually active adolescents. In pre-pubertal children, anogenital lesions may arise through auto-inoculation. However, a child with genital warts should be evaluated for possible sexual abuse, including the presence of other sexually transmitted diseases. This may require admission or referral to children's social care.

Criteria for referral
➤ Severe, widespread warts despite treatment for 3–6 months
➤ Significant warts in immunocompromised children
➤ Atypical appearance, site or age

MOLLUSCUM CONTAGIOSUM
Core messages
➤ This is a DNA poxvirus infection causing characteristic pearly, skin-coloured dome-shaped papules with central umbilication. Cheesy material can often be expressed from these papules (Fig 17.4 – *see* Plate section).
➤ The virus commonly spreads through skin-to-skin contact. Patients are advised to use separate towels and baths.
➤ Spontaneous resolution of the lesions usually occurs within 6–9 months; occasionally lesions persist for years.
➤ There is no permanent immunity to the virus, and re-infection may occur.
➤ The disease is self-limiting and treatment is not indicated in the vast majority of cases. In addition, treatment can be painful. If treatment is required (for example for cosmetic reasons, itching and discomfort):
  ➣ A brief, 6- to 9-second application of liquid nitrogen
  ➣ Papules can also be destroyed by expressing the plug with a needle or comedo extractor
  ➣ Laser therapy (pulsed dye laser) may be beneficial in multiple lesions.

🏳 RED FLAGS

- The genital area in children is commonly affected. In most cases the infection is not acquired by sexual transmission unless the individual is sexually active. However, child sexual abuse should be considered.
- When papules are widespread and large, immunosuppression such as HIV infection should be considered.

ACNE
Clinical features
➤ Acne is characterised by comedones (blackhead) or pustules (whitehead) which rupture, causing an inflammatory response (Fig 17.5 – *see* Plate section).
➤ An inflammatory response close to the skin surface causes papules and pustules, while a response deeper in the skin causes nodules and cyst formation.
➤ Sebaceous follicles are usually colonised by organisms, particularly anaerobic *Propionibacterium acnes* and *Staphylococcus epidermidis*.
➤ About 20% of neonates develop acne, predominately comedones, on the forehead and cheeks, resulting from placental transfer of maternal androgens.

Treatment
➤ Mild to moderate acne should be treated in primary care (Table 17.3).
➤ Patients should be discouraged from picking or squeezing the lesions.
➤ Treatment aims to:
  ➣ reduce the severity of the disease
  ➣ prevent long-term sequelae such as scarring
  ➣ reduce the psychological trauma on the individual.

Treatment should be assessed after 2–3 months and should continue for at least 6 months.

TABLE 17.3 Suggested treatment for acne in children

	Treatment	Tips
Mild		
Uninflamed lesions (mainly open and closed comedones)	Topical benzoyl peroxide	Apply once to twice daily, starting with lower-strength preparations
	Topical retinoids: Adapalene (Differin) Tretinoin (Retin-A)	Exposure to UV light, including sunlight, should be avoided
	Topical antibiotic*	For small area of pustules
	Salicylic acid (Acnisal) wash	Apply up to 1–2 times/day
		May cause irritation
Moderate		
More-extensive lesions	Topical therapy as above	
Mild scarring	Systemic antibiotic for 3 months: Lymecycline Oxytetracycline Doxycycline	In case of poor response use alternative antibiotic, e.g. erythromycin
		Oxytetracycline and doxycycline should not be used in children <12 years old

(continued)

	Treatment	Tips
Severe		
Nodulo-cystic scarring	Referral to dermatology for isotretinoin therapy	Refer urgently if the nodulo-cystic lesions are severe
Deeper inflammation		
Severe psychological reaction	Isotretinoin or co-cyprindiol (Dianette) may be considered	(*See* Red flags, below)
Treatment failure		
Maintenance		
	Topical retinoid or topical benzoyl peroxide	

* Topical antibiotics are probably no more effective than topical benzoyl peroxide. They may be indicated for children who do not wish to take oral antibiotics or who cannot tolerate them.

 RED FLAGS

- Isotretinoin can only be prescribed in secondary care; it is potentially teratogenic. Older girls should be on an oral contraceptive if the drug is used and they are sexually active or likely to become so during treatment.
- Girls with polycystic ovarian syndrome (PCOS) may not respond to isotretinoin, in which case co-cyprindiol (Dianette) should be considered.
- A pre-pubertal child with severe acne should be investigated for endocrine disorders such as congenital adrenal hyperplasia.

URTICARIA

Diagnostic features

➤ Urticaria is characterised by short-lived itchy wheals (Fig 17.6 – see Plate section), angioedema, or both. In angioedema the deeper layers of the skin and other tissues are involved (Fig 17.7 – see Plate section).

➤ Wheals usually last 2–24 hours in ordinary urticaria; up to 2 hours in contact urticaria and up to 1 hour in physical urticaria, except delayed-pressure urticaria which takes up to 48 hours to fade.

➤ Acute allergic urticaria is usually due to IgE-mediated type-I hypersensitivity reactions. Chronic urticaria lasting longer than 6 weeks is rare in children.

➤ NSAIDs should be avoided in aspirin-sensitive patients with urticaria.

AETIOLOGY

(*See* Box 17.7.)[3]

Investigations

The vast majority of cases of acute urticaria do not require investigation, particularly patients with mild urticaria responding to antihistamine. Those with severe, chronic urticaria or cases that do not respond to treatment may require the following tests:

➤ FBC, ESR (abnormalities may suggest auto-immune or collagen-vascular causes)

➤ TFTs and antibodies

➤ ANAs for suspected auto-immune causes

➤ LFTs

➤ IgE for cases of ordinary and contact urticaria
➤ Allergy testing (often requested by the parents)
➤ Physical challenge
➤ Complement C4 for hereditary and acquired C1-esterase inhibitor deficiency

---

BOX 17.7 Causes of urticaria

- Idiopathic
- Infections (viruses, bacteria, parasites)
- Dietary, such as fish, shellfish, nuts, eggs and food additives
- Drugs such as penicillin, aspirin, NSAIDs and angiotensin-converting enzyme (ACE) inhibitors
- Plants, e.g. stinging nettle
- Hereditary. Angioedema without wheals may be caused by angiotensin-converting enzyme (ACE) inhibitors or C1-esterase inhibitor deficiency which is usually inherited
- Urticarial vasculitis
- Physical urticaria (usually causing chronic urticaria)
  - › Dermographism (caused by scratching or firm stroking)
  - › Aquagenic (water contact)
  - › Delayed-pressure
  - › Exercise-induced
  - › Vibratory angioedema
  - › Cold contact
  - › Localised heat
  - › Solar
- Autoimmune urticaria, e.g. systemic lupus erythematosus

Management

(*See* Box 17.8.)
➤ Acute urticaria (lasting <6 weeks) is a self-limiting disease that usually resolves.
➤ Antihistamines are the mainstay of treatment. The use of sedating antihistamines is now less common because of their sedating effect and concerns about concentration and performance at school.
➤ Steroids and adrenaline are not indicated for the management of simple urticaria.

BOX 17.8 Management of urticaria

General
- Allergy testing in urticaria is generally not helpful except when specific drug (e.g. penicillin) or food allergies are suspected
- In the absence of any clue suggesting food allergy, elimination diets are generally not helpful

Acute

- Avoidance of known trigger
- Trial of non-sedating antihistamine:
  - › Loratadine
  - › Cetirizine
- If sleep is disturbed
  - › chlorphenamine (Piriton); sedating antihistamines are otherwise to be avoided
- Menthol 1% in aqueous cream helps to sooth itch

- Short-term use of prednisolone may be required if children remain symptomatic while on maximal doses of antihistamine. It is also indicated in severe acute urticaria or angioedema
- Addition of an H_2-blocker, e.g. cimetidine, may provide additional benefit in some cases
- Anti-leukotrienes (montelukast) and immunomodulating agents (cyclosporine, tacrolimus) are rarely used in primary care, but they may be helpful if used in combination with H_1 antihistamines
- Adrenaline can be life-saving in anaphylaxis and severe angioedema (*See* Chapter 5)

Referral to dermatologist should be considered for:

- Acute severe urticaria
- Failure of treatment
- Chronic urticaria lasting >6 weeks

RED FLAGS

- Cold urticaria is the most common form of physical urticaria. The cooling of the skin associated with evaporation on emerging from swimming water is hazardous and may be fatal.
- In any child presenting with acute urticaria, angioedema and anaphylaxis should be excluded by examining the ears, nose, throat and chest, and measuring the blood pressure and pulse.
- Urgent hospital admission is indicated if acute urticaria rapidly develops into angioneurotic oedema or anaphylactic shock. Adrenaline should be administered before referral.
- Urticarial reactions to H_1 antihistamines may occasionally occur, and this should be borne in mind when a patient's condition worsens while taking these drugs.

SCABIES

Diagnosis

(*See* Box 17.9.)

BOX 17.9 Diagnostic features of scabies
(Fig 17.8 – *see* Plate section and Fig 17.9 – *see* Plate section)

- Infants: bullae, vesicles and pustules affecting the palms, soles, face and scalp are common
- Older children: lesions are in the inter-digital spaces, wrist flexors, axillae, and groin. Bullae are uncommon

- Scabies should be suspected in any itchy papular rash when other family members are similarly affected
- Scabies can be confirmed by scraping the burrows with a needle and finding the mite or eggs (a low-powered lens may be required)

Treatment

(*See* Box 17.10.)

BOX 17.10 Scabies treatment

- Treat patient and all close relatives
- All bed linen and clothes should be hot-washed
- Topical scabicide:
  - › permethrin 5% cream (Lyclear Dermal cream) as a single application over whole body. *OR*
  - › malathion 0.5% aqueous solution (Derbac-M). Apply over whole body, and wash off after 24 hours.
- If residual rash/itch, use:
  - › crotamiton (Eurax) and emollients after treatment
  - › topical steroid also helps to reduce itch
- Pruritis does not improve immediately after treatment, but subsides slowly over several days. Persistent pruritis during this period does not mean treatment failure. If pruritis persists for more than 2 weeks after treatment, the patient should be re-examined for mites

---

IMPETIGO

➤ This is a contagious superficial bacterial skin infection usually caused by staphylococcal infection. It manifests as honey-coloured crusts, usually around the mouth and nose (Fig 17.10 – *see* Plate section).

➤ A pre-school child should not return to nursery or playgroup until the scabs have fallen off. School children can normally return to their classes after 3–4 days of topical treatment or 2 days of oral antibiotic treatment.

➤ Strict hygienic measures should be maintained, including regular washing of hands using a separate towel.

Management

(*See* Box 17.11.)

BOX 17.11 Treatment of impetigo

For localised, uncomplicated impetigo:
- Cleansing, removal of crusts. A mild antiseptic such as povidine–iodine may help to soften crusts
- Topical antibiotic such as fusidic acid or mupirocin (useful for methicillin-resistant *Staphylococcus aureus*, MRSA)

For widespread complicated impetigo:
- Oral flucloxacillin (first-line treatment)
- Cephalosporin
- Co-amoxiclav
- In case of penicillin allergy, use erythromycin

TINEA CAPITIS (RINGWORM)

Core messages

➤ Tinea capitis is caused by a superficial fungal infection which invades the keratin layer of the skin.

➤ There are four types of tinea: tinea corporis, unguium, pedis and capitis. Tinea capitis is the most common and important type.

➤ The infection is characterised by an erythematous and scaly circular plaque within which the infected hairs become broken just above the scalp (Fig 17.11 – *see* Plate section).

➤ The diagnosis can be confirmed using a Wood's light (blue-green fluorescence) or by culture of skin scrapings. A summary of management is shown in Fig 17.12.

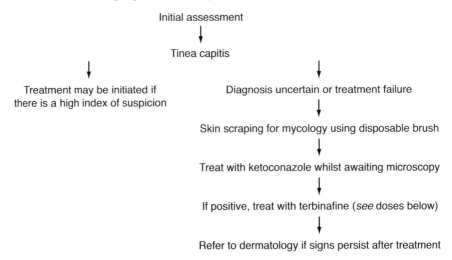

FIGURE 17.12 Assessment and treatment of tinea capitis

Treatment

➤ Topical antifungal treatment is sufficient for fungal skin infection, but scalp infection usually requires oral treatment with terbinafine or fluconazole. Griseofulvin is rarely used nowadays.

➤ Oral terbinafine is being used increasingly and has largely replaced griseofulvin. It appears to be safe and very effective. Treatment duration is usually 4 weeks. The dose is:

  ➤ 62.5 mg once daily for 10–20 kg bodyweight

  ➤ 125 mg once daily for 20–40 kg bodyweight

  ➤ 250 mg once daily for >40 kg bodyweight.

➤ Fluconazole (for treatment of *Trichophyton* species):

  ➤ Child 1–18 years: 6 mg/kg daily for 2– weeks.

PITYRIASIS ROSEA

➤ This is a benign, self-limiting rash of uncertain aetiology, possibly caused by the immune reaction to a viral infection. It is not contagious and does not spread to other people.

➤ The rash begins as a small, pinkish single 'herald patch' lesion on the chest, trunk or back (Fig 17.13 – *see* Plate section).

➤ 7–14 days after the 'herald patch', a generalised rash follows consisting of a pink or red, 2–10 cm diameter, scaly, oval-shaped eruption, which usually spreads across the chest and trunk following the rib-line in a characteristic Christmas-tree distribution. The rash usually resolves within 6 weeks, but it can take as long as 6 months.

➤ The rash is commonly mildly itchy; occasionally severe.

➤ No treatment is necessary for asymptomatic patients. Direct sunlight may hasten resolution. Options to treat severe itching include:

   ➢ Avoidance of fragranced soaps, bath with hot water, wool and synthetic fabrics

   ➢ Calamine lotion

   ➢ Oral antihistamine.

➤ Following resolution of the eruption, there may be post-inflammatory hypopigmentation or hyperpigmentation patches which resolve during the subsequent weeks to months.

PITYRIASIS VERSICOLOR

➤ This is a benign rash caused by yeasts of the genus *Malassezia* which are normally found on the skin.

➤ The rash is characterised by hypopigmented or brown well-defined round or oval spots with fine scales, which are mainly localised on the upper trunk and back (Fig 17.14 – *see* Plate section).

➤ Diagnosis can be established by Wood's light showing typical yellow fluorescence.

➤ Treatment is usually with topical antifungal medications: ketoconazole or clotrimazole (daily application for a few days followed by weekly applications), or topical selenium sulphide (Selsun). If there is no response to topical treatment, oral treatment with itraconazole may be required.

RED FLAGS

When itraconazole is used, particularly for longer than 1 month, liver function tests should be performed and patients should be monitored in regard to the following risks:

● Hepatotoxicity – although this has very rarely been reported, children and their parents should be told how to recognise symptoms of liver disease such as nausea, vomiting, abdominal pain or dark urine.

● Heart failure, particularly in patients with a history of cardiac disease and those receiving negative inotropic drugs, e.g. calcium-channel blockers.

REFERENCES

1. NICE guidelines, 2007. CG57: Atopic eczema in children: management of atopic eczema in children from birth up to the age of 12 years. www.nice.org.uk/CG57

2. S Gibbs, I Harvey. Topical treatments for cutaneous warts (review). The Cochrane Library 2009, Issue 1. www.thecochranelibrary.com

3. British Association of Dermatologists. Guidelines for evaluation and management of urticaria in adults and children. www.bad.org.uk

CHAPTER 18

Safeguarding children

The purpose of safeguarding children is to:
➤ protect children from maltreatment
➤ prevent impairment of children's health or development through maltreatment
➤ ensure that all children grow up in an environment of safe and effective care.

High-profile media coverage of Victoria Climbié and 'Baby P' has led to the 2010 government guidance document 'Working Together to Safeguard Children'. This promotes inter-agency cooperation and places the onus on health professionals to share concerns and refer or ask for advice if in doubt.

All clinicians working with children should be familiar with:
➤ NICE guideline CG89: When to suspect child maltreatment
➤ General Medical Council (GMC) guideline: Protecting children and young people.

Links to these documents are given at the end of the chapter.

GPs play a key role in recognising patterns of worrying behaviour, including multiple presentations at different visits, and being in contact with the whole family. We are in a key position both to recognise abuse and to recognise children at risk in the hope of intervening to support the family and prevent abuse occurring. GPs and trainees should have completed child safeguarding training to at least level 2 and be working towards level 3. This is available online from the Royal College of General Practitioners, or e-LFH.

The Children's Act 2004 makes the welfare of the child the clinician's first concern, and this takes precedence over maintaining confidentiality when these are in conflict. GPs will naturally want to maintain the doctor–patient relationship. To this end, any action taken should be discussed with parents/carers first and their consent sought where possible, unless this would put the child at risk of further harm.

GPs should be familiar with local referral arrangements, which is usually to Children's Social Care (formerly Social Services) who have the statutory responsibility for investigating suspected child abuse. There is a designated nurse and GP for child safeguarding in each area; they are available for advice when the best course of action is unclear. Each GP practice should also have a nominated safeguarding lead GP for advice.

Risk factors for child abuse are
➤ *Parental risks*
  ➢ Domestic violence
  ➢ Drug and alcohol misuse
  ➢ Mental health problems

➤ Deprivation
➤ Single-parent family
➤ Young age of parent
➤ Parent abused or neglected as a child
➤ *Child risks*
  ➤ Learning difficulties and physical disability
  ➤ Chronic illness
  ➤ Learning or behavioural difficulties
  ➤ Prematurity
  ➤ Poor infant hygiene

The **main categories of abuse** are:
➤ Physical abuse may involve hitting, shaking, throwing, drowning, suffocation, burning or scalding, poisoning or other forms that cause physical harm and injury to a child.
➤ Sexual abuse includes penetrative contacts (e.g. genital-genital or hand-genital), non-penetrative physical acts (e.g. masturbation, kissing, rubbing, or touching outside the clothing) and non-contact activities (e.g. involving children in looking at, or in the production of sexual images, or watching sexual activities). These activities are usually carried out by an adult or a significantly older child on a child by force, and before the age of legal consent.
➤ Emotional abuse indicates persistent emotional ill-treatment of a child likely to result in persistent and severe effects on the child's emotional development. This form of abuse appears to be the most prevalent form of abuse. Because of the absence of physical injuries, it tends to be under-diagnosed and underestimated. Emotional abuse can take many forms from failure to provide love, affection, security, emotional support to rejection and verbal assaults.
➤ Neglect is the persistent failure to meet a child's basic physical and/or psychological needs, likely to result in the serious impairment of the child's health or development. It usually involves failure by a parent or carer to provide adequate food, clothing or shelter, or to protect the child from physical or emotional harm or danger, or failure to ensure adequate supervision or access to appropriate medical care or treatment.
➤ Fabricated or induced illness (see below).

DIAGNOSTIC FEATURES OF CHILD ABUSE
Diagnostic features of child abuse include the following:

Physical abuse
➤ An injury that is unexplained
➤ An injury that is incompatible with the history or with the child's level of development
➤ Unexplained recurrent injury
➤ A delay in seeking medical help
➤ Certain skin manifestations including:
  ➤ Bruises on the cheeks, buttocks, genitals, and back
  ➤ Bruise marks shaped like hands, fingers or a belt
  ➤ Black eyes
  ➤ Cigarette burns, producing circular, punched-out lesions of uniform size

➢ Human bite marks

➢ Alopecia in which the hairs are broken at various lengths

➤ Unexplained causes of increased intracranial pressure, with signs of a reduced level of consciousness, bulging fontanelle. (Head trauma, including subdural haematoma, is the most common cause of death from physical abuse)

➤ Any fracture in an infant too young to walk. Fractures that are unusual or unexplained, such as spiral fracture from twisting rather than transverse from impact

➤ Unexplained intra-abdominal injuries

Emotional abuse

➤ Failure to thrive, particularly in infancy; developmental delay

➤ Change in behaviour, e.g. aggressive or withdrawn behaviour

➤ Poor interaction with parents

Sexual abuse

➤ Genitals: pain in the vaginal, penile or rectal area, discharge or bleeding

➤ Chronic dysuria, encopresis

➤ Bruises or bleeding near the genitals

➤ Sexually transmitted disease

➤ Sleep disorders, aggression, withdrawn, depression, poor school performance

Neglect

Maltreated infants suffer from greater developmental disability than children who were maltreated later in childhood. The child achieves more motor and developmental milestones during infancy than at any other period in life. In contrast to other causes of developmental delay, neglect-related developmental delay is commonly associated with the following features:

➤ Abnormal behaviour including avoidance, insecure withdrawal and inactivity

➤ Poor social interaction, including parental interaction

➤ Signs of neglect often present, including clothes that do not fit or are inappropriate, and poor hygiene

➤ Delay in seeking appropriate medical attention for illness or injury

➤ Significant improvement of milestones once the child receives adequate affection and care

Fabricated or induced illness (FII)

Fabricated or induced illness describes behaviours by a carer that may result in harm, including:

➤ Deliberately inducing symptoms by administering medication or other substances or by intentional suffocation

➤ Interfering with treatments by over-dosing, not administering medication, or interfering with equipment

➤ Claiming the child has symptoms which are unverifiable

➤ Exaggerating symptoms which may result in unnecessary investigations or treatments

➤ Falsifying test results and observation charts

➤ Obtaining specialist treatments or equipment for children which are not required

➤ Alleging psychological illness in a child

Fabricated or induced illness is associated with significant mortality (around 6%), long-term or permanent injury (7.3%) and long-term impairment of children's psychological and emotional development.

PRACTICE POINTS

When the possibility of abuse or fabricated or induced illness is being considered, it is important to:

- Take a detailed history from both the child (appropriate to their age and developmental level) and their parent or carer. Look especially for implausible, inadequate or inconsistent accounts of an injury.
- Distinguish between anxious carers whose children are genuinely sick and the rare case of carers whose behaviour risks causing harm to the child.
- Observe the child's demeanour and interaction with other family members.
- Consider full examination top to toe, with appropriate chaperoning and consent.
- Document the history fully – what was said and by whom. Likewise, examination and clinical findings – a body map diagram may be useful for multiple injuries.
- Consider discussing any concerns with the lead GP within the practice or organisation, or with the designated GP or nurse for the area.
- Gather information about the wider family, e.g. from health visitors or colleagues.
- Discuss concerns with the parent or carer. In the case of FII, consider how to support the perpetrator. About two-thirds of perpetrators may suffer from chronic somatoform or factitious disorder.

RED FLAGS

Indicators which should alert professionals to the possibility of fabricated or induced illness (FII):

- A carer reporting symptoms and observed signs that are not explained medically
- Physical examination and results of investigations that do not explain symptoms or signs reported by the carer
- The child has poor response to prescribed medication or other treatment
- Acute symptoms that are exclusively observed by/in the presence of the carer
- Following resolution of the child's presenting problems, the carer reporting new symptoms in different children.

REFERRAL

➤ If referral is considered appropriate, ask parents/carers for consent to refer to Children's Social Care unless the child's wellbeing will be endangered by doing this. The referral should still be made even without consent if there are significant concerns.

➤ Referral to Children's Social Care should be made initially by phone, followed by a written referral.

➤ GPs should not wait to confirm the diagnosis before referring to Children's Social Care, as delay may be detrimental to the child.

➤ GPs should discuss concerns with named and designated health professionals, including the 'responsible paediatric consultant'. The important key task is to determine whether the child is in need of immediate protection.

➤ In cases of serious injury or concern when parental consent is withheld, consider admission to hospital. If this is done, ensure that you communicate your concerns to the admitting team even if you are not happy to put these in the referral letter.

➤ Recent GMC guidelines emphasise the importance of GPs in child protection proceedings. Every effort should be made to attend case conferences, and where this is not possible a full report should be supplied.

In summary – everyone has a responsibility for safeguarding children and inter-agency sharing of information and concerns is crucial.

FURTHER READING

➤ NICE guideline CG89: When to suspect child maltreatment.
www.nice.org.uk/CG89

➤ GMC guidance: Protecting children and young people.
www.gmc-uk.org/guidance/ethical_guidance/13257.asp

➤ Royal College of Paediatrics and Child Health. Safeguarding children and young people. Intercollegiate document. September 2010.
www.rcpch.ac.uk/safeguarding

➤ National Society for Prevention of Cruelty to Children
www.nspcc.org/inform

➤ Royal College of General Practitioners. Clinical resources concerning safeguarding children.
www.rcgp.org.uk

➤ e-Learning for Healthcare, e-learning resources
www.e-lfh.org.uk/projects/safeguarding-children

Index

References to boxes, figures and tables are in **bold**.

CPD with Radcliffe

You can now use a selection of our books to achieve CPD (Continuing Professional Development) points through directed reading.

We provide a free online form and downloadable certificate for your appraisal portfolio. Look for the CPD logo and register with us at: www.radcliffehealth.com/cpd

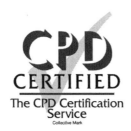